ANYONE, ANYTHING, ANYTIME: A HISTORY OF EMERGENCY MEDICINE

ANYONE, ANYTHING, ANYTIME: A HISTORY OF EMERGENCY MEDICINE

BRIAN J. ZINK, M.D.
Associate Professor
Department of Emergency Medicine
Associate Dean for Student Programs
University of Michigan Medical School
Ann Arbor, Michigan

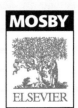
MOSBY
ELSEVIER

1600 John F. Kennedy Boulevard
Suite 1800
Philadelphia, Pennsylvania 19103-2899

This book project was partially supported by Grant 1 G13 LM007935 from the National Library of Medicine

Library of Congress Cataloging-in-Publication Data

Zink, Brian J.
   Anyone, anything, anytime : a history of emergency medicine / Brian J. Zink -- 1st ed.
      p. ; cm.
   Includes bibliographical references.
   ISBN 1-56053-710-8
   1. Emergency medicine--United States--History. 2. Emergency medical services--United States--History. I. Title.
   [DNLM: 1. Emergency Medicine--history--United States. 2. History, 20th Century--United States. WZ 70 AA1 Z78a 2006]
   RC86.7.Z54 2006
   616.02'5--dc22

                                                                                              2005041586

Acquisitions Editor: *Todd Hummel*
Editorial Assistant: *Martha Limbach*
Project Manager: *David Saltzberg*
Book Designer: *Steven Stave*

Dedicated to

Dana
For your strength and support

Korie
For your wit

Eli
For your depth

Ethan
For your smile

History, n. An account mostly false, of events mostly unimportant, which are brought about by rulers mostly knaves, and soldiers mostly fools.
—Ambrose Bierce, The Devil's Dictionary[1]

Barbara Tuchman once quoted a history professor with whom she studied to the effect that: "There is no history without a historian."[2] When I read this, it at first bothered me because it seemed to imply exactly what Bierce proposed in his dictionary. I felt that events do occur whether anyone records them, and it is not the historian who makes them happen whether anyone remembers them or not.

On more reflection however, it becomes clear that there can be no single memory of an event that isn't changed by its recording. In a complex series of events, there are multiple participants, and there must be multiple memories. Leibniz seemed to think that this totality of multiple consciousness was the reality that we know.

Reading this account of the history of emergency medicine, I realize that without Brian Zink's recording of these events, they exist in the multiple memories of the individual participants, but for no one else. Moreover, I was struck by how much I, as one of the participants, had forgotten or never knew. There were events of which I had never been aware, backgrounds that surprised me, and details of problem solving that I found either new to me, or totally different from my own memories of the events. That is not to suggest that others' memories were wrong and mine the only correct ones, but a more Rashomon-type occurrence of two people experiencing the same thing, but recalling it differently.

For many who now practice emergency medicine, many of the events, people, and problems have never existed. Perhaps this is just as well, and perhaps they don't "need to know" where we came from and how. But if for no other reason than simple curiosity, this account of our past is worth the read. It also helps in the solution of current problems to realize that not everything is novel or unsolved. As Santayana is quoted, those who don't understand history are doomed to repeat it.

I don't believe we thought of ourselves as making history, but rather simply living our lives and solving our problems. Fortunately we were young, because when you are young, nothing is impossible. I remember, memories triggered during the reading of this account, of my past, how easy I thought it would be. Here was the problem: how to take care of very sick patients in the emergency department. We needed people who were trained to do this. It never occurred to me that it was a complex problem, with multiple agenda. I was too young to know about power, turf, economics, hierarchy and pride of place. Nobody was solving the problem, and we thought we were filling a vacuum. Who would be concerned enough to prevent an easy solution?

Brian Zink has answered these, and many more questions. I am greatly impressed with the diligent and accurate record that he has created. I would not have thought it possible even after only thirty years to have forgotten so much of what happened, and I am truly grateful that he has produced this record.

It is a very curious experience to be a part of a history; it is like reading a novel in which you are suddenly one of the characters. It is hard to know what impression you make upon others, what are your contributions to the history, and whether this actually happened. It was certainly fun to be one of the "fools" of this history, and it was also fun to discover many of the contributions of so many other very effective people who created our field of emergency medicine.

I think that the readers of this history who lived through it, and were the ones to create these events, will be equally pleased with the account. Of course there will be some who will feel that their contributions were greater than are recorded. This however should be counterbalanced by those, and I am one, who will feel that their contributions were much less. For those readers who didn't live through these events, I believe that they will also be pleased with this account. It will enable them to understand the people who they may know only by name, and perhaps understand events that they didn't even know had occurred.

The most important reason for reading this history in my mind, however, is that there are still many of the problems that we thought we had solved that are still the battle ground for a new generation of emergency physicians. Some of these battles are being fought in other countries where emergency medicine is beginning to evolve as a specialty. Some are still being fought in our own country where there remain foes who would still prefer to see emergency medicine disappear. What should or would replace it is as vague and mysterious as it always was.

For those readers who will not know or care about the politics of the late 1960s and early 1970s, the book will still be a revelation about the emotions and feelings of the times. Perhaps it required a general need to rebel against traditions as was stimulated by the revulsion against the national policies on Vietnam. Perhaps the bureaucratization of training had reached a point where there had to be a revolution. Perhaps this is all part of a general evolution of systems and institutions, and emergency medicine in its own time will go through the same evolution. This book will stand as a wonderful picture of an important period in the practice of medicine in the United States. Like it or not, emergency medicine has changed our medical delivery system. There were important and difficult problems to solve, and this book is a great description of the solution that worked. This is not a case where individual tastes can produce a variety of solutions. There are simply no better solutions to the problems that were faced, and will continue to be faced.

The best reason for reading this book is to learn what that unique solution was, how it was arrived at, and who were the people who lived it. I can only hope that every reader learns as much, and enjoys what is learned as much as I did.

Peter Rosen, M.D.
Senior Lecturer in Medicine, Harvard University School of Medicine;
Visiting Professor in Emergency Medicine, University of Arizona School of Medicine;
Attending Physician, Emergency Medicine, Beth Israel/Deaconess Medical Center, Boston, Massachusetts;
Attending Physician, Emergency Medicine, St. John's Hospital,
Jackson Hole, Wyoming

REFERENCES

1. Bierce, Ambrose. The unabridged devil's dictionary. Athens: University of Georgia Press, 2000.
2. Tuchman, Barbara Wertheim. Practising history: selected essays. New York: Knopf, 1981.

One way to introduce the history of the field of emergency medicine in America would be to describe a critically ill patient with congestive heart failure who presented to an emergency room (ER) in the 1950s, and contrast the care this patient received with "modern" emergency care of congestive heart failure. Or perhaps we could look at the case of a young boy on his bike, struck by a car in the 1950s, and trace the emergency medical services (EMS) response and treatment—at that time almost non-existent—with the system of EMS, pre-hospital care, and emergency department trauma response that is common today. Other books on medicine and emergency care have shown this marvelous progress in medicine quite well, but this approach does not capture the special nature of the field of emergency medicine. Forty years from now, current emergency practice will undoubtedly look as primitive and outdated as the practice of the 1960s looks to us today. To me, the most fascinating aspects of the post-World War II history of emergency medicine relate to the strong link between societal changes and the development of this new profession.

One of the first things we find in looking back is that the knowledge of how to provide better quality emergency care in America far preceded the application of that knowledge by physicians and hospitals. Physicians from World War II and the Korean War had discovered improved ways to manage the critically injured and ill, but the systems and practice to do so did not develop in U.S. medicine for decades. Many advances in the treatment of cardiovascular diseases, infections, shock, and poisonings that arose in the 1950s or 1960s were not routinely used in emergency rooms until the 1970s.

A number of questions arise when the evolution of emergency medicine is explored. It is easy to see why the hospital emergency room became the main venue for the care of the acutely ill and injured, but why did it also come to serve as a major source of primary and non-urgent care for many U.S. citizens? Why, pre-1970, were the sickest patients, who presented to the hospital's community portal—the ER—attended to by the least-qualified physicians? Why would a radiologist, or dermatologist, who had minimal clinical skills or interest in emergency care, be forced by his hospital to work in the ER in the 1960s? Why did the field of emergency medicine develop outside of the traditional house of medicine? Why did the most powerful medical fields, internal medicine and surgery, strongly oppose the development of emergency medicine as an academic discipline, even when it was obvious to everyone that emergency care in the U.S. was substandard? How did emergency medicine move rapidly from being viewed as a dead-end career, to one of the most popular and competitive specialty choices for medical students? Why, despite all the attention on providing health care to all Americans, have emergency departments (EDs) continued to serve as the health care safety net for up to 15 percent of the population?

To answer these questions one must look outside of medicine, and consider the social and political scene in post-World War II America. Emergency medicine came about in a different manner than the traditional medical specialties. It was bred by new social and political conditions, borne out of service needs, and nurtured by a few maverick physicians. It developed as an outsider looking in—a populist favorite shunned by the medical establishment. The early leaders of emergency medicine were different from the leaders in other fields. They were less educated, less academic, more Midwestern. And as is the way with people who push the edges, and like to take risks, these nonconformist, pioneer emergency physicians were interesting characters. In their bold, tireless, and sometimes bumbling and fractious paths, one finds the story of emergency medicine in America—at first tenuous, one wrong turn away from dissolution, then gaining momentum, then taking off like a rocket to become a new and distinct medical specialty.

The four-year project which resulted in this book had its roots in conversations with my academic colleagues in 2000 and 2001. Three themes recurred as we discussed and considered our past. The first was that four decades after the first U.S. physicians began to practice full time in emergency departments, enough time had elapsed to compile a history of the field. The second was the observation that current medical students and resident physicians training in emergency medicine had lost the vital, direct connection to their past. The third realization was that a window of time existed to hear the story of emergency medicine directly from its founders. Almost all of the early leaders of emergency medicine, although aging, are alive and more than ready to tell their stories. Because no one seemed ready to do it, and for other reasons that are still not clear to me, I decided to embark on this book project.

The first decision was how far back to go. Physicians and healers have been providing emergency care since the dawn of civilization, but I knew that I had so much potential material and so many subjects to interview that it would be best to focus on emergency medicine in post-World War II America. Better historians than I can and will document the rest of the story. I also decided not to delve too deeply in to the history of the development of emergency medical services or pre-hospital care. This area has its own rich history, and warrants a separate work. One note on terminology; many emergency physicians feel that the term ER is disparaging, and prefer the term emergency department or ED. Therefore I have chosen to call it ER until the time when full-time emergency physicians began practice in 1961. After that, it becomes ED.

The three-year odyssey of oral history interviews for this book took me from southern California to Boston, from Florida to Seattle, and many places in between. The interviews included a fly-fishing float trip down the Snake River in Wyoming with Peter Rosen and Robert Dailey, and a personal guided tour of Ronald Stewart's beloved Cape Breton in Nova Scotia. I interviewed George Podgorny amidst the beautiful Persian décor of his home in Winston-Salem, North Carolina, and was treated to "real Carolina barbeque" for lunch. I had tea with the elegant and modest Frances Mills, wife of James Mills, Jr., at their home in Alexandria, Virginia, where it all began. I had a beer with R. R. Hannas in the Irish pub he bought and ran as a retirement diversion in Tucson, Arizona. I visited the "the Big County" in Los Angeles, and many other emergency departments across the country. All told, I recorded around one hundred hours of oral history, and was inspired, humbled, surprised, enlightened, sometimes frustrated, but always grateful to people who were willing to share not only their successes, but the stories of their mistakes, failures, and misjudgments. Only a fraction of what I recorded has made it in to this book. The recordings and transcripts will be archived in the Bentley Historical Library at the University of Michigan. I did not have the time to interview many physicians who were instrumental in developing the field, particularly on a regional level. Many local histories of emergency medicine have their own special features, and deserve to be recorded and told.

Along with the rich oral narrative, I needed the hard data of history, and this was generously provided by the American Board of Emergency Medicine (ABEM), the American College of Emergency Physicians (ACEP), the Society for Academic Emergency Medicine (SAEM), the National Academy of Sciences (NAS), and the Robert Wood Johnson Foundation. Mary Ann Reinhart of ABEM, Lisa McKinley of ACEP, Mary Ann Schropp of SAEM, and Diane Bollman of the Michigan College of Emergency Physicians were especially helpful in providing guidance as I researched the archives of these organizations. I am grateful to those I interviewed who shared their personal documents or photographs with me, including John Wiegenstein, R. R. Hannas, Ronald Krome, Frances Mills, Leonard Riggs, Phillip Buttaravoli, Richard Levy, and Kenneth Iserson.

The time and resources to sustain this project came from the Department of Emergency Medicine at the University of Michigan. A sabbatical in 2003 allowed critical time for research and writing. My faculty colleagues who were covering my emergency department shifts marveled at how many of my interview subjects seemed to live in desirable vacation destinations. Our chairman, William Barsan, M.D., has been a valued advisor, mentor, and friend. This project is supported by a Publication

Grant from the National Library of Medicine. I am also grateful to Joel Howell, M.D., Howard Markel, M.D., and Kathryn Montgomery, Ph.D., who have been kind and valuable mentors. I am also indebted to my secretary, Nancy Collins, who upon completing the transcription of the oral history interviews, promptly retired.

This book is a first attempt at compiling and analyzing the modern history of emergency medicine in the U.S. It is undoubtedly incomplete, and the material will need corrections and future revisions as more information becomes available. But, what started out as a project has become the most rewarding period of discovery in my career. I welcome dialogue and efforts by others to build on this fascinating story of the profession of emergency medicine.

Brian J. Zink, M.D.

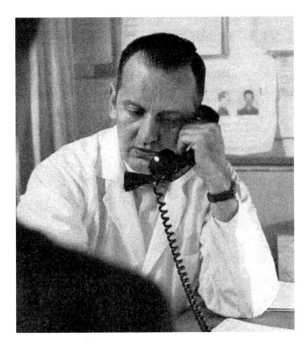

Figure 1. James Mills, Jr., M.D., the founder of the Alexandria Plan in the Alexandria Hospital Emergency Department, 1963. (From Medical Economics, July 15, 1963.)

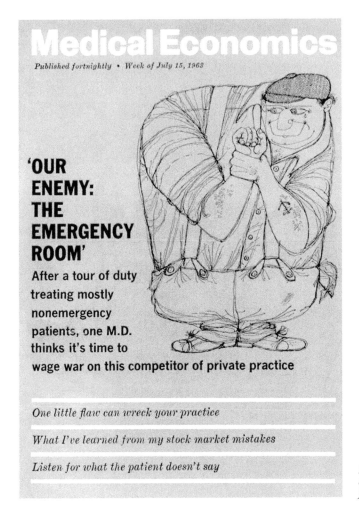

Figure 2. Disparaging cover article about emergency practice in Medical Economics, July 15, 1963.

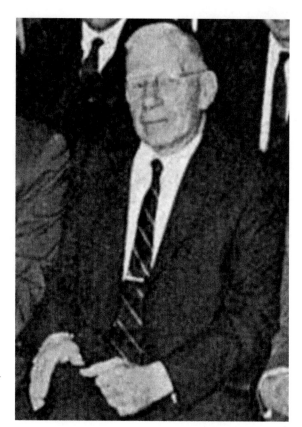

Figure 3. *Robert H. Kennedy, M.D., the "King of Trauma," at the age of 80. (Photograph from the* Bulletin of the American College of Surgeons, *March–April 1968.)*

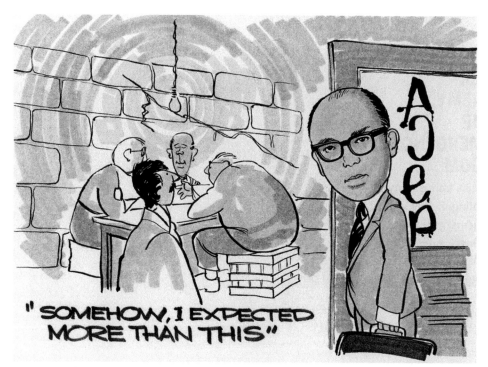

Figure 4. *Cartoon depicting the visit of Reinald Leidelmeyer, M.D., to the early American College of Emergency Physicians (ACEP) office in Lansing, Michigan, in autumn, 1968. (Cartoon commissioned by John G. Wiegenstein, M.D., 1978.)*

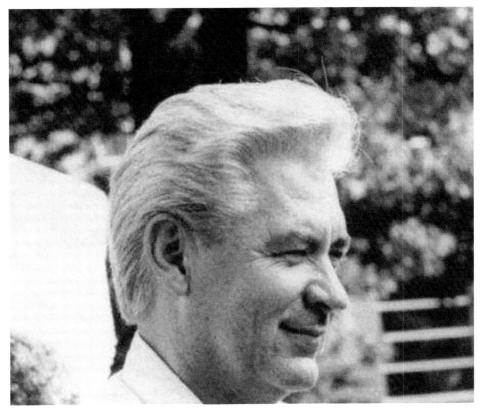

Figure 5. John G. Wiegenstein, M.D.: a founder and first Chairman (President) of the American College of Emergency Physicians. (Photograph from the Michigan College of Emergency Physicians archive.)

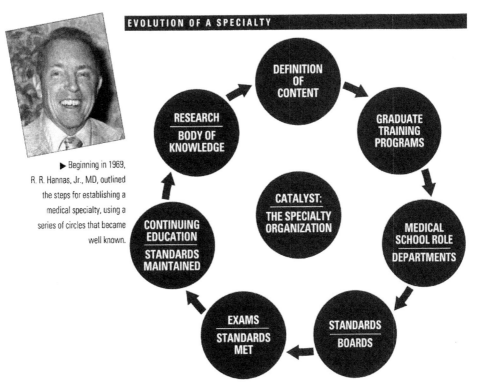

EVOLUTION OF A SPECIALTY

DEFINITION OF CONTENT

GRADUATE TRAINING PROGRAMS

RESEARCH
BODY OF KNOWLEDGE

CATALYST:
THE SPECIALTY ORGANIZATION

MEDICAL SCHOOL ROLE
DEPARTMENTS

CONTINUING EDUCATION
STANDARDS MAINTAINED

STANDARDS
BOARDS

EXAMS
STANDARDS MET

▶ Beginning in 1969, R. R. Hannas, Jr., MD, outlined the steps for establishing a medical specialty, using a series of circles that became well known.

Figure 6. R. R. Hannas, Jr., M.D., and his circle. (From "Twenty-five Years on the Front Line," American College of Emergency Physicians, 1993.)

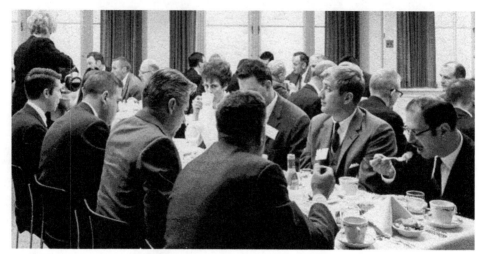

Figure 7. First national meeting of the ACEP, November, 1968. Lunch at Fairfax Hospital. (Photograph from Reinald Leidelmeyer, M.D.)

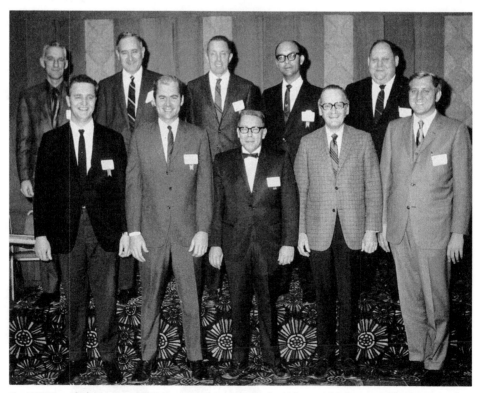

Figure 8. ACEP Board of Directors, 1970. Front row from left: *Rupke, Wiegenstein, Rogers, Mills, Haeck.* Back row from left: *Graves, Nakfoor, Hannas, Leidelmeyer, Rathburn. (Photograph from Reinald Leidelmeyer, M.D.)*

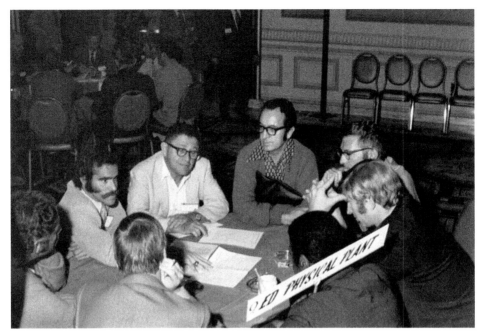

Figure 9. *ACEP members attend round table discussion session at the ACEP Scientific Assembly, early 1970s. (Photograph from the American College of Emergency Physicians archive.)*

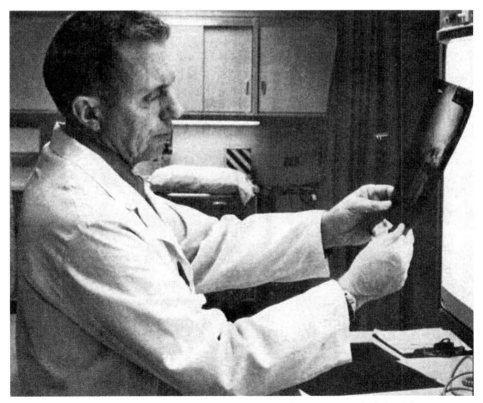

Figure 10. *R. R. Hannas, Jr., M.D. Experienced in practice and medical organizations, he helped show emergency medicine the path to take to specialty recognition. (Photograph from The New Physician, December, 1974, p. 22.)*

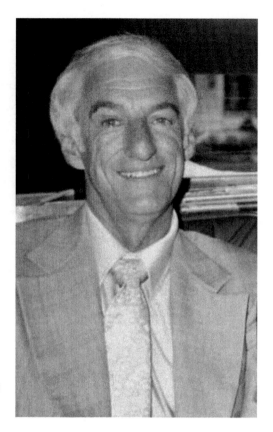

Figure 11. Harris Graves, M.D., ACEP founding member and President, 1975–1976. (Photograph from Leonard Riggs, Jr., M.D.)

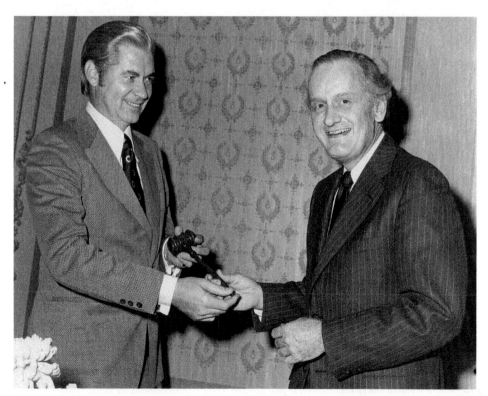

Figure 12. John G. Wiegenstein, M.D., passes the gavel as ACEP President to James Mills, Jr., M.D., in 1972. (Photograph from the ACEP archive.)

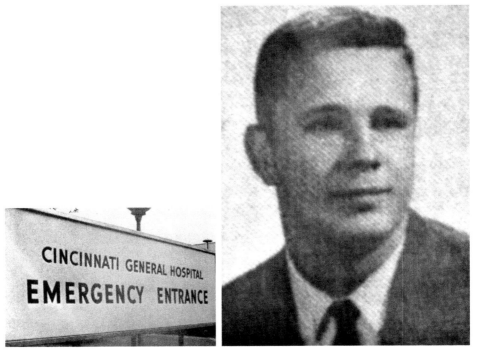

Figure 13. Bruce Janiak, M.D., 1970, the first emergency medicine resident. (Photographs from the University of Cincinnati Department of Emergency Medicine archive.)

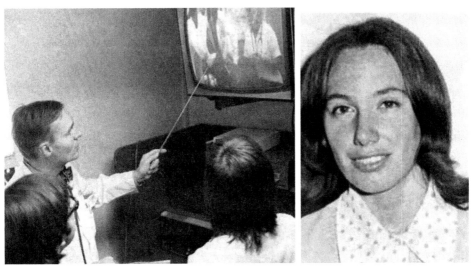

Figure 14. Left: David Wagner, M.D., who started the Medical College of Pennsylvania emergency medicine residency. Right: Pamela Bensen, M.D., his first resident. (Wagner photograph from The New Physician 1974;23:29; Bensen photograph from JACEP 1977;6:86.)

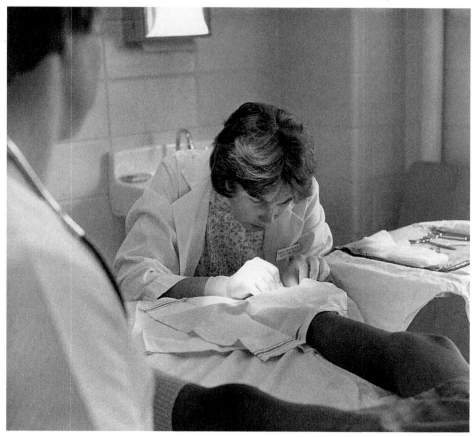

Figure 15. Pamela Bensen, M.D., the first emergency medicine resident at the Medical College of Pennsylvania, provides wound care, 1971.

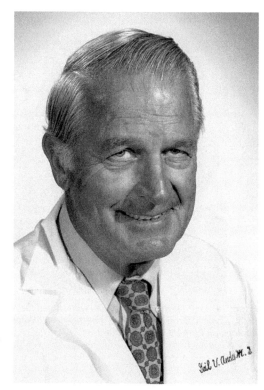

Figure 16. Gail V. Anderson, Sr., M.D., the first Chairman of an academic department of emergency medicine at a U.S. medical school—the University of Southern California. (Photograph courtesy of Gail V. Anderson, Sr., M.D.)

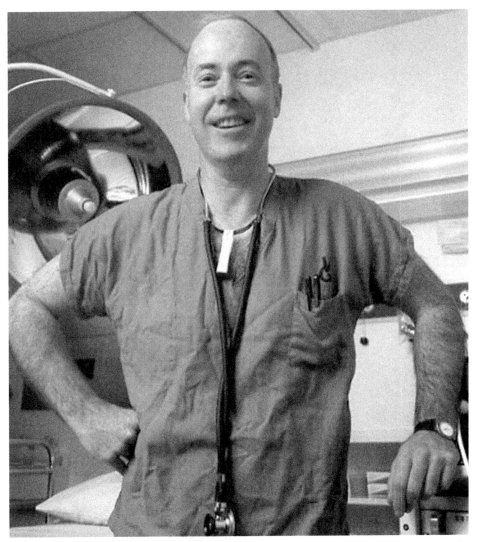

Figure 17. *Ronald Stewart, M.D., an early emergency medicine trainee at the Los Angeles County/University of Southern California program, who played a major role in the development of emergency medical services in the region.*

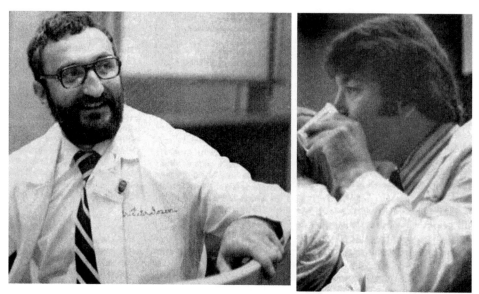

Figure 18. Left: *Peter Rosen, M.D., who started the emergency medicine residency at the University of Chicago. Right: Harvey Meislin, M.D., one of his first residents. (Photographs from* The New Physician, *December, 1974, pp. 23–25.)*

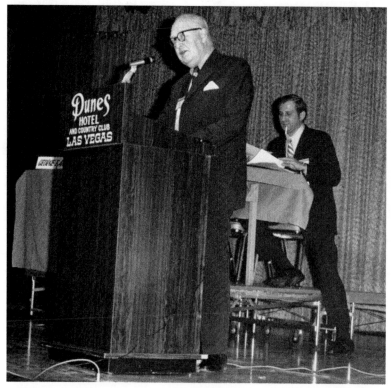

Figure 19. *Oscar Hampton, M.D., American College of Surgeons, who opposed the development of emergency medicine as a specialty, speaking at an ACEP meeting in 1972. William Haeck, M.D., is in the background. (Photograph from the ACEP archive.)*

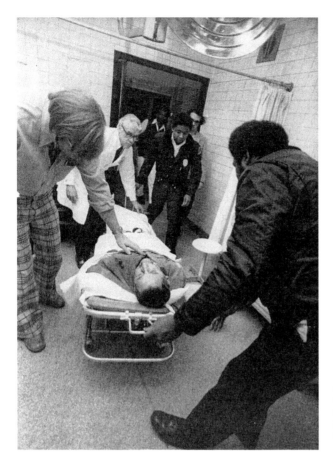

Figure 20. Robert Wolfensperger, emergency medicine resident (left), and program director, Dr. Allen Klippel (white coat) *assess a patient in the St. Louis University Hospital ED, 1973. (Photograph from* Medical World News, *Feb. 1, 1974, p. 39.)*

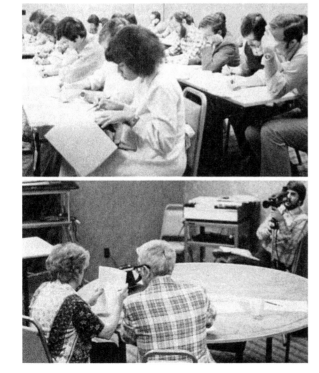

Figure 21. Emergency medicine residents and practicing physicians at the American Board of Emergency Medicine Certification Examination Field Test in 1977. (Photographs from JACEP 1977;6[12]:89.)

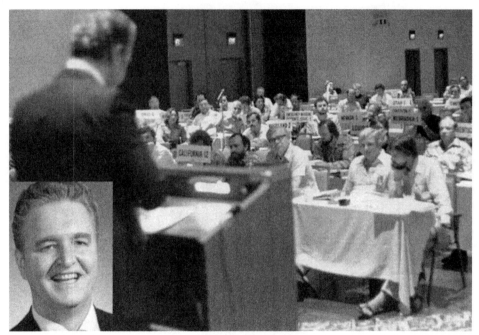

Figure 22. *John Rupke, M.D., tries to appease "The Young Turks" at the ACEP special Council meeting, April, 1978, Tarpon Springs, Florida. (From "Twenty-five Years on the Front Line," American College of Emergency Physicians, 1993.)*

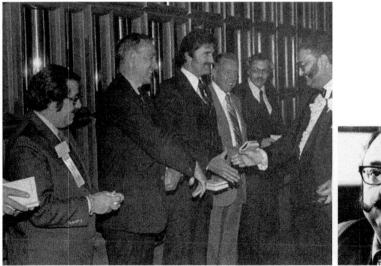
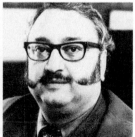

Figure 23. *Left: George Podgorny, M.D., ACEP and ABEM President, congratulates his colleagues (from left, Ron Krome, David Wagner, Karl Mangold, R. R. Hannas, Jr., Carl Jelenko III) after emergency medicine is approved as the 23rd medical specialty board by the American Board of Medical Specialties. (From "Twenty-five Years on the Front Line," American College of Emergency Physicians, 1993.) Right: George Podgorny, M.D. (From the American College of Emergency Physicians archive.)*

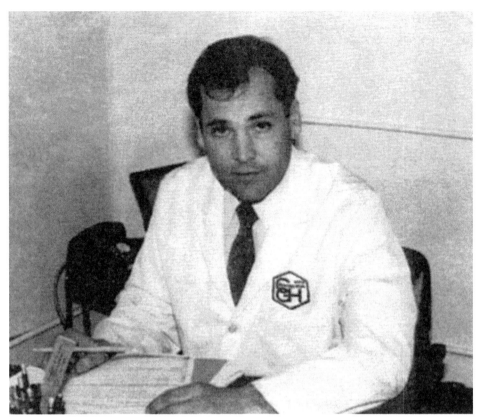

Figure 24. Richard Levy, M.D., circa 1978, returned from a vacation in Fiji to resurrect the Cincinnati emergency medicine program. (Photograph from the University of Cincinnati Department of Emergency Medicine archive.)

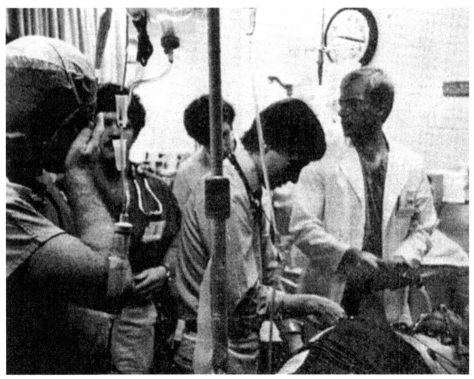

Figure 25. William Barsan, M.D., as an emergency medicine resident in the Cincinnati General Hospital ED, 1977. (Photograph from the University of Cincinnati Department of Emergency Medicine archive.)

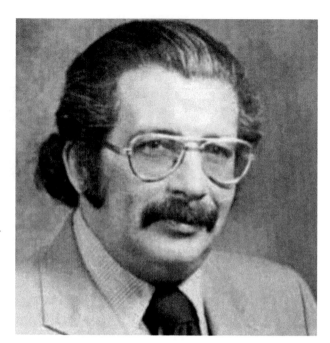

Figure 26. *Ronald Krome, M.D. Krome served as President of the American College of Emergency Physicians (ACEP), University Association of Emergency Medicine (UAEM), American Board of Emergency Medicine (ABEM), and editor of* Annals of Emergency Medicine, *providing a crucial link between emergency medicine practice and academic organizations. (Photograph from JACEP 1976; 5:1003.)*

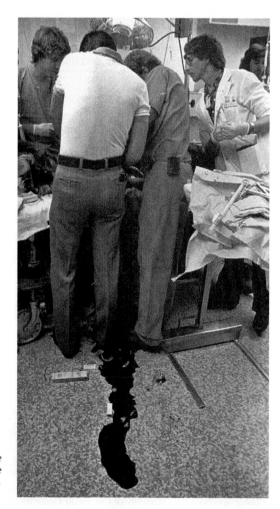

Figure 27. *Denver General Hospital. Emergency medicine residents manage a trauma patient. (Photograph from Eugene Richards,* Knife and Gun Club, *Atlantic Press Monthly Books, 1989.)*

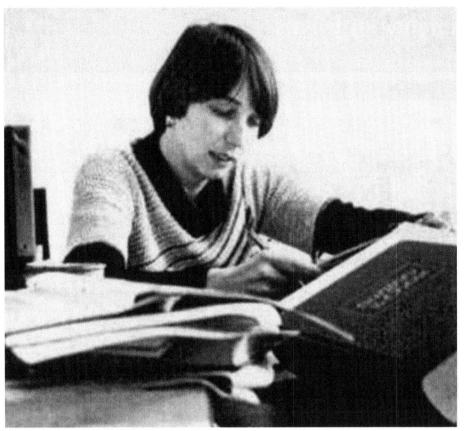

Figure 28. *Judith Tintinalli, M.D., prepares the first Study Guide in Emergency Medicine. (Photograph from JACEP 1977;6:87.)*

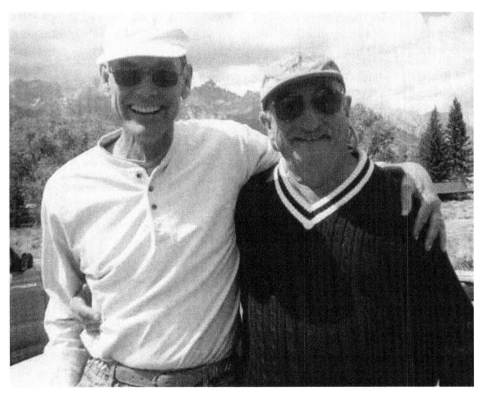

Figure 29. *Robert Dailey, M.D. (left) and Peter Rosen, M.D. (right), Grand Teton National Park, August 2002. (Photograph by Brian J. Zink, M.D.)*

Timeline of Events in the Development of Emergency Medicine in the United States, 1954–1989

Year	Event
1954	Robert H. Kennedy, M.D., "Oration on Trauma"—E.R. is "the weakest link."
1954	Thomas Flint, Jr., M.D., writes *Emergency Treatment and Management*, first "modern" textbook of emergency medicine.
1961	James Mills, Jr., M.D., and colleagues incorporate to establish the "Alexandria Plan" full-time emergency practice in Virginia.
1961	"Pontiac Plan" part-time emergency practice group incorporates in Michigan.
1965	Medicare and Medicaid legislation enacted.
1966	American Medical Association publishes *Emergency Department: A Handbook for Medical Staff*.
1966	National Academy of Sciences/National Research Council Report publishes *Accidental Death and Disability: The Neglected Disease of Modern Society*.
1968 (August)	John Wiegenstein, M.D., and seven other Michigan physicians form the American College of Emergency Physicians (ACEP).
1968 (November)	First national meeting of emergency physicians in Arlington, Virginia, organized by Reinald Leidelmeyer, M.D.—ACEP approved as the national emergency medicine organization.
1969 (February)	ACEP organizational meeting held in Chicago—supported by the AMA.
1969 (November)	First ACEP Scientific Assembly, Denver, Colorado.
1970 (February)	ACEP Workshop Meeting, New Orleans, Louisiana.
1970 (March)	University Association for Emergency Medical Services (UA/EMS) forms.
1970 (July)	Bruce Janiak, M.D., becomes the first emergency medicine resident at the University of Cincinnati.
1971	First academic Department of Emergency Medicine at the University of Southern California.
1972	First issue of *Journal of the American College of Emergency Physicians*.
1973	AMA hosts the Workshop Conference on Education of the Physician in Emergency Medical Care—"Blue Book" meeting.
1973	Emergency Medical Services (EMS) Act passes.
1973	Emergency Medicine Foundation created.
1974	Emergency Medicine Residents Association (EMRA) forms.
1974	ACEP forms the Committee on Board Establishment.
1975	Society for Teachers of Emergency Medicine (STEM) forms.
1975	AMA approves a permanent Section Council for Emergency Medicine.
1975	Liaison Residency Endorsement Committee forms.
1976	American Board of Emergency Medicine (ABEM) incorporates.
1976	Health Professions Educational Assistance Act provides funding to train emergency medicine residents.

1977	American Board of Medical Specialties votes down ABEM application as a primary Board.
1977	ABEM Certification Exam Field Test.
1978	ACEP Special Council Meeting to discuss modified conjoint Board proposal for ABEM.
1979	ABEM approval by ABMS as a modified conjoint Board.
1980	First ABEM certification exam administered, and first Board-certified emergency physicians are approved.
1982	Residency Review Commission for Emergency Medicine established.
1983	Emergency medicine first participates in National Resident Matching Program.
1989	ABEM is approved as a primary Board by the ABMS.
1989	University Association of Emergency Medicine and Society of Teachers of Emergency Medicine merge to form the Society for Academic Emergency Medicine (SAEM).

1 Seeds of Emergency Care

The Fifties: Happy Days for Some

The period from the end of World War II to the 1960s in the United States is regarded as one of economic prosperity and social stability. The mid-1950s has been described as "prosperous, stable, bland, religious, moral, patriotic, conservative, domestic, and buttoned-down."[1] After World War II unified the country, the energy, industry, and sense of purpose devoted to winning the war was transferred to developing a new, modern, urban/suburban, fast-moving America. The millions of veterans who returned from World War II ambitiously worked on new suburban communities, shopping malls, and super highways. Over the next decade society became much more mobile and less parochial. Business and the media became more national in scope—by the end of the 1950s, McDonald's restaurants were popping up in many cities around the country and television sets were present in most homes.[1] The 1950s are often viewed as a placid and harmonious time, but beneath the surface were ripples of uneasiness and discord.

After paying a dear price to defeat fascism during World War II, America found a new antagonist. The dominant foreign preoccupation, which also became a domestic obsession, was to halt and eradicate communism. Strong ideology meant strong economics as huge arms build up and United States involvement in the Korean War acted as a prolonged stimulus to the American economy.[1,2] But, Cold War politics, like a boogeyman in the closet, affected the psyche and sometimes the structure of people's lives. The same children who first played with Barbie dolls were introduced to Bert the Turtle, a government cartoon figure who instructed how to "duck and cover" in the event of an atomic bomb attack. Mothers stocked up on food and supplies for the family bomb shelter.[3,4] The activities of Senator McCarthy against perceived American communists created fear, uncertainty, and then embarrassment for the country.

Americans were also struggling with persistent racial inequalities. Although the 1954 Brown v. Board of Education Supreme Court ruling against segregated education in the South is heralded as the first significant step toward ending segregation, it was met with significant condemnation. In 1956, 101 members of Congress signed the "Southern Manifesto," expressing sharp disagreement with the Brown v. Board of Education ruling, and calling for the impeachment of Earl Warren, the Supreme Court chief justice.[5]

One of the biggest inequalities in 1950s American society was the economic disparity between the well to do and the poor, regardless of race.[2] The American dream of climbing from poverty to a better lifestyle was not realized on a large enough scale to prevent the existence of a poorly educated, downtrodden class of people. This underclass lacked the political power and resources to gain attention and help their condition at the federal level.[6] Nowhere was this more noticeable than in health care. In this pre-Medicare and pre-Medicaid era, health insurance was nonexistent for most poor Americans. With no ability to pay for medical care, and no obligation from private doctors to treat them, the poor typically did not seek medical care unless they were very ill or seriously injured.

American medicine was not quiescent in the 1950s. Spurred on by an infusion of federal funding for medical research and hospitals, significant advances were seen in treating disease. Perhaps the greatest medical triumph of the 1950s was the development of the polio vaccine. The work of Jonas Salk was followed closely by the media, and the announcement that the vaccine worked was trumpeted in the news.[7] Advances in the treatment and prevention of other infectious and medical diseases and the improvements in surgical care of trauma that came out of the Korean War made the public more aware of the potential for technologic and scientific progress to result in real improvements in health. Society pushed medicine, and medical discovery pushed society, toward a new type of health care.

One of the components of medical change of the post World War II period was an increased public reliance on hospital emergency rooms (ERs). In other medical fields, scientific discovery and academic growth often preceded or occurred with clinical demand. This was not the case with emergency care. As patients began to flock to ERs in the 1950s, the medical expertise and a system for providing quality emergency care were sorely lacking. Medicine was put into the position of having to catch up to public demand, but the professional solution to the ER problem did not arise until the 1960s. Some of the physicians who would provide the solution and would later have significant roles in the founding of emergency medicine were in their formative years or were starting their careers in the 1950s.

R. R. HANNAS, M.D.: THE EX-MARINE, GENERAL PRACTITIONER

From 1952 to 1965, the rural Oklahoma town of Sentinel was fortunate to have as one of its two physicians a wiry, energetic, former Marine who had graduated from Harvard Medical School. Although Ralston R. (R. R.) Hannas, Jr., was Ivy League–trained, he was a salt-of-the-earth Midwesterner. His father was an educated poultry man who became the editor of the *American Poultry Journal*. As a young man, R. R. was attracted to the order and discipline of military life. Following his undergraduate studies at Purdue University, where he was involved in the ROTC, he turned down his acceptance to Harvard Medical School to enlist in the Marine Corps in 1939. Hannas was stationed in the Pacific theater in World War II. Although he "never had to fire an angry round" in the war, he organized troop movements and support and was viewed as a strong leader by those under his command.[8] By the end of the war, at age 26, he had risen to the rank of Lieutenant Colonel. Perhaps his most important contribution to the Marines, and one that foreshadowed his organizational skills in the world of medicine, was his role in developing a program to facilitate the return of Marine Corps veterans to civilian life.

After his military service, Hannas reapplied to Harvard Medical School and was accepted into the entering class in 1946. He now had a wife and young children to support, and struggled to keep financially solvent. He asked his father's advice on raising chickens in order to help feed his family.

> ...he said get some New Hampshire Reds...that is the best breed for that area, they will do fine. I bought a hundred of them about the second month I was there. I made a little incubator in the basement, I got 95 to maturity, and at a certain point, when they were fryer stage, I just cut them in half and then I killed the poor half and dressed them myself and got them frozen, put them in a locker. We ate those the rest of my 4 years in medical school. The others laid eggs for us...I built my own chicken house in the backyard, I had a half an acre.[8]

Hannas received the Maimonides Award from Beth Israel Hospital, recognizing him as the student who worked the hardest during medical school, both on his studies and in his various jobs. He and his wife suffered a tragedy when their 5-1/2–year-old daughter, Margaret, developed an infectious illness and died. Hannas felt the horrible irony of "going to medical school to learn to cure and treat people and you can't do it in your own family."[8]

Following an influential medical school rotation at Boston Children's Hospital, Hannas decided he would become a pediatric surgeon. He did his internship at the University of Kansas Medical Center and then another year of training in Surgery. By the end of his second year, he was so far in debt that he realized he would need to go into practice to support his family. He worked with the state of Oklahoma to find a general practice position and joined a practice with another physician in the tiny town of Sentinel. He loved the tough and self-sufficient nature of the people of Southwest Oklahoma. He made house calls up to 50 miles from Sentinel: "If they called you, by God, you had better go!"[8] As a general practitioner who also had surgical training, Hannas did just about everything that a physician of those times could do for his patients.

> I can think of some experiences that were just unbelievable. I got called over to Rocky. Rocky was a little town 6 miles east of Sentinel…probably a town of about 500. I got called over to see this lady…she had this pain in her left side down here and she was in her 70s…anyhow, I went over and checked her and she was tender. I probably drew a blood sample and took it back with me, I gave her something to settle her down a little bit, probably 50 mg of Phenergan or something like that, which stopped them all. I got called the next morning—well, then I could feel like an ass. There is something going on here. It was palpable, but it was tender, but it wasn't a mass. So I brought her over to the hospital, got her typed and cross-matched, and we had a list of donors. Called a donor in, drew the blood myself, a couple of pints, from two different people. So, got her prepped, put a tube down, took her into surgery, gave her a spinal, opened her up. She had herniated a loop of her small intestine through the tubo-ovarian ligament. So it got through there, and it got caught, and it was getting gangrenous, so I calmly proceeded to excise the bad segment and get them out from under there and…and put her together. She didn't bat an eye during the procedure or after the procedure. I'm sure she went home in 4 or 5 days, something like that. You do it by yourself, what the hell, you can't wait for 5,000 guys to come in and help you. Those were the experiences that I will never forget. Then the same lady a few years later, they moved from Rocky up to Dill City, and she fell and busted her hip. I brought her down and pinned that. You know, you just did it. But, you had to have training. I had the training and when I was in my surgery residency, when I was on orthopedics… a couple of my best friends were orthopods, and, I said, "God damn it, you've got to teach me how to do these things or you are wasting my time!" They did. It was great. I really helped, but you had to do it.[8]

This ability to handle almost any medical problem in any patient would later serve Hannas well in his emergency medicine practice.

THE GENERAL PRACTITIONER: AN ANCESTOR TO THE EMERGENCY PHYSICIAN

R. R. Hannas's scope of practice was not unique in that era of medicine. Until the late 1960s, many general practitioners (GPs), most of whom had only a rotating internship, provided medical, minor surgical, obstetrical, and pediatric care. They had far fewer options for diagnosis and treatment of even common illnesses than exist today, but they were readily accessible and the first, and often only, point of care. But, despite this central role in American medicine, GPs were threatened as early as the 1930s by the movement to advanced training in medicine and medical specialization. GPs who trained in the early 1900s attended medical schools of varying quality and received little clinical instruction. Most went from medical school directly into practice, without the benefit of an internship or residency.

The Flexner report of 1910 helped to improve and standardize basic medical education. By promoting alliances between medical schools and hospitals, the Flexner report also played a role in creating the infrastructure for internships and residency training.[9–11] By the end of the 1920s, a 1-year internship was considered standard preparation to be a GP. A year of internship was required by the Surgeon General in World War I for a medical school graduate who wished to enlist in the Army Medical Corps.[11] Internships were largely unsupervised and viewed as a way for the medical school graduate, who had received primarily book knowledge, to gain practical clinical skills through long hours of immersion in hospital work.[11] By the 1930s, internships were a standard part of medical training, and in the Depression, they were even more valued. Rosemary Stevens notes,

There was every incentive for the intern or resident to stay on in his hospital post, where he at least had board and lodging, rather than to brave the financial uncertainties of private practice.[11]

When the early medical specialties of surgery, ophthalmology, otolaryngology, and internal medicine declared themselves and began to organize in the 1920s and 1930s, GPs found themselves competing with physicians who had residency training, certification, and better access to hospitals. For example, as the field of surgery evolved toward more complex, longer, intraabdominal procedures, it began to surpass the skills of the average GP, who had training only in simple surgical techniques. The GP who performed surgeries was now being scrutinized more carefully for competence, and some hospitals began to consider American College of Surgery fellowship status in granting privileges to perform surgery.[11]

The nature of general practice changed during this time. By the late 1920s, most physicians were delivering care from their offices, clinics, or hospitals. The number of house calls dropped greatly, especially in urban and suburban areas.[11] Most physicians at this time recognized the need to be affiliated with a hospital to have a successful practice. This was even more essential for the specialist than the GP. A Chicago physician, Quentin Young, M.D., described the demise of house calls:

The house call became the hostage and ultimately the victim of high tech. You'd say to the patient, who would describe a high fever, coughing, headache, and something severe, "Go to the emergency room." There you had the equipment for a proper exam. That was the beginning of subverting the emergency room into an alternative, very costly, primary care setting.[12]

GPs were in an undesirable and untenable position from the mid-1930s on as specialty training and organization increased. There was movement toward establishing some type of requirements and certification for GPs, mainly from the National Board of Medical Examiners (NBME) and the American Medical Association (AMA) and its Committee on Medical Education, but this fizzled after the advent of World War II. As Stevens describes it,

...a logical solution...would have been for the specialty certifying boards to come together, pool their resources, and offer a structure for graduate education and certification in all fields and branches of medicine, including general practice. Logic, however had little to do with the case.[11]

GPs had an identity crisis—they were a mixed group of practitioners with varying qualifications and types of practice and no clear voice in the world of medicine. In the 1920s and 1930s, training in general practice was viewed as a prerequisite for all medical practice. By the 1950s, general practice training was no longer considered the foundation for specialist training.[11,13] In 1947, GPs officially organized, with the formation of the American Academy of General Practice (AAGP). This was preceded in 1945 by a General Practice Section in the AMA House of Delegates. A proposal for a certifying board in general practice was submitted by the AMA's Committee on Medical Education to the Advisory Board for Medical Specialties in 1945, but was regarded as a bit premature and was turned down. The AAGP decided not to petition for a certifying board, and instead focused on helping GPs get hospital privileges and postgraduate or continuing medical education.[11]

Medical specialists had a mutually beneficial relationship with hospitals and came to dominate hospital care by the 1950s. GPs were not as likely to gain hospital appointments as specialists and began to fight for greater access to hospitals. The issue of hospital appointments became a legal one in 1945 as the GPs claimed restraint of trade. Hospitals and specialty organizations became more cautious about rules and policies that restricted hospital appointments to specialists.[11] This relaxation of qualifications for hospital appointments made it easier for GPs to work in hospitals. It may also have contributed to the permissive attitude in hospitals that later allowed the hiring of poorly qualified physicians to staff hospital ERs.

The shift in the proportion of American physicians who were general practitioners in the middle decades of the 1900s was remarkable. Pre–World War II, three of four physicians classified themselves as GPs. By 1955, this had decreased to two of three. In the first half of the 1960s, specialists became more common than GPs, and by 1966 only 31% of physicians were GPs.[9,11] As general practitioners felt the pinch from specialists, their survival as a medical group was threatened by reduced numbers of medical students choosing general practice as a career. Medical students, who were educated primarily by specialists, came to realize that greater prestige and incomes could be gained through residency training as a specialist. Even those students who entered medical school with plans to be GPs often were seduced to specialty practice.[14] The nature of general practice was also changing—less surgery and obstetrics, fewer house calls, but more patients per day. Those GPs who had hospital privileges also had to take care of increasingly complex hospitalized patients. By the mid-1950s,

> *The traditional family doctor was under siege and found he could not be the 24-hour-a-day, 7-days-a-week, 365-days-a-year bonesetter and pill roller to the thousands who rang his office phone.[15]*

It is notable that in a 1957 article in *Time* magazine describing a physician survey on house calls, the physician who reported the most house calls—77 in a week—was 70 years old. Most younger physicians were making far fewer calls and were increasingly steering their patients to their offices or the hospital, where better resources for diagnosis and treatment existed. There was a conflicted sense of responsibility in the medical world. On one extreme a Montana physician said in the survey:[16]

> *A doctor's justified in refusing at any time he doesn't want to serve the patient. We're no more obligated to give service than is the grocer.*

A more traditionally rooted Michigan physician is quoted as saying:

> *Nothing about medicine is as impressive to the layman as our willingness to get up and go out at midnight. Doctors must maintain their reputation on this score.[16]*

Another change in the way GPs practiced stemmed from how many physicians came to view their professional lives. In the early decades of the 20th century, physicians were viewed by their communities like clergymen—educated, selfless, always available, and more likely to comfort than cure. The post–World War II era brought increased business and increased incomes to physicians. The same advances that spurred specialization made medicine less accessible to the layman, but created a public that was more in awe of the physician as a professional scientist–healer.

In the prosperous years of the 1950s, physicians, like other Americans with the means, came to value and place more emphasis on leisure and family time. Some physicians began to refuse to provide around-the-clock coverage and would not take calls at night. This caused some public outcry, as examples of physician unavailability leading to poor patient outcomes hit the newspapers and magazines.[17,18] Physicians began to look for ways of alleviating the 24-hour-a-day commitment that went with some general and specialty practices without abrogating their duty to serve their patients.

In some communities, physician groups set up 24-hour physician exchanges to serve emergency calls. In Louisville, Kentucky, the Jefferson County Medical Society started an emergency call plan in the mid-1950s. Patients needing emergency attention would phone JU4-6357 and one of 25 physicians on call would promptly call the patient back and handle the case by either visiting the patient at home or seeing the patient in the ER. A magazine article describes how the system worked:

> *…an emergency panel doctor was called at 3 AM to see a man with fever, sore throat, and stiff neck. The doctor found him semiconscious, diagnosed meningitis, put him in the back seat of his car, and rushed him to a hospital.[17]*

Most of the physicians who participated in the emergency call plan were young and just starting to build their practices. By the late 1950s, physician exchanges were widespread, and it was claimed that no community in the United States with a population of more than 20,000 was without this type of plan.[17,18] Dr. Frederick W. Carr, a GP in Knoxville, Tennessee, took this concept a step further. In 1954, as a recent medical graduate, he became a total "night man." With his station wagon loaded with medical supplies and medications, he worked solely from 6 PM to 6 AM taking referrals from other doctors and answering medical emergency calls that came in through the doctor's telephone exchange. This practice was welcomed by the Knoxville medical community.[19]

Even as they changed with the times, or were forced into different roles by the pressures of medical specialization, the GPs of the 1940s and 1950s became the ancestors of both family practice physicians and emergency physicians. Some GPs, like R. R. Hannas, left their practices to become emergency physicians. In the early years of emergency medicine, they encountered the same issues that GPs had faced for decades—less training than their specialist peers, huge clinical demand, the perception of being less skilled and less in touch with modern medical science and procedures, and lacking a platform in the world of academic medicine. However, the early emergency physicians learned from the hard lessons of their general practice ancestors and made residency training, the creation of a specialty board, and academic development priorities in their quest for specialty recognition.

The Potent Effects of Wars on 20th Century American Medicine

Military experiences had a profound influence on many of the men who would enter medicine after their service. R. R. Hannas had not yet entered medical school when he was in the military, but came to admire his defense battalion doctor, Orrin Levin, who worked in Boston and later became a mentor when Hannas attended Harvard Medical School.[8] The number of physicians who served during World War II was staggering—by 1944 the number of physicians in the medical departments of the U.S. Army and Navy was 52,000, and the number of physicians left home in civilian practice was around 94,000.[20] As would be expected from an institution that values rank and classification, the Army's medical department emphasized the importance of advanced training and specialty certification for World War II physicians by reviewing and categorizing nearly 22,000 medical officers as A, B, C, or D. The more prestigious A and B classifications were given to those physicians who were board certified, had completed a residency, or had extensive experience in a medical specialty. GPs were considered less qualified and were usually assigned to group D.[10,11,20]

Military medical practice and research during World War II had a major affect on American medicine. For the first time, antibiotics were used on a widespread basis to treat infections in soldiers and to prevent postoperative infections. Army researchers and physicians discovered preventive measures for typhoid fever and perfected a vaccine. The treatment of shock and multiple-trauma casualties was improved through a better understanding of the role of blood and fluid resuscitation. Psychiatric conditions in soldiers were also studied, and new treatment strategies were developed.[21] In terms of a systems approach to battlefield casualties, a more rapid response and transport to field hospitals allowed wounded soldiers to receive emergent treatment in time for it to make a difference. Clinical research in the military was conducted on a larger scale, and was arguably more sophisticated, than research at U.S. medical schools. The improvements in military health systems and medical advancements in the 1930s and 1940s led to a marked decrease in morbidity and mortality for soldiers in World War II compared with those in World War I. The mortality rate for wounded soldiers in World War II was 4%, compared with 8% in World War I. For other medical problems, the improvements were even more striking. The mortality rate of pneumonia was 28% in soldiers of World War I, but was reduced to less than 1% in World War II. Overall, the annual death rate per 1,000 soldiers for nonsurgical diseases was 0.6 in World War II compared with 15.6 in World War I.[20,21]

The military experience for most U.S. physicians was not just service, it was also a valuable training experience. Especially for those who had minimal training prior to their military stint, the knowledge gained about the diagnosis and treatment of acute medical and surgical problems was considerable. The application of this knowledge improved civilian medical practice. Physicians also gained an appreciation for how a medical care system that utilized multiple health providers for disease prevention, triage and acute management of injuries and illnesses, and convalescence could function. This appreciation contributed to the shift in American medicine away from a physician-centered approach to a health system approach.[11,13,22] Even nonphysician soldiers became accustomed to an approach to medical care that did not revolve around one physician. Robert Rathburn, M.D., who was one of the founders of the American College of Emergency Physicians, noted that the hundreds of thousands of servicemen returning from World War II were

> ...oriented toward this kind of...sick call medicine...In the army when you were sick, you didn't call a doctor, you showed up at sick call, got your shot or your aspirin, and that was that.[15]

After World War II, military policies continued to influence American medicine. The Veterans Administration (VA) required that all physician specialists working in the VA system have specialty board certification.[9] The military also encouraged specialty training through the GI Bill. This educational program for World War II veterans provided a residency subsidy of up to 4 years with a living allowance. Hospitals, both academic and community, also received a subsidy for offering residency positions to general infantrymen (GIs).[11,23,24] General practice physicians and veterans who were considering careers in medicine had received a clear message from observing military medicine that specialists were a higher class of physicians. Many nonspecialist physician veterans took advantage of the GI Bill to become specialists. The result was that thousands of physicians pursued specialty training in the post–World War II years. The number of residency positions increased from 5000 in 1940 to nearly 19,000 by 1950. By 1955, over 25,000 resident physicians were training to become specialists.[9–11]

The Korean War continued to emphasize specialist-delivered medical care, particularly in the management of battlefield casualties. Advances in drug therapy, surgical procedures, and technology that had their roots in World War II, and had been refined in the next decade, were applied during the Korean War. For the first time, surgical specialists were used in field hospitals. Deaths from hemorrhage due to vascular injuries and the limb amputation rate were reduced dramatically by the end of the Korean War. New methods of getting casualties to field hospitals were also used in Korea. Battlefield triage systems and helicopter transport of injured soldiers to nearby hospitals (MASH units) became commonplace. Over 17,000 wounded soldiers were evacuated by UH-1 (Huey) helicopters during the Korean War. This improvement in wartime emergency surgical and medical services further reduced morbidity and mortality in battlefield casualties.[21,25] Although the incorporation of these principles into U.S. civilian emergency care would take another two decades, the lessons that military physicians learned in Korea directed greater scrutiny on the care of acutely injured and ill patients. Another insight gained by some physicians from their Korean War experience was that it might be possible to develop a medical career around the care of trauma victims.[9,10,26,27]

Although military medicine in World War II and the Korean War was extremely important to the development of medicine in the second half of the 20th century, it was not the primordium of American emergency medicine. Even the Vietnam War, as will be seen in subsequent chapters, did not have as much effect on the field of emergency medicine as one might imagine. Wartime advances in management of shock and multiple trauma focused new interest in these areas, but the treatment of shock and injuries remained in the domain of surgeons. A few of the founders of emergency medicine, like R. R. Hannas, served in World War II or the Korean War, but they do not usually credit their war service with their eventual interest in emergency medicine. In terms of emergency medical systems (EMSs), World War II may have been the first venue where a functioning system of triage, transport, and acute attention to casualties resulted in improved outcomes, and Korean War EMS took this to a new level. The significance of this was not lost on physicians and other health care providers, but the dissemination of the principles of EMS to the civilian world was very slow. In Great Britain, emergency medical services in the civilian sector were acutely needed during the German attacks of World War II, and the knowledge gained from the this experience helped to organize British EMS years before the same process occurred in the United States.[28]

A key concept to come out of the comparison of World War I with World War II care was the important role of professional experience in the early triage and management of battlefield casualties. In World War I, the task of triage and directing initial care in the "sorting tent" was given to the most inexperienced medical officers. In World War II triage and early battlefield casualty management was the job of experienced medical officers, and it is generally accepted that this was part of the reduction in morbidity and mortality seen in World War II casualties. The obvious analogy of an inexperienced intern in a busy ER being like an inexperienced medical officer in battle was not drawn in the medical literature until 1958.[29] The large scale utilization of trained, experienced physicians in emergency care would not be realized until at least 30 years after the end of World War II.

DAVID WAGNER, M.D.: A QUAKER DISPOSITION AND A LIBERAL HEART

David Wagner was born in 1931, a Depression-era baby, and was brought up in the small midwestern city of Jackson, Michigan.

> ...I was born to a rather liberally focused, well-educated, dirt-poor minister...as part of an era when money was scarce and progressive movements were rampant. My father was active very early on in Michigan labor movements with Walter Reuther and...was an activist cleric, you might say.[30]

Wagner's father was an Evangelical Reform minister, but his parents were very influenced by the Quaker philosopher D'Elton Trueblood. They encouraged David to attend Earlham College, a small Quaker school in Indiana. His parents could not pay for his entire education, but Wagner remembers his father's generosity when he went away to college:

> ...when I went to college there wasn't any money. He went to the upper drawer of the desk, I can still see it, which was our bank, that's where all the money was, so I could always know how much we had—it was always there. He pulled out $600 and said, "You know, that's all I've got, but here it is...go to college."...I never got another penny from home and I was able to find ways to get through college and subsequently medical school without going to a well that didn't have much in it. Looking back, that was a wonderful thing.[30]

At first, Wagner did not do well at Earlham College,

> I really goofed around the first couple of years, and then all of a sudden there was a moment when I told myself that you had better get your act together. I got a bead on medicine...and then went from near the bottom of the class to graduating with some nice credentials and getting on into medical school.[30]

Wagner tried to get into medical school at Washington University in St. Louis, but was wait-listed. He interviewed at the University of Missouri in 1952 but found that some of the interviewers expressed their displeasure at having to enroll black medical students for the first time. This did not sit well with Wagner: "...so when I got an acceptance there I made a point of sending them a letter and saying 'thanks, but no thanks, you're not the type of school that I want to go to'." Wagner was accepted to St. Louis University Medical School. Only about 10% of the student body was non-Catholic, but Wagner found the experience of being a religious minority to be interesting and enriching.

After medical school, Wagner did an internship at the Milwaukee General Hospital from 1956 to 1957. In Milwaukee, he discovered a medical care system for emergencies that was unique in the 1950s and gave him an early taste of emergency medicine:

> Milwaukee at the time had an Emergency Hospital down in center city Milwaukee...all the emergencies from the towns went there for initial triage and treatment. They had a second floor in which people who needed to be hospitalized were hospitalized. This would be considered today a broad-based holding unit...you were there for 24 hours and then dispersed to the hospital of your choice. It was way ahead of its time, and I stumbled on to that in the first month or two of my internship.[30]

Although the concept of an emergency center was new, the Emergency Hospital had the physician-staffing pattern of the times. The least experienced doctors, the rotating interns, were in charge of the emergency area. But, Wagner was attracted to this environment,

> I liked it so much that I juggled my internship to go back and do another couple [of] months of that...you were on 12 then off 12, then on 24 and off 24, and you worked with the medical resident who was in charge of the upstairs. As you look back it was pretty scary, but it was the typical model.[30]

Military service was a requirement for young men in the 1950s, but Wagner's Quaker beliefs were not compatible with serving in the military. Fortunately, an alternative existed in the Indian Service. After his internship, he and his new wife moved to New Mexico where he served a 2-year stint at the New Mexico Indian Service Hospital. The clinical experience was enriching and rewarding, and Wagner developed a new passion outside of medicine that affected his career path. As he now tells medical students who seek career counseling,

> ...You wind up making...what turn out to be life-defining issues on very serendipitous, flimsy bits of information...Well, I had gotten the skiing bug. I had discovered skiing in Santa Fe at the Santa Fe Basin, and I was nuts for skiing. I just wanted to ski more than anything else in my life. My wife sort of went along with me...So we looked around the country and said, "Where can we ski?" We decided the Northwest was going to be it, because they could ski up there 11 months of the year...I said, "What are we going to do in the Northwest?" ...I didn't want to be a psychiatrist and I didn't want to be a pediatrician. They had an opening in a surgery position, and I said, "I'll take it!" That is how I made the decision to go into surgery. It was clearly because I was absolutely nuts to go skiing. Of course, we didn't get to ski a lot....[30]

Wagner went from the Indian Service Hospital to the general surgery residency at the U.S. Public Health Service Hospital in Seattle, Washington in 1959. During his 4 years of surgery training, he developed a strong interest in pediatric surgery, and did a pediatric surgery fellowship at St. Christopher's Hospital for Children in Philadelphia. In 1964, he and his wife went back for a year to New Mexico where he was a surgeon at the U. S. Indian Service Hospital in Gallup. Although they enjoyed the experience, he and his wife decided to move back to Philadelphia and settle where their children could attend Quaker schools. Wagner settled into a practice of pediatric and general surgery.

The Central Role of the Hospital in the Advent of Emergency Care

Without the development of a strong hospital system, hospital-based medical specialties like emergency medicine would not have evolved. It is difficult to imagine the practice of medicine without the hospital as a major part of the picture, but in the pre–World War II era hospitals played a less dominant role in medicine. Many city hospitals arose from 19th century almshouses, and in the early 1900s, they were more able to minister to the poor and address social problems than they were to provide health care.[31] A number of factors contributed to the rise of hospitals in the United States. The first was the advancement of medical science and the clinical application of scientific discoveries in the hospital setting. Post-Flexner medical schools became more science-based, and had a better infrastructure for conducting laboratory and clinical science. In the World War II years, the federal government provided a strong stimulus to all types of scientific research, including medicine, through sponsored research programs. Academic hospitals transitioned from being places of humane care and convalescence for mostly incurable conditions, to places of application of new scientific discoveries in medical diagnosis and treatment. The ability to diagnose and monitor diseases with new technologies such as x-rays, electrocardiograms (ECGs), and laboratory blood tests, coupled with the ability to treat diseases with antibiotics and other drugs, meant that the hospital was now a place for potential cure, rather than a place to go to die.[9,10,22,32] The health care workforce changed dramatically during this time. In 1900, physicians accounted for 35% of those in health occupations. By 1967, this had decreased to 9%, as the number of nurses, technicians, and ancillary hospital staff greatly increased.[33] Having the rudiments of diagnosis and treatment readily available at hospitals changed the way that people reacted when confronted with an acute medical problem. They now considered going to the hospital instead of their physician's office when they were acutely ill. In 1964, an Ohio physician described how his office practice had changed as hospitals developed.

> *Thirty years ago my office was much better equipped to handle accidents than our hospital emergency room was. I had a nurse, lab technician, x-ray, fluoroscope, ECG, closet full of plaster and splints, Kirschner drills and wire, all kinds of operating sets, facilities for anesthesia, etc. Today I have no x-ray, no ECG, no lab technician, and my office is not cluttered up with splints, plaster, and Vincent tubes for transfusion, etc. Were I to do the procedures I formerly did in my office I would be held for malpractice simply because we now have adequate and better facilities in the hospital emergency room.*[34]

The shift of diagnosis and treatment from the doctor's office to the hospital also meant that the physician could see more patients in a day and did not have to bear all the costs of new medical devices and equipment. The number of patients seen per week by a physician in general office practice doubled in the period from 1935 to 1955. Therefore, it was not just the access to technology that made hospitals the focus of care, it was also the movement toward specialist care and the convenience and efficiency of consolidated resources in the hospital. Another effect was the geographic localization of health care. Hospitals, as the centers for diagnosis and treatment, became like magnets for physician practices. By the 1950s, many physicians relocated their offices out of their homes or their immediate communities to be adjacent to hospitals. Some enterprising hospitals built outpatient clinic buildings and rented space to physicians. This clustering of physician practices around hospitals lead to the logical next step—physicians began to band together and work in group practices.

As hospitals became the focal points of health care, the federal government began to provide large-scale support. The Hill-Burton Act of 1946 allocated federal funds to help build hospitals, especially in rural and smaller communities. This legislation was the result of haggling between those legislators who wanted a full, national health care plan and those who wanted a hands-off approach by the federal government toward health care. In the end, giving money to build hospitals was the best compromise. Between 1946 and 1968, the Hill-Burton initiative, established as a cooperative program between voluntary hospitals and the states, spent over $10 billion on hospitals. The number of U.S. hospitals increased 21%, from 4,523 in 1946 to 5,736 in 1965.[10] Some of the Hill-Burton money went to renovate existing hospitals and to build new emergency departments.[10,22] Despite this huge level of federal support for hospital construction and renovation, many communities in the 1960s still lacked an adequate number of hospital beds, and many municipal hospitals, once the palaces of medical care, were in a sorry state of disrepair.[35] Hospital development had not caught up with the demographic shifts of the 1950s and 1960s—suburbanites were often without a nearby quality hospital. The regulation and accreditation of hospitals became formalized in 1952 with the formation of the Joint Commission on Accreditation of Hospitals (JCAH)—this was a nongovernmental program developed by the AMA, the American Hospital Association, the American College of Surgeons, and American College of Physicians.[10] The Hill-Burton legislation increased the number of hospitals, and along with the shift in specialist care, created an "if you build it, they will come" phenomenon in hospital emergency departments that was evident by the mid-1950s.

The Milwaukee Emergency Hospital, where David Wagner did some of his internship training, was an early attempt by the Milwaukee County hospital system to address care in the inner city. The Milwaukee County Board has a history dating back to the 1840s of providing care for those who cannot pay for medical care. The original county hospitals, including a 600-bed facility constructed in 1927, were built about 6 miles west of center city. Two explanations are given for this location—first, the hospital was built where the population was centered at that time, and second, the county administrators were trying "to get these unfortunate folks out of sight, and perhaps as a result, also out of mind."[32] By the 1930s, the city's poor expressed a growing displeasure with the remote location of the County Hospital. This prompted the construction of what came to be known as Milwaukee Emergency Hospital in the center city. This hospital opened in 1929 and served as a receiving hospital for acutely ill or injured residents of Milwaukee. Patients might be transported to the Emergency Hospital by the Milwaukee County ambulance service in Cadillac hearses that were customized to serve as ambulances. Indigent patients were attended to, and might even have surgery at the Emergency Hospital, but were then transferred out to the County Hospital if they required a longer hospital stay. Those who had the ability to pay were initially treated at the Emergency Hospital and then transferred to a private hospital.

Although the Milwaukee County system for providing emergency care to indigent patients in the 1930s to 1950s was ahead of its time, and may have planted a seed in David Wagner's mind about emergency care, it was more of a triage system than an early model for emergency medicine. As will be seen later, by the mid-1950s some hospital administrators and professional hospital organizations began to publish articles about ER service. However, the physician component was still missing. In the 1950s, emergency care in Milwaukee and elsewhere in America was provided by the least trained physicians. County boards and hospitals could ensure access for their citizens, but they could not ensure quality emergency care.

The concept of emergency hospitals in cities carried through to the 1960s and was proposed in the National Health Forum on emergency care in 1962. By then, however, the Milwaukee Emergency Hospital had become inferior to the County Hospital for the management of trauma patients and critically ill patients. With improved ambulance transport, not much rationale could be found for taking critically ill patients first to an Emergency Hospital that was inadequate to care for them, and then transferring them several miles to the County Hospital. Three surgeons who had worked for decades in the Milwaukee County Hospital system wrote a very negative review of the Milwaukee Emergency Hospital in the *Journal of Trauma* in 1963. The title was provocative: "The Trauma Patient vs. Emergency Care." The authors cited that most emergency patients in the Emergency Hospital were not trauma patients, sicker patients were not well managed, and a full range of medical backup to handle emergency cases was lacking in the Emergency Hospital. "Emergency care is every physician's responsibility" became an often-quoted statement from this article by surgeons who felt the burden of an increasing number of trauma victims and saw no involvement in the emergency department by their medical colleagues.[36]

City hospitals were the default centers of care for black and other minority patients, regardless of their ability to pay. In Chicago, black patients who were cared for at Cook County Hospital in the 1950s and 1960s actually had higher incomes and were more likely to have health insurance than white patients, but they were forced to use the public hospital because of their race.[31] In the South, the problems of poor-quality hospital and emergency care were felt even more acutely by blacks, who were not allowed access to the normal medical care received by whites. Most hospitals in the South were segregated by race—in some cities separate hospitals existed for blacks and whites, in others the hospital itself had white and black wards. In Memphis, middle-class blacks resented having to go to the charity wards of municipal hospitals for care, and this spurred the building of the E.H. Crump Hospital in 1956. Named for a prominent black politician, the hospital would become a state-of-the-art academic facility for black patients, staffed by black doctors. Although this was a partial solution to the problem of health care for blacks, it perpetuated medical racial segregation in Memphis.[37]

JOHN WIEGENSTEIN, M.D. (1930–2004): FROM SEMINARY TO AVIATION TO MEDICINE

John Wiegenstein, was born in 1930 in a farm cabin in Missouri, and like David Wagner, was raised during the Depression. Wiegenstein's grandfather, who had a large farm in Fredericktown, gave his son and new wife the cabin to help them get started. The birth was not officially recorded, and years later Wiegenstein had to ask the doctor who delivered him to provide an affidavit so that he could obtain a birth certificate.[38] John's father was a foreman for the Missouri highway department, and the job required travel to construction sites around the state. John and his sister spent much of their preschool years living in various Missouri motels and hotels. The family settled back in Fredericktown where John attended a Catholic grade school with eight students in his class. He then entered the St. Louis Preparatory Seminary, a 6-year program for those aspiring to priesthood. Overall, he enjoyed his seminary experience and performed well enough to earn a scholarship to American University in Rome for 3 years of study in philosophy. By that time, Wiegenstein was starting to have second thoughts:

> I was asking a lot of questions in class about why we go to hell. Religion has to be rational and it didn't seem to me that some parts were rational. They made appointments for spiritual counseling, and I decided I'd had enough…I didn't feel I had the vocation…The Seminary had Polish nuns and they started looking good to me, I thought that was a bad sign.[38]

Wiegenstein turned down the scholarship and left the seminary. He consulted a pastor on what he should do next. The pastor looked at John's excellent math and science grades and advised him to study engineering at the General Motors Institute of Technology in Flint, Michigan. Wiegenstein soon discovered that engineering was not for him, nor were brief studies of business and economics. He and a friend decided to pursue the military and enrolled in the Aviation Cadets program in the United States Air Force. Wiegenstein was excited to learn how to fly, but realized that military aviation also was not his calling. He had just married, and he and his wife were thinking about starting a family. After getting his pilot's license, Wiegenstein had to undergo a 60-hour flight check by the Air Force. If he "washed out" and did not pass this check he could be released from the military after his 2-year commitment. Wiegenstein "gave them a ride they'll never forget," washed out, and at the age of 19 returned to Flint. He took premedical courses at the University of Michigan and borrowed the $20 application fee to apply to the University of Michigan Medical School. He was accepted into the entering class of 1956.[38]

Wiegenstein's medical school academic record was undistinguished, although he was a class leader and vice president of his graduating class. He worked nights as a cab driver and at the information desk of the hospital. He often nodded off during his morning classes, and ended up failing pathology. In his clinical years, he worked a different night job—as the covering ER physician at Beyer Memorial Hospital in neighboring Ypsilanti. Wiegenstein was hired by the hospital administrator and was pleased to be paid $1.50 per hour. He recalls one of his experiences:

> I got a lot of lacerations. People in Ypsilanti had a tendency to have slasher fights and so I got lots of training—no training! I had foreign bodies that were embedded in a cornea and I'd call the ophthalmologist and he'd say, "Well, just flip it out."

I'd say, "No it's too deep, I tried with a Q-tip."

"Well, do you know how to curette this?"

I said, "I'm going to leave you on the phone while I do this. I don't want to perforate this guy's cornea."

"He's tough, don't worry about it!"

In other words, they forced you into doing these things. Good experience I suppose, but not well directed.[38]

EMERGENCY ROOM PHYSICIAN STAFFING: PRE-1960

Like many of the pioneers of emergency medicine, John Wiegenstein got his first experience in an ER as a largely unqualified physician provider. Why would a hospital in a well-populated area have to resort to staffing its ER with medical students? Why were some of the sickest and most emergent patients being attended to by the least qualified physicians? The answers to these questions lie in the peculiar physician demographics of post–World War II America and the evolution of hospitals and access to care.

The emphasis on scientific development during World War II helped to spawn huge federal and private corporate initiatives in medical research. As Kenneth Starr notes, the four major federal postwar programs—medical research, mental health, the VA, and community hospital construction—boosted the resources and capabilities of the medical profession and institutions, but did not threaten their sovereignty.[9] The rapid growth of the National Institutes of Health (NIH), with generous grants to academic medical centers to carry out the work of the NIH, shifted the focus of medical schools from merely educating students to building biomedical research programs. More medical students became interested in academic and scientific careers, and the faculty ranks of medical schools swelled. The growth in the percentage of physicians who practiced as researchers, teachers, or as employees of governmental or other institutions was accompanied by attrition in the ranks of general practitioners. The number of U.S. doctors in private practice per capita declined from 108/100,000 people in 1940 to 91/100,000 people in 1957.[9,13]

At the same time that the numbers of GPs and physicians in private practice were declining, the number of people who were presenting to hospital ERs for care was increasing. The first data on ER visits began to appear in the mid-1950s. In 1954, an estimated 9.4 million patients were seen in U.S. hospital ERs, and by 1965, it had tripled to 28.7 million patients.[39] A 1956 study of 90 Eastern and Midwestern hospitals found a nearly 300% increase in ER visits from 1940 to 1955.[40] At the same time, hospital admissions and nonemergency outpatient visits were increasing at a more modest rate.[40-44] At Hartford Hospital, ER visits went from fewer than 2,000 per year in 1938 to almost 22,000 per year in 1957.[43] The first assumption by health and hospital experts was that the relative physician shortage during World War II had caused an increase in ER visits. However, the rate of increase was higher after the war than during the war. From 1940 to 1945, ER visits increased by only 8.4%. From 1945 to 1950, the increase was 60%, and from 1945 to 1950 was 64%.[40] This growth in ER patient volumes was not primarily attributable to population growth or shift. Hospitals reported a marked increase in ER visits even when the local population served had remained the same. The rise in ER visits continued unabated in the 1960s and 1970s. By today's standards, the hospital ER patient volumes of the 1950s seem small. For example, the 22,000 ER patients that Hartford Hospital treated in 1957 is only about one fourth of what a similar teaching hospital of today handles. But, in the 1950s, hospitals and the medical profession were not prepared for any increase in ER visits.

A common method of ER staffing for smaller and midsized nonacademic hospitals in the 1950s (and even until the 1970s for some) was to have a nurse assigned to the ER who would assess patients, make triage decisions, and then call an appropriate physician to deliver care.[22,45] Physicians were not obligated to provide this care, and some with busy practices found emergency patients to be a significant distraction from their regular duties. Several phone calls might be made by the nurse to find a physician who could care for an emergency patient. In critical cases, the time spent trying to locate a physician could be fatal. By 1960, most larger hospitals began to staff their ERs with physicians, residents, or medical students like John Wiegenstein, but finding willing and able providers was very difficult.[38,46,47]

Some of the medical students hired by hospitals may have been better trained and qualified than the physicians who were often hired to staff ERs. Since emergency practice was not considered a real occupation for a physician, only those without a regular job were available to be hired. Hospitals sometimes resorted to hiring troubled, transient, or aged doctors work in the ER. Some were alleged to have alcoholism, drug abuse, or criminal records. Emergency practice was not something that any self-respecting physician would do for a living—it might be part of a physician's career journey, but it was never a destination.

The debate about the U.S. physician workforce had been ongoing since the end of World War II. The large influx of veterans who entered medicine or did residency training under the GI Bill increased the number of physicians in the United States and this led to a feeling that the number of medical school graduates was adequate and should not be increased. There was no master plan on physician supply at the federal level, or in the medical professions. The prevailing philosophy in medicine was that private practice was also "...taken to mean professional privacy—the privilege of a responsible profession to regulate its members and to dictate its destiny...."[11] This philosophy was put in to action by the AMA and effectively minimized public or governmental input in to the supply and practice patterns of physicians from 1945 until the 1960s. In 1951, the AMA's Committee on Medical Education recommended that the number of internships be reduced. Hospitals vigorously opposed this, and no restrictions were put in place—in fact, the number of internships and residency positions continued to increase in the 1950s. The Hill-Burton legislation had resulted in an increased number of hospitals, but little thought had been given at the federal level to how these hospitals would be staffed with health care providers.[10] The transition of medicine to a more business-oriented, profit-driven enterprise meant the application of corporate principles, and one of these was finding cheap labor.

The lack of a coherent policy on physician workforce between medical schools, the federal government, and the growing health care industry created an intern deficit in the 1950s. In 1957, American medical schools were graduating fewer than 7,000 medical students per year while hospitals were seeking to fill more than 12,000 internship positions. Foreign medical graduates and physicians began to immigrate to the United States in large numbers to fill this gap. The United States was not always a favored place to do postgraduate medical training. In the early 1900s, it was common for U.S. physicians who aspired to greater clinical knowledge and exposure to the science of medicine to seek additional education in Germany or other European nations.[22] However, by the end of World War II, massive U.S. federal support of medical science had helped to build strong biomedical research and medical education systems. American medicine and biomedical research were viewed worldwide as state of the art. Doctors from other countries began to look to the United States as the best training environment.[11,48] Prior to the 1950s, most foreign physicians who emigrated to the United States came from Northern European countries where medical training was more similar to American medicine. In the 1950s and 1960s, the swell of immigrant physicians arose from Asia, Latin America, and the Middle East. Twenty percent were from the Philippines. Public concern about the number of foreign doctors and their qualifications and expertise spurred the creation of the Educational Council for Foreign Medical Graduates (ECFMG) in 1956. The ECFMG developed an exam, first administered in 1958, to test medical knowledge and English competency. As hospitals and residency programs began to require successful completion of the ECFMG exam for foreign interns and residents, a temporary slowing in the numbers of foreign medical graduates available for intern and residency positions was seen.[49] This had some effect on the origination of emergency medicine practice in the United States, as will be seen in Chapter 2. By 1965, one fourth of all interns and residents in the United States were foreign graduates.[50] The prior medical training of these new immigrants was inconsistent, and their education once in the

United States was often hampered by limited English language comprehension. The flood of international physicians in to the United States was perpetuated by the 1965 amendments to the Immigration and Nationality Act. Foreign physicians were given preference for immigrant visas, presumably because of the shortage of U.S. physicians. The control of foreign physicians in to the United States, like all of the major decision-making in American medicine, was spastic, with the AMA, federal and state governments, hospitals, and political groups all having influence on the process.[48,49]

Unlike today, in the 1940s and 1950s, many smaller community hospitals offered internships. Interns were a key element in the symbiosis of hospital and private physician. They provided cheap labor, while ostensibly receiving quality training. This allowed hospitals to keep their beds full and patients moving through the hospital system without having to rely on busy community physicians for basic patient care. Private practice physicians were freed of many hospital tasks and could spend their time seeing patients in the office or doing surgery.[11,51] While most academic medical centers could compete for U.S. medical school graduates through the National Residency Matching Program, which was established in 1952, community hospitals and inner city hospitals were less favored by U.S. medical graduates. These hospitals often turned to foreign medical graduates to fill internship and residency positions.

Interns and residents played a big role in ER staffing in the 1950s. In Shortliffe's 1956 survey of 90 hospitals with a range of 150 to 1,000 beds, 71% of hospitals reported staffing their ERs with house officers, and 21% used private physicians.[40] Academic medical center ERs were routinely staffed by interns, with occasional supervision by resident physicians, and even less often by the presence of a faculty-teaching physician. This type of junior-level staffing met the needs of many large urban teaching hospitals.[52] As community hospitals were finding it harder to fill their internships with U.S. medical graduates, they were facing increasing ER patient volumes.[40,43,46]

Many foreign physicians were assigned to the ER as part of their internships. At some community and inner-city hospitals, the percentage of foreign interns and residents was so high that patients might have come to assume that only foreign doctors worked in the ER. Although many of these new immigrants were strong students in their native lands, they were often struggling to learn English, may have had inferior medical training, and were not provided with adequate supervision as they worked in U.S. hospitals.[48] As a result, the rest of the medical profession and the public came to perceive the ER as a place of poor-quality medical practice—a place where, as Frances Mills, who lived in this era notes, "...the great unhappiness with the ER at that time was that people couldn't understand the doctors, they were all foreign."[53] Kenneth Iserson, an emergency physician who worked on a Rescue Squad in Maryland in the 1960s describes Holy Cross Hospital at that time

> ...there were a few emergency docs working there, and if they spoke English that was good. It was clear that most of them would have had trouble working any place else.[54]

After their internships, foreign physicians were usually less competitive for residency training, or for quality jobs in communities. Many found employment in the most undesirable positions of those times. Starr describes three groups of physicians in 1960 America—academic physicians (including interns and residents); private, office-based community physicians; and physicians working in rural or inner city areas or state institutions. This third group included physicians who worked in ERs.

> Smallest in number, lowest in prestige, these were often older general practitioners or, increasingly, younger foreign medical graduates. They were the most professionally isolated of physicians, though some worked in the shadows of the great medical centers.[9]

By the early 1960s, some concerns were developing about the number of foreign physicians in the United States, and that too few U.S. physicians were being trained.

In New York City, 11 of the major municipal hospitals had house staffs that were entirely composed of foreign medical graduates.[50] Hospitals in Chicago, Los Angeles, and other large cities had a similar reliance on foreign physicians for ward and emergency coverage. Dr. Ray E. Trussel, commissioner of hospitals in New York City, described the situation in the Harlem Hospital in the late 1950s:

> A state of crisis developed...A large number of interns and residents had to be removed from patient care responsibilities because they had failed the examinations given for foreign medical graduates. I was requested immediately to conduct an independent survey. The conditions found were incredible. Injured and sick patients were sitting on benches because there were no more beds...Patients were lying in bed with fractures 5 days old, which had not been set....[50]

This example, which helped to bring about a reorganization of New York hospitals starting in 1961, demonstrates the pattern of blaming foreign medical graduates for the ills of the health care system of the late 1950s. It was easier to attribute poor care to the poorly trained and qualified foreign physicians who, out of their own desperation and that of hospitals, came to staff the ER, than to admit that organized medicine had failed to notice or address the marked increase in emergency visits and was providing no leadership in developing emergency care in the United States. Foreign medical graduates were convenient scapegoats, but they were not the root of the problem. In 1958, the ECFMG educational requirement made it more difficult for some foreign-trained physicians to become interns or residents. In 1959, the State Department ruled that foreign medical graduates who were training as interns and residents could stay in the United States a maximum of 5 years. Many foreign graduates circumvented this restriction by marrying American citizens. In 1963, Congress finally passed legislation to increase the numbers of U.S. health professionals, and medical school enrollment significantly increased.[9,48]

Two of the pioneers of emergency medicine in the United States were foreign born, but unlike most foreign-born physicians who came to work in ERs, Reinauld Leidelmeyer and George Podgorny had advanced training before their emergency medicine careers.

REINALD LEIDELMEYER, M.D.: FROM DUTCH RESISTANCE TO AMERICAN MEDICAL PRACTICE

Reinald Leidelmeyer was born in The Netherlands in 1924. As a young man, he and his family experienced the hardship of the German occupation of The Netherlands. He remembers, "...my mother made a diary of the starvation winter. We lived on 400 calories a day, which consisted of sugar beets and tulip bulbs, and no other food."[55] Leidelmeyer joined the Dutch Resistance to the Nazis in the later years of World War II and was arrested and sent to a prison camp. He recalls,

> I was a young guy, actually five of my high school friends were executed, and my physics teacher was executed. I have pictures of it...I was walking with a stack of papers, underground papers, one day in one of the back streets and I was suddenly surrounded by five German Gestapo police on bicycles, guns and all. I was taken to the Gestapo headquarters. We were put in a cattle car on a train, only at night, we traveled very slow—finally 2 or 3 days—I got to Germany. I became an interpreter that day because I could speak four languages...It probably saved my life...at some point they asked for gardeners. I said I am a gardener, I wasn't but...they took me apart and my jobs were, among others, getting water out of the electrical company's basement where the generators were and I had to get in with a shovel and a bucket get a layer of water out of the floor everyday. Then they took me to the public park in a nearby town also, and I had to clean the public latrines.[55]

Leidelmeyer, in the prison camp for about 3 months, was released when the war was ending and walked back home to Holland.

The only thing I remember of that is that I crossed the Dutch border and a little old lady gave me fried potatoes, which I had not seen for God knows how long, and a little further somebody with a horse and buggy picked me up and took me to a Sanitary Red Cross Station and they deloused me and from that moment until I reached my house I have no memory. Anyhow, when I came home, the war was just about over and the Americans and the British came over very low flying and throwing food because the population was starving. The next day I got diphtheria. There were no medicines. My mother finally found a doctor who had one ampule of serum left, which she shot in my leg right here. For years I had a numb spot here, it was a bubble. It was 20 cc I'd say. But, I survived.[55]

When the Dutch universities reopened in 1945, Leidelmeyer enrolled in medical school at Leiden University and graduated from a 6-year program. He then did 2 years of a rotating internship in Dutch university hospitals before coming to the United States in 1953. He did a rotating internship in Richmond, Virginia, and passed the Virginia state medical boards. Ironically, a year after he came to the United States he was drafted in to the Army and became the Commanding Officer of a dispensary in Germany. After 2 years in the Army, he did further training in internal medicine and pulmonary diseases in a tuberculosis sanitarium affiliated with the University of Virginia. He became somewhat bored with limiting his practice to tuberculosis and pulmonary diseases, so he moved to Fairfax, Virginia, and set up a general practice in 1960. Fairfax Hospital, a new, state-of-the-art facility had just been built and the administration staff was determining how to staff its ER. Reinauld Leidelmeyer would become the solution to that problem.

GEORGE PODGORNY, M.D.: A BOY FROM PERSIA BECOMES A CAROLINA SURGEON

George Podgorny has an interesting heritage. As the only child of a Czech father and Armenian mother who had separately fled to Iran in the aftermath of World War I, George was born and raised in Iran. His father was in charge of physical education and physical training at the military academy in Tehran and was head of the Iranian Olympic Committee. One of the duties for Podgorny's father was to try to train the unathletic son of the Shah. George was a playmate of the young Shah to be and remembers riding horses and playing games with the royal family.[56]

George was interested in medicine, but his parents believed that universities in Iran would not provide their son with an adequate education. In the mid-1950s, the United States welcomed foreign students to study in American colleges. This was part of U.S. efforts to curb the spread of communism. The rationale was that by teaching foreign students the merits of capitalism and democracy, they would promote this type of society when they returned to their countries of origin. This policy did not account for the seductive influence of America on foreign visitors, and many of those who trained in the United States, particularly those in postgraduate medicine, did not return to their native lands.

Podgorny used a private U.S. agency to learn about U.S. colleges and universities. In a catalog from Maryville College in Tennessee, he saw a familiar name— Commodore Fischer. Fischer was a Presbyterian missionary and historian who had taught at Tehran University. George had played soccer with Fischer's children in Iran. He contacted Fischer and arrangements were made for Podgorny's admission to Maryville College. George's mother, who was a writer, had just published a book— she wrote in Armenian—and the proceeds from the book were given to George so he could come to the United States and start college in 1958.[56]

George majored in biology and chemistry with the intent of going to medical school. He did well, but was not always encouraged by his faculty.

I applied to med schools, and you know you have to have some letters of recommendation from college professors. I went to one of my advisors, who was a chemistry professor, for whom I was an assistant in the lab, and who professed a great deal of affection and interest for me…and he said, "What are you going to do?" I said, "Well I am planning to go to medical school." He said, "You'll never get in and you'll never make it."[56]

Podgorny persisted and was accepted to three medical schools. He was familiar with Bowman Gray Medical School from a college friend and decided to enroll there. He began medical school in 1958. He was drawn to the surgical fields. As a second-year medical student he learned how to suture on a rabbit, then sought some more experience.

> *I started hanging out in what was then called the emergency room. People working there were interns…and not only clinical interns, but radiology interns were there, pathology interns were there, people who hardly knew anything, so to say, about medicine any more than a senior medical student would because their internship was not clinical. These people were extremely unhappy. So, I offered to suture and though it probably wasn't appropriate being a sophomore medical student, they just didn't want to suture. I became the suturer as a sophomore medical student.*[56]

Podgorny decided to do a residency in surgery, and based on his positive experiences in medical school and the strong surgical training at North Carolina Baptist Hospital, he stayed in Winston-Salem for his internship and surgical residency. He started internship in 1962, completed a program in general and thoracic surgery, and then served 3 additional years as a chief resident in general surgery and thoracic and cardiovascular surgery. He finished in 1969, and ironically, after this extensive surgery training, he never practiced as a surgeon. Rather, he found himself drawn to the field of emergency medicine.

Academic Medicine and Emergency Care: Pre-1960

Emergency medicine was not on the radar screen of academic medicine in the 1950s. Although the ERs of medical school hospitals and urban teaching hospitals were providing care to large numbers of emergency patients, these venues were the forgotten stepchildren of medical academia. Medical schools traditionally have advanced a tripartite mission of clinical care, teaching, and research. Despite being an area of the hospital where critically ill patients presented for care, where interns and residents were assigned to learn, and a rich site for clinical research, the ER rarely figured into the mission of academic medical centers until the 1900s. As patient volumes and the percentage of admissions increased, the ER was generally viewed as an annoyance, not an opportunity.

The academic disinterest in what was happening in the ER can be better understood by seeing where interests were greatest during this time. Specialty medicine was burgeoning in the 1950s, in both the medical and surgical subspecialties. Technology was making new procedures possible, and general medicine and broad-based skills were not as valued in the academic setting. Many of the prominent areas of emergency medicine such as trauma care, acute cardiac disease, and toxicology would not emerge as major areas of medical scholarship until the 1960s or later.

This is not to say that all academic physicians were unaware of emergency care. The first "modern" English language book on emergency care was produced by the British physician C. Allan Birch in 1948 and had five subsequent editions through 1960.[57] This book focused on medical rather than surgical emergencies, and the first chapter describes an "emergency bag" with the emergency medications and tools of those times for "every physician who is liable to be called in an emergency…."[57] In 1949, two American academic physicians from the State University of Iowa College of Medicine, Stuart Cullen, M.D. (chairman of anesthesiology) and E. G. Gross, M.D. (head of pharmacology) wrote the *Manual of Medical Emergencies*, which was also limited to medical emergency conditions and did not address surgical issues. Cullen and Gross dedicated the book to "the general practitioner who is expected to see all, know all, and do all in the field of medicine and who, to his everlasting credit, fulfills these expectations admirably."[58]

The first comprehensive post–World War II book on emergency care in the United States was written by Thomas Flint, Jr., M.D. and published in 1954. The book, *Emergency Treatment and Management* was favorably reviewed in the *Journal of the American Medical Association* and consisted of an alphabetical listing of emergency problems from abdominal pain to wartime emergencies. Most conditions such as allergic reactions, cardiac emergencies, and head injuries were addressed in a few concise paragraphs. Some of the other topics covered in the book demonstrated that patients were presenting for emergency care with problems that were less acute. Flint included sections on bunions, "ingrowing" toenails, insomnia, and gonorrhea. The section on poisons—the most extensive in the book—accounted for 115 of 300 pages. Unlike the preceding authors of emergency books, Flint included injuries and trauma in his text. Flint was probably the first to use the term *emergency physician*. He notes that the term is used:

> ...to designate the physician in charge of the patient in the emergency room, department, or private office. In large hospitals, this physician may be on a full-time basis; in smaller units he may have numerous other duties, or be on part-time emergency call. Too often he is an intern, resident, or general practitioner of very limited experience in the management and treatment of acute conditions.[59]

Flint was the Director of the Division of Industrial Relations for the Permanente Medical Group and Chief of the Emergency Department at the Kaiser Foundation Hospital in Richmond, California. As would be expected for this time, he did not speak of emergency medicine as a distinct medical area or career option. However, the Kaiser Hospital was quite progressive in having named Flint as its emergency chief and referring to an "emergency department" rather than an ER.

Emergency care received very little attention in medical school curricula in the post-Flexner era, and this was bemoaned by physicians who were interested in accidents and injury. Robert H. Kennedy M.D., the surgical director at New York City's Beekman–Downtown Hospital, who became a major advocate for improved trauma teaching and care, noted in 1937:

> There has been no organized effort to train the medical profession in first aid. The medical schools which [sic] give any instruction in this subject are a rare exception. The result is that the average medical student on receiving his degree knows less about it than a first-class Boy Scout.[60]

Eighteen years later, in 1955, Kennedy, who served from 1939 to 1952 as chairman of the Committee on Trauma of the American College of Surgeons, lamented that the words he had written in 1937 were still true—the medical profession had made little progress in the treatment of traumatic injuries and the quality of prehospital care.[52] At Hartford Hospital, a large teaching facility outside of the large shadow of the Boston world of medicine, two physician administrators, Ernest C. Shortliffe, M.D., and T. Steward Hamilton, M.D., were witnessing a boom in emergency visits and wrote an article called "The ER and the Changing Pattern of Medical Care," which was published in the *New England Journal of Medicine* in January 1958.[40] This paper was a compilation of historic data on ER use, current survey data from Hartford Hospital and other hospitals on ER visits and responses to survey questions about what caused the ER boom and what should be done about it. It was a watershed publication for emergency medicine, both in terms of bringing attention to the developing crisis in the ER and because it was printed in the world's premier medical journal. The closing sentences of the paper suggest that Shortliffe and Hamilton were thinking about the physician component of emergency care:

> Plans should also be made for modernization of staffing patterns in emergency rooms. As load and complexity increase it is increasingly important that these areas be well staffed with professional personnel of adequate training and mature judgment.[40]

The editors of the *New England Journal of Medicine* also seemed concerned about the lack of trained physicians in the ER. In an accompanying editorial to the Shortliffe article, they state:

> There is nothing to take the place of a physician experienced in the treatment of emergency-ward patients, medical or surgical. The public is increasingly demanding

good facilities for emergency-ward care, but in the last analysis the experience and judgment of the physician who directs this care is the indispensable sine qua non.[29]

The problem was that there were few "indispensable" physicians to dispense to ERs in most hospitals.

Some other physicians and organizations appreciated the need for emergency medical services. As early as 1947, the AMA had a National Committee on Emergency Medical Services. The focus for this group was primarily disaster preparedness and civilian defense in the event of a war on U.S. soil. The routine emergencies experienced by civilians did not receive much attention in the world of organized medicine in the 1950s, except from hospitals and their administrators. Because hospitals were dealing directly with the increase in ER visits, they were more attune to the problem and began discussing how to deal with it.

In 1953, Charles Lindquist, M.D., the chief of emergency service at Santa Monica Hospital and surgeon in charge at West Los Angeles Emergency Hospital wrote a paper entitled "Hospital Facilities Required for Emergency Care."[61] This paper described the components needed to make a functioning "emergency department" in a large hospital and spoke of the importance of a good emergency department to the public and professional impression of the hospital. He wrote the following equation, in capitals, which was well ahead of its time: "GOOD EMERGENCY CARE = GOOD PUBLIC RELATIONS." Lindquist was thus one of the first people to look at the ER as a positive part of health care, rather than as a burden.[61] Other publications also instructed the reader on how to run a good emergency department, with tips on architecture, ancillary services, supplies, and staffing. In 1957, the *Journal of the American Hospital Association* devoted the entire March 16 issue to the ER. The hospitals described in the articles were community or small teaching hospitals, not big academic medical centers.[45,62] This publicity for the ER did not make much of an impression in academic medicine, which was in a frenzy of scientific discovery.

In the research world, the fruits of basic science research were generating a great deal of excitement and interest amongst clinicians. The announcement in 1955 of an effective polio vaccine demonstrated how well-supported basic science research, with large-scale public participation in clinical trials, could result in a victory of medical science over a terrible disease.[9] The fact that polio was more likely to strike middle-class and upper-class white children made it easy to rally the public to finance the fight against this disease. Although the public obviously benefited greatly from the victory over polio, academic medical centers also benefited from the large grants that funded research on the disease and the prestige that came from being part of the effort. On the basis of the successes in battling infectious diseases, academic medical centers and faculty focused on building strong biomedical research programs, laboratories, and clinical research units. Considerable rewards would go to the medical schools that could compete well for federal and foundation research support. Between 1955 and 1960, Congress increased the funding of the NIH from $81 million to $400 million.[9,11,13] In this realm of specialty medicine, with a new focus on research, the academic ER, with its interns and large numbers of indigent and minority patients, was easy to ignore.

Because the ER was a place where interns and residents learned on their own, a faculty member who spent much time in the ER might be perceived as taking a step backward. This view of the ER as the kindergarten of academic medicine was coupled with the lowly reputation of ER physicians who worked in nonacademic hospitals. A faculty member who had a sincere interest in what was happening in the ER would have to battle a negative stigma that was deeply rooted. Faculty members who were put in charge of running academic ERs were usually junior level, and the ER job was not their primary focus. The fields of surgery and orthopedics had demonstrated some interest in emergency care through trauma management and emergency medical services. "Surgery men" were often appointed to run academic ERs. Two of these individuals— Peter Rosen and Ronald Krome—were just finishing medical school and starting their surgical residencies at the end of the 1950s. Although trained as surgeons, Rosen and Krome, along with David Wagner, would have a huge impact on the development of academic emergency medicine.

PETER ROSEN, M.D.: THE STREET FIGHTER
FROM BROOKLYN

Peter Rosen may have a genetic predisposition to his legendary toughness and stubbornness. His father was a general practice physician in Brooklyn. Rosen recounts a story of his 5 foot 6 inch, 300-lb father who one day wanted to make some firewood by chopping up a railroad tie with an ax. When the ax became stuck in the railroad tie, Rosen's father lifted the tie above his head. It then disengaged and fell on his foot. He screamed, cursed, and hopped about, then proceeded to chop the tie into pieces. He carried the wood inside and lit a fire in the fireplace, not realizing that railroad ties are soaked in creosote to retard rotting, and this produces a thick black smoke when burned. The Brooklyn fire department soon arrived, entered in their usual manner by chopping through the front door, and extinguished the fire of the erstwhile woodsman. Peter Rosen, a self-ascribed "street fighter from Brooklyn," would often mirror the persistence and outrage of his father and would go on to start more than one fire in his academic career.[63]

In 1951, Peter Rosen enrolled at the University of Chicago, where he honed his critical thinking abilities and became comfortable expressing his opinions.

> I remember one night in the dormitory, I picked up a book of Picasso prints and... I had never seen anything like it, it was his "blue" period. I looked at this and I said, "What is this painting all about?" The house head said something that nobody had ever said to me before in my life, "Well, what do you think?" It was kind of like a light switch went on in my brain. I started free-associating to the painting and I guess I've been doing it ever since.[63]

Those who later opposed him in the development of academic emergency medicine would wish the house head never asked Rosen that question. Rosen struggled to get into medical school and attributes some of this difficulty to being Jewish.

> I actually didn't get into medical school the first year I applied. It was very hard to get into medical school at the time I was doing it—probably even harder than it is right now. I think there was something like nine applicants for each place and virtually every medical school had a Jewish quota, and that wasn't to ensure that they had Jews! So, I didn't get accepted the first year I applied. Then I spent a year at Columbia basically taking more courses and reapplying. I got into medical school by sheer luck. I was placed on the waiting list at Washington U. and some poor bastard detached his retina. His bad luck was my good luck.[63]

Rosen attended Washington University Medical School in St. Louis, Missouri, from 1956 to 1960. At the end of medical school, Rosen did not have a strong feeling of what branch of medicine he would pursue. He hated the Surgery department at his medical school and did not like internal medicine much better. He thought that ophthalmology might be a nice combination of surgical and medical practice, and planned to do an ophthalmology residency at the University of Chicago after his required internship. He started his internship at the University of Chicago Hospital by rotating on the surgery service, thinking that because he did not like surgery, he would do it while he was fresh and get it out of the way. On his first morning he went to the operating room and got to do an appendectomy: "In the first 10 minutes of my internship I got seduced into general surgery." Rosen abandoned his plans to do an ophthalmology residency and instead started a general surgery residency at Highland Hospital in Oakland, California, in 1961.[63]

RONALD L. KROME, M.D.: FROM THE TOUGH
STREETS OF BALTIMORE TO DETROIT

Ron Krome was born in 1936 in the "Jewish ghetto" in Baltimore. His father was part owner of a bar, a bartender, and a numbers runner. Krome remembers being instructed to sit quietly in the car while his father made calls on people who were placing their bets. Krome had the classic urban, ethnic upbringing—a modest, but close-knit community and stickball in the streets. He was good in English in high school and despite his humble background decided to go to college.

> I was the first one in my Dad's family to have gone through college. Actually, I was probably the first one to graduate high school on my Dad's side.[64]

Krome started out in 1956 at small, conservative, rural Westminster College in Maryland. Freshman students were required to wear beanies, and when Ron was home on break, his father, who thought the beanies were hilarious, would wear Ron's beanie while he tended bar. Krome expected to do well in freshman English at Westminster, but his compositions were not getting better than Cs. He didn't seem to be able to find stimulating topics about which to write until he saw an article about the anti-Communist fervor that had swept the country in the mid-1950s, and by that time was being challenged.

> I was thumbing through Life magazine…and there was a big story about the big anti-Communist senator…McCarthy, and how…he wanted the book Red Riding Hood—to change the name—he was out to get the Boy Scouts because they were too socialistic. It was so stupid. I sat down, wrote, didn't correct it, didn't edit it, and turned it in. I figured, what the hell, I ain't doing well anyway. I got an "A" on it and I said to my roommate, I figured out what this lady likes, and the rest of the semester I did much better…I did my term paper on gamma globulin and spelled gamma globulin wrong, I think it was something like 30 or 40 times. I was consistent, I got an "A."[64]

After a year at Westminster College, Krome realized that his family would not be able to afford the expensive tuition for another 3 years, so he transferred to the University of Maryland. He developed an increasing interest in medicine and science and decided to apply to medical school. Krome's father died before he interviewed for medical school, and one of the faculty interviewers at the University of Maryland Medical School questioned how Ron would pay for medical school since his father was deceased. Krome was a quick learner.

> I had another interview and I had the same question, and I said, "My father was independently wealthy and left me money." I don't know if that contributed to me getting in or not…All the premeds would talk about what gets you in, what you have to say and that you have to be careful—had to know things like who discovered penicillin. I didn't know that in college, I knew it by the time I went for my interview… at that time there was a Hungarian uprising so, one of the questions he asked me was how was that connected to Lawrence of Arabia? I don't know why, I think—Lawrence was out of the movies. I said I'm not sure what happened but it had something to do with the Ottoman Empire. That impressed the shit out of him…you go through school and you pick up little things that you know are going to be of no value…so we talked about Ottoman Empire and Lawrence of Arabia.[64]

Krome went to medical school at the University of Maryland from 1957 to 1961. Two of the most influential, dynamic faculty members were the chief of surgery, Scott Buxton, and R. Adams Cowley, a surgeon who would later help to build the famous trauma institute at the University of Maryland. Krome was attracted to the big personalities and prestige of the academic surgeons. He remembers how surgeons were the main presence in the Maryland ER:

> Maryland's emergency room in those days was a typical university emergency run by interns and students. Surgeons were more or less responsible for everything that happened in ER…my first job was as a surgery tech behind the ER—that was how you got started. There were some pediatricians and some internists but I would guess about 85% to 95% that were surgically trained.[64]

Krome had an experience that current medical students do not have to face—he was drafted into the military during his sophomore year. At the time, college and graduate students could receive a military deferment if, scholastically, they were in the upper percentage of their class. Krome's college grades were good enough to get in to medical school, but in his senior year they slipped below the cut off, and he became eligible for the draft during medical school.

> *I knew that I was going to get caught the next year. I got a letter from the draft board, you've got to report, you are 1A, come down. So I went to my dean of students, …he said, "They haven't sent a student to the military since the Civil War." Some time later, I got a letter that said report for your physical. I go back to the dean and I said they ain't kidding now. He said, "Don't worry about it, we've never lost a student yet." So I go for my physical and I'm coming around the last stop—you don't see a doctor until the end. He goes over your whole form and it was my bacteriology professor. So he said, "What are you doing here?" So I told him the story and he said, "You are going—this ain't no time to kid! …You gotta get back to Dean Smith. I'll make you 4F for 3 months for athlete's feet." I said okay, so I go back to Dean Smith and say, "Dr. Jones was there, he tells me you're going you have to get me out of this." He said, "You know, Krome, you just worry too much," and he walked out. So now I'm really getting antsy. The next letter I get says come with 3 days of clothes for your next physical…I can't not report—that's called draft dodging! So I go with 3 days of clothes up to Fort Meade and I get my physical and I get to the end when they review everything to see what they are going to make you, and there the guy says, "You have a student deferment. It just came through." I could have killed him![64]*

So, Krome deferred his military service through medical school, but would be required to serve 2 years after his internship. He later volunteered for the Public Health Service. By his third year of medical school, Krome had decided to train in surgery. He took a 10-day trip between his junior and senior years to tour residency programs. He drove an old Fiat through the East and Midwest, visiting many of the traditional surgical residencies. At that time, many surgical residencies had a "pyramid" system. Residents were initially accepted in to the programs, but only a portion was allowed to complete the program. In some surgical residencies, a resident could put in 3 years and still be cut in the fourth year. Krome decided, "That wasn't going to be for me." He eliminated programs that had a strict pyramid system. His priority was getting good clinical training in surgery with a modicum of supervision. He decided to do his internship at Detroit General Hospital, a busy, urban center where "…house officers ran it but you had faculty there at least making rounds two or three times a week with you." Krome received a salary of $300 a month. This was considered excellent pay. In fact, up until 1960, some surgical residencies provided room and board, but no additional salary. Krome began his internship in Detroit in 1961.[64]

Health Care and the ER of the 1950s: The Perspective of Patients and Communities

The ERs of the 1950s, and many of the people they served, were in the same boat—disenfranchised, lacking a voice, and largely ignored by the "powers that be." The concept of the little man working hard—the American way—and getting ahead in life was more pipe dream than reality. The "power elite" in the United States concentrated major resources and influence in the hands of a small group of politicians, businessmen, and military figures.[6] The post–World War II economic boom had earned enormous profits for industry, and health care had emerged as one of those industries. But, the boom did not erase the disparities between rich and poor in terms of income and access to quality health care.[1,2,5] Poverty had not been addressed in any systematic way by the federal government, and health insurance for the poor was still a decade away.

Health insurance for working people had emerged as a viable concept by the early 1900s, and was promoted by both Winston Churchill and Theodore Roosevelt. In the late 1930s, a voluntary prepaid health insurance program called the White Cross was instituted in Boston. In this plan, patients had a primary care doctor with a system of referral to specialists if needed. The plan seemed to work well, but was disrupted by World War II and never regained its function after this.[11]

Those who pushed for health insurance in the United States would have a formidable opponent—the AMA. Although it at first seems paradoxical that the AMA would oppose health insurance, one must remember that the AMA functioned from its early days as an interest group for physicians. Patient advocacy was not its primary objective. As the position and wealth of physicians expanded in the early 1900s, the AMA aggressively used its growing political influence to protect the incomes and autonomy of physicians.[9] As Stevens notes, "Health insurance was seen not only to threaten the individual practitioner but also to divide the hard-won unity of the profession."[11] Strong lobbying by the AMA helped to keep compulsory health insurance from being included in Roosevelt's 1935 Social Security Act. Since both would benefit from hospital insurance payments, the American College of Surgeons and the American Hospital Association opposed the AMA and favored voluntary health insurance plans for workers.

Health insurance for children, the elderly, the disabled, and the unemployed was more of a problem. As early as 1936, calls for a national health care plan were heard from physician groups with a more socialistic orientation. By 1938, the federal government was looking closely at a national health care plan by convening the National Health Conference. Perceiving this as a bigger threat than employer-based insurance, the AMA voiced its support for voluntary hospital insurance and began a vigorous opposition to national health insurance.[9,11] President Roosevelt became supportive of a national health care plan, but his enthusiasm for national health care was opposed by a rise in the political power of conservatives in Congress. President Truman also advocated for a national health care plan, but in the end was defeated by powerful adversaries and new political developments.[9]

As Starr details, from the early 1940s to 1950, national health care reform plans were advanced three times, but died each time. When Congress began to propose modifications of the Social Security system to include health care coverage in 1943, the AMA once again fought to preserve the status quo. The most influential AMA members were urban, mostly Eastern, private practice physicians, who would stand to lose both autonomy and income if they were required to provide care under a national insurance plan. Businesses, especially the pharmaceutical industry, were also opposed to national health insurance, as was the national Chambers of Commerce.[9]

Whether based on fundamental beliefs, or as a political tactic, "the conflict was intensely ideological."[9] The rise of communism and socialism in other countries became a threat to American democracy, and opponents of national health care used this to their advantage by calling the proposals "socialized medicine." Proponents of national health insurance were insinuated to have communist leanings, and the more the communist threat grew, the stronger the argument seemed to be. The resources of the AMA and its alliance of industries were vastly greater than the patient and community groups that supported a national health insurance plan. In 1950, just before the Congressional elections, the AMA spent $2.25 million on its campaign against national health insurance. Widespread advertisements in newspapers and on the radio warned of the how socialized medicine would damage the American way of life. This effort has been referred to as the first major special interest victory in American politics. The other major factor and distraction at the federal level was the Korean War. By 1950, communism was a looming threat, and Korea only intensified the concern. The increasingly conservative government had to focus on stopping communism, and any domestic plan that was labeled as "socialistic" became dead in the water.[9]

The labor movement gained strength after World War II and through collective bargaining was a strong stimulus for employer-subsidized health insurance. In 1940, only 9% of U.S. civilians had insurance for hospitalization; by 1950, it had risen to 50%, and by 1966 to 81%.[11] The Eisenhower administration (1953–1961) pushed for private health insurance companies to cover all working Americans. Blue Cross and Blue Shield became the major private health insurance provider, covering nearly half of those with insurance by 1955.[11]

In the late 1950s, Congress also addressed health care for the elderly and those on public assistance. The Forand Bill of 1957 was the first to propose hospitalization, surgery, and nursing home benefits for those receiving Social Security. It was opposed by the AMA and Eisenhower administration, but it brought attention to the plight of the elderly. The Kerr-Mills Act passed in 1960. This was a compromise to the Forand Bill that used federal matching grants to the states to help fund medical care for the elderly poor. Although the amount of federal funding for state run health care programs increased almost tenfold from 1950 to 1960, these programs did not catch on and were not widely utilized.[9,11] The presence of at least some type of funding for hospital care for those on public assistance, with the concurrent lack of funding for outpatient physician visits, contributed to the movement of patients toward the hospital when they had medical problems.

Part of the post–World War II industrial boom was an urban–suburban population shift. Starting with the infamous William Levitt "Monopoly piece" suburban housing developments in Long Island, New York, in the early 1950s, the suburbs became the preferred place to live for educated, employed, middle class, white Americans. The population of suburbs grew 50% from 1950 to 1960.[1] The rapid shift of people created a crisis for many cities as their tax base and local commerce started to vanish. Into this urban void streamed thousands of less educated, poorer, minority, or immigrant citizens who were employed by the big industries—auto manufacturing in Detroit, steel in Pittsburgh. These workers were more susceptible to economic fluctuations, their jobs were less secure, and they had a lower margin for error.[5] Whereas many of the workers had health insurance, some of their dependents and the unemployed did not.

As the northern and midwestern industrial cities became essentially segregated from their suburbs by race and income levels, health care disparities were also evident. Private hospitals treated white, employed patients almost exclusively, whereas municipal hospitals treated poor whites and almost all minority patients. In 1957, only 3% of patients in private New York City hospitals were nonwhite, compared with 38% in municipal hospitals. These hospitals were not uniformly of poor quality, but had fewer resources and were disproportionately faced with the difficult problems of indigent urban populations—alcohol and drug addiction, violence, and diseases of neglect and abuse.[2,10,22]

An even larger problem than hospitals for poor inner-city residents was finding access to basic and preventive health care. GPs had joined the flight from inner cities to the suburbs, and the remaining GPs tended to the more affluent urban population. Municipal medical clinics were overrun and poorly staffed and supplied. By the late-1950s, the ERs of municipal hospitals and urban academic medical centers became the default medical care of the underclass. The health care paradigm of the urban poor became "if you are sick, wait and see if it gets better, if you get sicker, go to the ER." Most urban hospitals had at least marginal facilities to care for ER patients, but the best they could do to staff their ERs was to provide interns or hard-luck physicians who could not find employment elsewhere.

By 1960, the path leading to a national health care plan was blocked with too many political obstacles. One can contemplate how things might have played out if national health insurance had been enacted in the 1940s in the United States as it was in Great Britain. One strong feature of national health care plans is primary care providers who control access to other health care resources. A national health care plan in the United States might have given more people access to primary and preventive care and reduced the number who presented to the ER for care. However, this would have solved only part of the demand for emergency services. Professional interest and increased utilization of emergency services also developed in Great Britain and Canada—countries with a national health care program.

JAMES MILLS, JR., M.D. (1920–1989): CHIEF OF STAFF WITH A PROBLEM

James Mills, Jr., was born in St. Louis in 1920. He had a middle-class upbringing, but was reared during the Depression. His father, who was a vice president of an insurance company, thought that engineering was a field with good job prospects and encouraged his son to become an engineer. Mills enrolled at the University of Michigan in 1938, but did not like engineering. He returned home and attended the University of Missouri until 1941. Just before the attack on Pearl Harbor, Mills was commissioned in the Navy, and, like R. R. Hannas, served during World War II in the Pacific theater, but was not involved in major fighting. Mills took a course in 1944 at the postgraduate School at the Naval Academy in Annapolis, where he met and married his wife. He then received orders to go back to sea. In 1945, he and his wife were driving to California so Jim could ship out when they heard the war was over. Mills had begun to think about medicine as a career while he was in the Navy, and the G.I. Bill made it financially possible for him to go to medical school. He went back to the University of Missouri to take science requirements and in 1946 entered Washington University Medical School in St. Louis. Following his general rotating internship at St. Louis County Hospital, Mills contemplated doing a residency, but he was 31 years old and eager to start earning a real income. In 1953 Mills moved his family to Alexandria, Virginia, near his wife's hometown. Alexandria was a growing community less than 10 miles from the nation's capital.

It did not take long for Mills to establish a bustling general practice. He was "…full of piss and vinegar…," but at the same time "…had an idea toward being buddies with the rest of the world."[46] Mills became a respected and influential physician in Alexandria. Within 5 years, he was on the Executive Committee of Alexandria Hospital. Mills "…was always a kind man, and took a generous viewpoint toward other people…," and his service in the community reflected this.[53] He was on the Board of Directors and served as vice president of the Alexandria Community Health Center and was later the chairman of the Voluntary Services Study for the Hospitals and Clinics Section of the Health and Welfare Council of the District of Columbia. His partner, John McDade remembers, "…sometimes it used to get under our skin because he was such a social worker…he was a beautiful man, he was one of the great guys of the world."[46] Mills was also getting a bit weary with all his activities. His wife notes: "…his life was so busy and there were such demands on it, and he had so little free time, and then there was this complaint with the emergency department."[53]

One of the most vexing problems for suburban Alexandria Hospital was how to provide physician staffing for the ER. More and more patients were presenting to the ER for care, but many physicians who were on staff at the hospital were not eager to come to the ER to see their own patients or other patients. Both general practice physicians and specialists had busy practices and responding to the ER could leave office patients waiting for hours, or for a surgical specialist, could disrupt the operating schedule.

Alexandria Hospital, like many community hospitals, offered internships in the 1940s and early 1950s, and could conveniently use interns to staff the ER. In the days before ERs became busier, an intern could manage in this unsupervised setting by telephoning patients' physicians or consultants when he had a question. As the medical and surgical specialties emerged and more medical students chose specialty training beyond internship, the attractiveness of community hospital internships faded, and many community hospitals could no longer provide ER staffing with interns. This was the case with Alexandria Hospital. Those hospitals near medical schools settled for the next best thing—senior medical students. John McDade, who was also a general practitioner in Alexandria in the 1950s, recalls medical students from Georgetown University Medical School working unsupervised in the Alexandria Hospital ER. Some students would be in over their heads with a sick patient and would call for help. Others would flounder, and McDade would find out later about bad outcomes of ER patients.[46]

At the Alexandria Hospital ER, the number of patients was rapidly increasing, and the use of medical students in the ER was producing complaints from the medical staff. Also, the medical school dean began to object to students moonlighting in ERs. In 1960, James Mills became president-elect of Alexandria Hospital Medical Staff. The problem in the ER was of a pressing nature, and a committee was formed to address it. With his new position, his interest in social problems, and his ability to work with others, Mills was a clear choice to be chairman of the committee. As McDade describes it:

> *So he became the chairman. Then he really started to think about it in earnest—what could we do to fix this problem? It came to him, he said he was asleep one night, and he just woke up and he said, "I bet I could do that…."*[46]

The idea that came to James Mills in his sleep in 1960 would profoundly affect American medical practice.

Emergency Care in Pre-1960 America: A Problem Needing a Solution

Although the period from the end of World War II to 1960 is characterized as staid and conservative, the remarkable changes in the way Americans lived, coupled with the rise of hospital and specialty medicine, spawned a crisis in emergency care. Howell and Buerki in 1957 noted that unlike their prewar ancestors, post–World War II Americans came to

> ...take for granted that hospitals have emergency service at all hours where any problem, surgical, medical, or psychiatric can be treated...In time, the hospital emergency service may find its scope extended to meet many general medical and surgical problems, which the patient, at least, will deem urgent.[62]

The factors that created the crisis in the ER became more pronounced in the late 1950s, and most would continue unabated until at least the early 1970s. These factors have been alluded to, and were nicely summarized by M. L. Webb, M.D., D.P.H., in a doctorate thesis for the Johns Hopkins University School of Public Health (Figure 1.1). The most influential factor, in terms of increasing ER patient volumes, was the public's preference or need to seek care in a hospital setting when an emergency, real or perceived, arose. This primacy of the hospital over the private physician's office, when coupled with the decreasing numbers and availability of general practice doctors made it inevitable that ER visits would increase. The biggest increases occurred when other factors came in to play. Inner cities with larger indigent populations, increasing drug abuse and violence, and an exodus of doctors, experienced the greatest increase in ER visits, but even in fast-growing, affluent suburbs, the ER became the default venue for care when medical demand outstripped supply.

The American public did not realize how poorly prepared most ERs were for this expanded role. Even if they had, it is unlikely that any organized public outrage about emergency care would have occurred. As Howard Zinn noted, in the post–World War era:

> America was relatively calm. Neither the Korean War, nor McCarthyism, nor the continued humiliation of blacks, nor the increasing diversion of the country's wealth

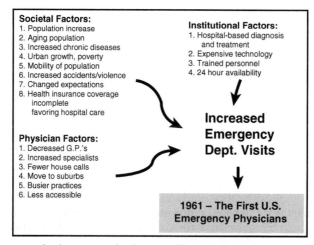

Figure 1.1 Factors involved in increased utilization of hospital emergency departments. Adapted from Webb ML: The Emergency Medical Care System in a Metropolitan Area. Doctoral thesis, Johns Hopkins University School of Hygiene and Public Health, 1969; published in: Emergency services: The hospital emergency department in an emergency care system. Chicago, 1972, American Hospital Association.

to the nuclear arms race aroused any widespread movement of opposition. Amidst the general complacency, based on middle-class prosperity, on lower-class fatalism, on agreement that communism was the great enemy, and on faith in the two-party system, only a few flurries of dissent were visible.[2]

The crisis in the ER was mostly out of the public eye. The coverage of emergency care by lay periodicals of the 1950s was generally laudatory, with accounts of accident victims being saved and healed by earnest physicians and surgeons.[65] A 1954 picture story in *Coronet* magazine related 12 hours in the ER through photos and breathless captions such as, "The fight goes on, the effort unstinting. People meet with accidents…a man may even be a police case. But in Emergency, a life is a life." The final photo is of a middle-aged, white male physician peacefully reclining on a stretcher, with the caption: "Near dawn, the doctor steals a moment of sleep—until the next cry for help."[66]

This rosy view of emergency medicine at a time when mounting evidence was indicting ERs as places of low-quality and inefficient care demonstrates the high regard that the public had for the medical profession in the 1950s. It was not until the 1960s that the public became more aware of and vocal about the problems in medicine in general and the ER in particular. In 1960, *Harper's* magazine published a special supplement called "The Crisis in American Medicine" that harshly questioned the training, politics, and practice of medicine, but emergency care was not mentioned.[67] A slew of lay articles on health care followed the *Harper's* series, with some very critical of emergency care.

Those few in the medical profession who saw the problem in the ER were able to characterize it well. In November of 1954, Robert H. Kennedy, the New York surgeon, was invited to give the Oration on Trauma at the American College of Surgeon's Clinical Congress in Atlantic City, New Jersey. In this address he talked about the clinical problems and deficiencies in trauma care and posed some questions to the audience:

In the emergency room in your hospital, who examines an injured patient first? May it be the most junior intern, who has never seen a traumatic case before, or an indifferently trained foreign physician with language difficulty? Have you prepared and posted a directive which will give these junior men an idea of what instances require the immediate notification of a surgical resident? …Will the attending notified be at the most junior level or a senior man with experience? …Do you know from personal inspection what goes on in your emergency room in the middle of the night or do you stay away due to a subconscious fear of what you might see? …There is little doubt in my mind that the weakest link in the chain of hospital care in most hospitals in this country is the emergency room's attention to the injured.[52]

Kennedy's use of the term "weakest link" to describe the ER was picked up and promoted in the previously mentioned paper by Shortliffe et al.[40] in the *New England Journal of Medicine* in 1958 and included in the title of a paper published by Shortliffe in *Hospitals* in 1960.[47] Intended by its authors to be a call for change in the ER, instead "weakest link" became a label associated with emergency care and those who practiced in ERs. Despite their eloquent description of the problem, neither Kennedy, Shortliffe, nor the other early advocates for better emergency care would personally play much of a role in the solution. For all the hand-wringing about the lack of proper physician staffing in ERs, no one seemed able to come up with a viable method for getting dedicated physicians to provide emergency coverage.

Academic medicine, with its large intern and resident workforce and the presence of many specialty physicians, was insulated from the problems in the ER. Hospital leaders from the nonacademic side first addressed emergency care issues because the problems were more visible in this setting. In the 1950s, the most forward-thinking and best-functioning ERs were not in the most lauded academic teaching hospitals or at the places where medical discovery was greatest. The strongest 1950s-era ERs were in places like St. Luke's Hospital in Racine, Wisconsin, or Kaiser Foundation Hospital in Richmond, California, or Hartford Hospital in Connecticut. The key players in the world of academic medicine would be content to ignore emergency care for two more decades.

The long, slow process to make emergency care an equally strong link in the chain of health care started in the 1960s and was led in part by the people who have been introduced in this chapter. These men, who would each play a role in the creation of emergency medicine were not born into rank or prestige, and their medical education and early career experiences did not put them in a position to be power brokers in American medicine. Men like Hannas, Wiegenstein, Mills, and Wagner were Midwesterners from relatively modest backgrounds. Podgorny and Leidelmeyer came from other countries and did residency training in the United States. Krome and Rosen were Easterners, but were not from wealthy or influential families, and came to the Midwest to train. Only Hannas went to an Ivy League school, but he never felt comfortable with the Ivy League aura, and ended up in Oklahoma. As these physicians were developing, a new demand for emergency services was coursing in the commons of American life. As commoners in the world of medicine, the early leaders of the profession of emergency medicine would grow in concert with their fledgling field.

2 Pioneers of Emergency Practice

…the American people expect more from us…For the world is changing. The old era is ending. The old ways will not do.
>
> John F. Kennedy, presidential nomination acceptance speech,
> July 15, 1960

The decade of the 1960s was one of turbulent sociopolitical winds that shook and tore the fabric of American life. The themes of the decade were youth and change, and they came in like a lamb and left like a lion. In 1960, one half of the American population was younger than 25 years old. On inauguration day, January 20, 1961, the oldest man to be president, Dwight D. Eisenhower, turned over the reins to John F. Kennedy, who became the youngest elected president. The Kennedy administration set a tone of involvement and social responsibility. Before he was sworn in as president, Kennedy delivered a speech in his native Massachusetts with the famous line: "For of those to whom much is given, much is required." This was followed by his inaugural invective: "…ask not what your country can do for you—ask what you can do for your country."[1] The early days of the civil rights movement were also filled more with hope than angst, as exemplified in Martin Luther King, Jr.'s "I have a dream" speech in the summer of 1963.[2]

The early 1960s had a fresh feel, and the radicalism that would characterize the latter half of the decade had not emerged. The new ideas embraced a community-based, more inclusive democracy and increased individual expression and freedoms. The country was at peace, and the economy was strong, with unemployment below 5% and an average growth rate from 1960 to 1965 of 5.3% per year. It was a good time for the government to focus attention on domestic programs and enact change.[3]

The Alexandria Plan

Less than 10 miles from the Capitol, James Mills, Jr., M.D., was also working on a change. As the president-elect of the Medical Staff at Alexandria Hospital, Mills had chaired the committee that was deciding how to solve the emergency room (ER) problem. The boom in Alexandria's population and shifts in the public's attitude toward emergency care led to a large increase in ER patient volumes in the latter half of the 1950s. By 1961, Alexandria Hospital had 190 beds, 10,500 admissions per year, and an emergency department census of approximately 18,000 patients per year.[4,5] Alexandria Hospital had used a traditional method for handling emergency cases in the 1950s. The tiny ER was staffed by around-the-clock nurses who triaged patients. For patients who had a private physician, the nurse would contact that physician to direct care. For patients who had no doctor or were indigent, the house staff would be called to assess the patient. Private physicians could request that the house staff see their patients, give the nurse orders, and depending on the time of day and severity of the condition, would come to the ER to see the patient. The approach of the triage nurse was much like a secretary trying to limit access to a busy executive—cases that were not deemed emergent were sometimes sent away or were sent to the waiting room for hours. Physicians were only called in for the sicker patients. The medical staff and hospital directors began to hear more complaints about service in the ER and were concerned that this was hurting the hospital's image. A negative public image for Alexandria Hospital would have been especially concerning to hospital administrators at this time, as the neighboring community of Fairfax, Virginia, was building a new, larger, state-of-the-art hospital that was due to open in 1961.

The problem was compounded after the institution of the Education Council for Foreign Medical Graduates (ECFMG) exam in 1958. This made it more difficult for minimally trained foreign physicians to obtain intern and residency positions and caused a temporary "deficiency" in foreign physicians. Throughout the 1950s, Alexandria Hospital had relied on interns and medical students, many of them foreign medical graduates, to staff its ER. In response to increased demand, local physicians had expanded their practices and were seeing more patients per day. By having interns or residents in the ER see their patients who might present there, community physicians could reduce the amount of time they had to spend in the hospital and ER. But by the end of the decade, the cheap labor provided by the house staff was evaporating. In 1959 to 1960 only nine residents and no interns were hired to fill 20 approved positions.[4] Although they had been valuable in the ER, resident physicians were even more essential in providing medical ward service, and the limited workforce was deployed there, leaving the ER horribly understaffed.[4,6–8]

Mills and his committee had explored a number of options for the ER. First, they tried to adjust resident staffing, but as the pool of interns and residents decreased, this became unfeasible, and the unwritten rule was that residents' first priority was ward care. The hospital administrator, Charles Goff, in remarking on the number of emergency cases somewhat disingenuously noted, "The residents couldn't possibly have handled them without giving up virtually all their other training."[4]

Mills's committee next proposed a rotating system of the private medical staff to provide coverage, but specialists and those not comfortable with handling general emergencies balked at this idea. A proposal was made to have only generalists staff the ER, but the generalists felt that the problem should be shared by all medical staff and they would be unfairly burdened. The options seemed to be exhausted, and administrator Goff recalled,

> We even considered bringing in senior medical students or enlisting licensed Public Health Services men, but we decided that such solutions were either legally or ethically suspect. It looked as though we might have to close down the emergency room entirely.[4]

Goff apparently was not aware that senior medical students had been used for ER staffing at Alexandria Hospital earlier in the 1950s.[7] None of the available options seemed viable, especially because Mills and his colleagues knew that the logarithmic growth in ER cases was not going to cease. In 1960, Mills became president of the Medical Staff and was under great pressure to do something. John McDade, who would be one of the original Alexandria four, recalls,

> We had a staff meeting at the hospital, a medical staff meeting, and one of the things that was talked about was, what are we going to do about this stupid emergency room? Nobody knew. Jim was sitting home one night and he got the idea, "I bet if we got some practicing physicians in there and we could take this thing over somehow, we'd have to work it out, but somehow take it over, we could do the job. We could do a good job and we could probably do somebody some good."[7]

The impetus for Mills to change his life came not only from problems in the ER. He was also becoming a bit weary in his busy general practice. By all accounts, he was an excellent and well-loved family doctor and had built a very successful, but demanding, practice. The population of Alexandria was growing rapidly, and there were too few general practitioners to meet the basic medical needs of the community. A loose system of cross-coverage existed so that the general practitioners (GPs) would not be on call every night, but the workweeks still averaged 60 to 80 hours.[4] Mills and his wife Frances had three children, and he tried to be a conscientious father and husband. He wished he could spend more time with his children.

> *One night I came home after 1 AM from a working day that had started that morning at 7. I remember thinking that as a chronically tired and overworked GP, I wasn't being fair to myself, my family, or my patients. It came to me that in emergency service, with regular hours, I would be able to practice much better medicine. If I could get three other good men to join me, we'd have a team that could provide top-notch treatment at all hours, and each of us would have reasonable free time to keep up with medical advances and spend time with our families.[9]*

A combination of professional and personal factors moved Mills toward his innovative idea. It is unlikely that the pressure he was getting from the hospital and medical staff and his dissatisfaction with his hectic practice would have driven Mills to develop his plan without one more factor—he liked working in the ER. When Mills provided coverage for the ER as one of the rotating medical staff or saw his own patients in that setting, he enjoyed the acute care, the variety of cases, and the pace. It also seems likely that Mills's social consciousness was stimulated by the subset of patients who were indigent or suffering from diseases of abuse and neglect. The patients Mills encountered in the ER would have been different from those in his private practice. Alexandria in the 1950s had essentially become a bedroom community for the federal government, and most of Mills's private patients were employed and well off. ER patients were more often poor, uninsured, and from minority groups. Mills may have found in ER practice a way to bring his concerns for the poor directly into his professional life (see insert, Figure 1).

Mills's generous and sympathetic view toward the less fortunate in society also factored into his view of how "emergencies" should be defined and handled. By 1960, two opposing viewpoints had developed on emergency care. It had become obvious that many patients who presented for emergency care were not critically ill or injured, and many believed that the solution to the ER problem lay in preventing these nonemergent cases from being seen. The other view, espoused by Mills and some of his peers, was that "what may not be emergent to the physician may certainly be emergent to the patient."[10] One emergency physician articulated it well when it was suggested to him that a patient with a hemorrhoid did not need emergency care and could wait until morning to see a doctor: "That may be true, but it depends on the situation in which you see the hemorrhoid—whether as the possessor or the beholder."[11]

This view, that the patient defines the emergency, could be seen as self-serving for the emergency physician, but it also reflected the practical aspects of what happened when people became sick or injured. The early emergency physicians understood that people present with symptoms and problems, not diagnoses, and what may at first glance seem trivial and nonacute could turn out to be a true emergency. No triage system could effectively or correctly screen out all nonemergent cases, and unless physicians could truly commit to being available 24 hours a day, emergency medical care could not be provided around the clock except in the ER. Mills expressed his views on this subject in a written description of the Alexandria Plan,

> *Much futile discussion is spent defining "emergency," "true emergency," or worse, "urgent emergency." The patient's point of view is properly quite different from that of the physician or of the emergency department nurse. The wisest course seems to be to accept the patient's definition of an emergency (which is also Webster's), "An unforeseen combination of circumstances which calls for immediate action." The solution is the assignment of priority in dealing with large numbers of patients, and in having reserve facilities for seriously ill patients.[8]*

After conceiving the plan for full-time emergency practice in the middle of 1960, Mills had three significant hurdles to jump for it to become reality. A calculation of the manpower needed to staff the ER full time led him to believe that a group of four physicians would be sufficient. His first step would be to convince three other generalist physicians to join him. Second, he would need to convince the rest of the medical staff that this was a good idea. Third, he would have to find someone to take over his practice.

Mills first approached John McDade about his idea for an emergency group. McDade's training was in pathology, but he had given this up to go into general practice just down the street from Mills.

> *I was doing a pathology residency at Temple. It was ugly, I was bored. I wanted to treat people not corpses. I really like pathology, I really enjoyed it, and I learned a ton in that year. But, I wanted to have something to do with live people.*[7]

McDade remembers that Mills was welcoming and helpful when he came to Alexandria, and they were soon covering for each other. Mills respected McDade as a clinician, and he was a logical person to approach with his new idea. As McDade recalls,

> *I was in the elevator going up to make rounds, Jim got on and he said, "Let me ask you a question." I said, "Okay." He said, "What do you think about taking over the emergency department and running it like a private practice?" I said, "You know I always liked the emergency department." At Temple, first time through, it was the first rotation in our internship…And then the last rotation was also the emergency department… I think there were six of us on that rotation, what we decided was to give somebody a week off because we were getting tired at that time. In those days, it was 36 on and 12 off and you are blasted. So, we decided for this time, if we could give one guy a week off we'll do it, and we did. It was great fun. I loved it. The first time around in the emergency department, it was kind of a test. The last time was our last rotation, it was duck soup, and we loved it. So, I said to Jim, "You know I liked the emergency department when I was in med school and when I was interning, let's think about it. I'd be glad to talk to you about it, let's kick it around a little bit." So that is what we did.*[7]

McDade was soon convinced, and Mills had to find two more people. It is thought that he asked about four or five others to get two takers. The other two were William J. (Jack) Weaver, Jr., and C. A. (Babe) Loughridge, both respected Alexandria internists who were well known to Mills and McDade. Weaver had also helped to cover for Mills and McDade when they were in general practice.[7] Mills invited the other three to discuss the details, and at meetings that were held in his living room they developed a general plan and set of principles. McDade recalls that they developed a list of rules,

> *…that we were going to observe when we got into the emergency department. We never changed one. The reason why we never had to change one was because these were all in practice. We went through our own practice and thought now what would we like to see done? How would we want to see this run? That is what we did. We kicked it around. We met four or five times and just kicked it around and those are the primary rules that are in the American College of Emergency Physicians for putting together an Emergency Department.*[7]

The rules were an interesting combination of the ethics of emergency practice and practical elements.[6] They were very mindful of the other physicians in the community—the emergency practitioners would contact a patient's private doctor to seek permission, they would seek specialists' help when a problem was too complex, they would only see a patient once, and would refer the patient to their regular doctor. As savvy, experienced, and well-regarded members of the Alexandria medical community, Mills and his new partners crafted a practice model that would be minimally threatening and potentially very helpful to other physicians. When they took their plan to the Alexandria Hospital medical staff and Board of Directors, and the City Council, there was little opposition. Everyone knew that the problem in the ER was getting worse instead of better, and it did not hurt that the mastermind of the emergency coverage plan was the president of the medical staff. The colleagues he recruited were not desperate men looking for work. A *Medical Economics* article later noted,

> *If the four had been fresh from training, their offer might have been less surprising. But they were experienced men in their mid-30s and early 40s, with established practices and prestige in the community.*[4]

The plan was approved without changes to start in June of 1961.

The third hurdle, giving up their successful general practices, was the most emotionally troubling for Mills and the others. Mills later noted, "We had to terminate those relationships for the plan to succeed… It wasn't easy to give up the practices we'd built over the years."[4] The break with patients had to be unequivocal and complete. This was the element that separated Mills, McDade, Weaver, and Loughridge from other physicians who had previously spent some time in ERs and some who would do emergency practice in other plans in the 1960s—they were totally relinquishing their regular practices and going full time in the emergency department (ED). Mills sent a letter to his patients announcing that he would no longer be their regular doctor. The reaction from patients was intense. Mills's wife Frances remembers being told by a friend, who was a patient of Mills, that people were "running in the streets" in response to the announcement.[12] When their emergency practice commenced, some patients tried to reestablish their connection with Mills when he saw them in the ER. He was quoted in 1963,

> The other day a woman I've known for years came in and asked if she couldn't keep coming to see me as she used to do at my office. I said no, as we always do in such cases. We follow the same routine in the emergency room with our former patients as we do with strangers.[4]

Mills's transition was helped greatly when he found a physician who was interested in opening a practice in Alexandria and took over Mills's office building and his practice. The other three physicians made similar arrangements for their general practices.[12]

Mills and his partners were then clear to start staffing the ER, but needed to develop their formal contract with Alexandria Hospital. They chose the term "emergency department" (ED) instead of "emergency room" in the official language. With the help of an attorney, Mills and his partners set themselves up as independent contractors with Alexandria Hospital. The 5-year contract, dated June 26th, 1961, listed each of the four physicians and gave them the authority to "take charge of, conduct, manage and operate the emergency department at the Alexandria Hospital."[8,13] This included the "responsibility for the technical supervision" of the "employees or servants" who worked in the ED, but the hospital would retain the "administrative and executive control of these employees." The physicians were each paid a salary by Alexandria Hospital for professional services, but could bill private patients for their services with the fee scale "normally observed in the City of Alexandria by other private physicians."[13] The hospital provided billing services at a cost of 15% of billings. A portion of the emergency physician's salary came from the hospital's compensation from the county for providing indigent care. The contract specified that Mills's group was responsible for obtaining their own malpractice insurance policy with minimum coverage of $100,000/$300,000 per year for each member. Each physician was guaranteed 1 month of vacation per year, with 1 week for scientific meetings, conventions, and assemblies. The hospital did not provide any retirement benefits for the physicians, but did provide hospitalization coverage if they became ill. The contract specified that the physicians while on duty could not leave the hospital. It allowed Mills's group to hire other licensed physicians to work in the ED, but stated that the group, not the hospital, would be responsible for paying these individuals.

The Mills group decided that they would split the work into 12-hour shifts, with one physician on duty at a time. The physician would work for 5 consecutive days, and then have 5 days off, then work another 5 days and have 5 days off during which he would provide backup by being on call if the ED became too busy for one person to handle. The shifts were noon to midnight and midnight to noon. The choice of five consecutive days on duty with a large block of time off may have come from McDade's fond memories of the time during internship when he and his cointerns arranged their ED schedules to have a week off. This type of work schedule was unlike anything in medicine at the time. Few, if any, full-time American physicians could expect more than a 2-day weekend off, and this was not common. To have a 5-day stretch off at least twice a month was unheard of. The counter to this was that five consecutive 12-hour workdays as a single physician staffing a busy ED were very challenging.

Mills's wife Frances remembers, "It was very concentrated. When he was on duty there was very little time for anything else. But then, then there were the 5 days coming up!"[12] Mills later noted,

> We're better able to plan our family life than when we were at the patient's beck and call. That's one big personal benefit supplementing the professional satisfaction of filling a medical need that wasn't being adequately met in the community before.[4]

The Alexandria Plan appears to have been a success from its inception. Having experienced generalist physicians on duty full time was such an improvement over the previous level of care that an immediate impact was noticed. Critical cases were handled better, patient waiting times were reduced or eliminated, and community physicians and specialists received better information and consultation on their patients who presented to the ED. Complaints from the public decreased. The physical space for the ED was not ideal. It consisted of three rooms in the basement: 450 square feet for an annual volume of 18,000 patients. Equipment was of very poor quality. Patients who were brought in by ambulance were wheeled down a ramp, and lying on their backs, they would have viewed a cramped hallway with a very low ceiling and exposed pipes. Since radiology was on the fifth floor, sending patients for x-rays was an ordeal. John McDade recalls the early work in the basement ED,

> When we started down in that little basement, there was one big room with two stretchers in it and one small room with one stretcher and then there was the GYN [gynecology], that was it. It was at the end of a little hall. In order to get in there you had to come down a steep slope into the basement. That is the way things got delivered. It wasn't too much later we said. "We are going to have to do something about this." They are bringing these sick patients down this silly slope to get to us. We were seeing all kinds of things…A house burned down on Prince Street and it was a fairly large house…the people that lived there were all black…We had seven dead children, several burned children, two or three dead adults and a couple of badly burned adults. That's the worst day I had in that section of the hospital. I had three nurses and…we just took them in as they came in, if they were pronounced, they were pronounced, then we put them in the GYN room and one of the nurses went in there to try to take care of that and then we took care of everything else that came in. It was a bear. But, it was just that way down there…if you had 10 patients that were waiting, obviously you only had four places to treat them. Three places, really, because the fourth was GYN, which we used for more than one thing.[7]

Mills pushed for better and larger space, and wanted to get up to the first floor. At the time Alexandria Hospital was finally doing away with its black ward. Like many hospitals in the southern United States, Alexandria Hospital remained segregated into the late 1950s. Black patients were seen in the ED, which was integrated, but if they required admission, they went to the black ward on the first floor. Just after Mills and his group began their ED practice the hospital decided to integrate, and 3,000 square feet of space on the first floor became available. It was renovated and outfitted for emergency care, and about a year after they started, the first full-time emergency physicians moved into a real ED with 19 beds.[7]

Although the original Alexandria plan passed through administrative channels without any dissent, many community physicians were concerned about the effect that the ED contract physicians would have on their practices. Some of them voiced concerns at hospital medical staff meetings. McDade remembers,

> …when we started out, we had a lot of enemies. People were certain that we were going to take over the medical practice in the hospital. We had a lot of people suspicious of us. So suspicious. Mostly the surgeons that were involved with the emergency department. Things like compensation—stuff like that. So we said when we first started, okay we are not going to do any of that. We are going to take care of the emergency department and we are going to do this for the benefit of the medical staff. We decided we were going to have three audiences. Three people that we were going to

take care of—patients, the hospital, and the medical staff. We were going to give them all the same top-door service. That was the whole purpose when we went into it.[7]

Mills later noted,

We had to avoid even the slightest suspicion of patient stealing. And there's been none. There's no continuous therapy in the emergency room. No patient is seen more than once for the same complaint.[4]

Within a short time, the suspicions of the community physicians lessened, and most became, if not supportive, at least tolerant of their ED colleagues. A survey of local practitioners several months after Mills's group started was overwhelmingly positive. A reporter from *Medical Economics* also questioned Alexandria doctors in 1963. A local physician noted,

The case is usually one I can ask the doctor in charge at the emergency room to handle for me. I'm confident he'll give the patient all the care he needs. So the patient's own doctor isn't needlessly disturbed from his rest. And I haven't heard of a single instance of case-lifting.[4]

Mills and his partners thrived in the new contract. They worked 15 shifts in most months, and their workweek averaged about 42 hours if they did not get called in when they were on backup duty. Compared with private practice, this was a big decrease in hours, even if the hours were more irregular and demanding. Mills and his colleagues had estimated that they would make a bit less money in the ED. Their private practices had not been overly lucrative, but because of the choice location their incomes were higher than the average GP. In the ED, the physician's salary came from a standard $5 fee assessed to each patient and the subsidy that was paid to them for indigent care by the hospital. The Mills group soon found that although they were not grossing as much money as they did in private practice, their income was the same, or slightly higher, due to the lack of practice overhead. The billing for Mills's group was done by the hospital, with a collection rate of around 50%. The hospital ED charge was also $5, and the combined $10 bill was higher than patients typically paid for an office visit. If a patient presented to the ED, was assessed but not treated by the ED physician, and then referred to his or her own doctor, no ED bill was assessed.[4]

Part of achieving success in the new venture was not stepping on the toes of physicians in the community, but even more important was acquiring rank and power in the hospital system. Mills was already in a powerful position as president of the medical staff when he hatched the Alexandria Plan, but he encouraged his partners to take an active role in the hospital and medical community. They became chairs of the important committees in the hospital and began to have considerable influence. John McDade recalls,

One of the plastic surgeons…came into the emergency department after a medical staff meeting and said, "You know, I think I understand now why you guys have got this place under your thumb." I said, "What do you mean under our thumb?" "Every time there was a report to be given you gave it. It was either Mills, Weaver, or you or Loughridge, were giving all the reports for the staff." I said, "Well, we just like to be helpful."[7]

As the word of competent ED care spread in the community, and local physicians realized they could refer their patients to the ED without fear of losing them, the Alexandria Hospital ED volume increased. In the first 5 years after Mills and his colleagues started, ED visits doubled from around 18,000 to 36,000 per year. The ED practice became more taxing, and Mills and his colleagues had to call in backup more often. They also were finding that covering each other for vacations, conferences, or other obligations meant some periods of very heavy work that may have exceeded their hours when they were in private practice. Mills realized that they could no longer function as a foursome, and their incomes were high enough to hire some part-time help. Fortunately, they had a pool of young, but well-trained physicians to draw from in the Washington area. Mills had spent time at the postgraduate school in Annapolis when he was in the Navy, and from these connections he was able to hire military physicians to work part time in the ED. Another source was physicians who were doing fellowships at the National Institutes of Health. These part-time physicians were required to obtain Alexandria Hospital medical staff privileges. Mills was very conscious that the quality of physicians who provided part-time coverage would not be substantially below that of the regular doctors.[6-8]

The Alexandria four were the first group of American doctors to engage in full-time emergency practice. It is likely that a sprinkling of other physicians across the United States were at that time employed by hospitals and working in EDs on a full-time basis. What separated the Alexandria group from the other emergency practitioners was that Mills had developed a formal plan and contract, with buy in from the hospital, medical staff, and city. Rather than being physicians who just ended up working in an ED, Mills and his colleagues proactively set up the first viable system of emergency care for a community, with the control of the system resting in a physician group. Emergency medicine would go on to become a specialty of teamwork, and it is notable that the distinguishing feature of the pioneers of emergency practice was the formation of a group that would work together as a team to solve the problem in the Alexandria ED. The other factor that separated Mills's group from others who may have been doing full-time emergency practice in the early 1960s was the notoriety and exposure that would come to the Alexandria four.

Why did it happen first in Alexandria, Virginia? In reviewing the factors that created the crisis in the ED (see Figure 1.1), it is clear that many of the leading societal and physician factors were prominent in the Alexandria community. The population was increasing and the federal government administrations were changing over in late 1960 and early 1961, bringing in many new government workers and staff who often had no family doctor. A small, but growing underclass also lacked medical coverage. The practices of Alexandria area GPs and internists were saturated. Specialists were plentiful, but often not readily accessible. The Alexandria Hospital, despite its ancient ED, was a fully equipped hospital, using all the latest technologies, and was viewed favorably by the community. The rise in ED visits and the low quality of care created public complaints, and being in a competitive market, the hospital took these seriously. These emergency care problems were not unique to Alexandria, but unlike other U.S. cities in 1961, it had a solution. In hindsight, it is easy to see that Mills's plan was a logical way to solve the problem, but at the time, it was remarkably innovative. Group practices were uncommon, and were discouraged by the American Medical Association (AMA). Mills knew that although his collection of physicians functioned like a group, he would not be able to start out with a group contract. As a result, the four physicians each functioned as an independent contractor for Alexandria Hospital.

The 16 rules developed by the Alexandria group anticipated and answered almost every potential problem and concern that would be raised by the medical community and the public. When a controversy occurred, Mills could usually refer back to the approved rules to bolster his stand. For example, some community physicians objected to the Alexandria ED group seeing workmen's compensation patients who did not have a private physician in the ED. Previously, these patients might have been seen in the ED by an on-call physician or referred to private physicians. Because these were, by definition, paying patients, the community physicians viewed this as lost business. The Alexandria Plan rules stated that all patients who did not have a private physician were to be treated by the emergency physicians. Mills cited this during the argument, and the conflict dissolved. Mills later noted that within a couple of years these same physicians started to refer their workmen's compensation patients into the ED to be seen.[6] Alexandria was the birthplace of American emergency medicine because conditions were ripe for change and because of the talent of an experienced physician who was adventuresome enough to embark on a new career, but politically astute enough to craft an organized plan for successful emergency practice.[8]

Mills and his colleagues were aware that they were doing something new and exciting, but they were not prepared for the huge amount of attention that would be focused on the Alexandria ED. For the first year they worked hard and received local acclaim for their system. Then their reputation spread. The journal *Medical Economics* got wind of Mills experiment in the ED and sent a reporter in early 1963 to interview Mills, his colleagues, hospital administrators, and even community physicians about their system. The result was an article called "Practice Limited to the Emergency Room," and included photos of Mills and his group. The article, published in July 1963, was quite comprehensive, providing details of the group's contract, work hours, and comments from administrators and community physicians. Although the article had a positive tone, it was directly preceded in that issue by another article entitled "Our Enemy: the Emergency Room." This title was featured in bold on the cover of the journal, next to a cartoon of a laborer holding up his injured index finger and shedding a tear (see insert, Figure 2). The article was written by a psychiatrist, using the pseudonym Roswell Porter, who had been consigned by his hospital to work in the ED three or four times a year. "Porter" expressed dismay and disgust at patients who presented to the ED with what were viewed as nonemergent conditions. The author believed emergency care constituted a "threat" that "destroys our professional liberty."[14] He listed patients he had seen while working in the ED—a 3-year-old girl who injured her eye by falling on a stick, a 9-year-old with an injured foot, a 62-year-old with an ankle fracture, and a 13-year-old girl who came in with vomiting and turned out to be pregnant. In each case, the psychiatrist claimed the case was not a true emergency, and it "could have received as good or better medical service at a local practitioner's office." The article concludes with a diatribe against hospitals and emergency care,

> *Doctors on hospital staffs should refuse to be exploited any longer. We should agree to continue serving in emergency rooms only if patients admitted for treatment are true medical emergencies… Hospitals shouldn't be permitted, under the deception of maintaining an emergency room, to lie, cheat, and falsify the truth to compete with private practitioners.*[14,15]

The placement of this emotional opinion piece on the cover of a widely read journal, and directly before a well-researched article on the Alexandria Plan, demonstrates how the medical world did not quite know what to make of emergency practice in 1963. But despite having second billing in the journal, it was the Alexandria Plan article that drew attention from the medical world and public. Although Mills was not promoting or concealing what he was doing, the *Medical Economics* article effectively let the cat out of the bag. By the end of July, reporters and photographers from *Time* magazine were in the Alexandria Hospital ED interviewing Mills and his colleagues and snapping more than 500 pictures. A possible cover story was mentioned, but the result was a 2-page article in mid-August, without photos, featuring Robert Kennedy, the New York surgeon who was advocating for better emergency care, and a brief but accurate description of the Alexandria Plan. Earlier in 1963, *Virginia Medical Monthly* had requested that Mills write an article about his emergency group, and this was published in October as a 2-page article entitled, "A Method for Staffing a Community Hospital Emergency Department." The article described 15 months' experience at Alexandria Hospital and focused on the relationship between the ED physicians and the medical community.[16]

Television came next—McDade remembers huge television cameras being set up in the Alexandria ED when Mike Wallace interviewed Mills for a report on emergency care for the CBS Morning News. One of Mills's relatives in California phoned the Mrs. Mills, asking, "Is that our Jim Mills?"[7,12] By 1966, other popular magazines had caught onto the buzz generated by the Alexandria Plan, and articles on emergency care were published in the *Reader's Digest*, *Atlantic Monthly*, and *U.S. News and World Report*.[9,17,18] Most of the articles, while citing the problems of staffing busy EDs had a hopeful outlook, viewing the Alexandria Plan as an improvement over what had been previously offered. And although organized medicine was conflicted on the issue, the public and many physicians wanted more, not less, access to quality emergency care. John Knowles, M.D., who had witnessed the changes in the Massachusetts General Hospital emergency ward between 1951 and 1965 noted in a 1966 article in *Atlantic Monthly*,

> *The chief reason for the ever-expanding use of the emergency ward is simply that it is the best possible place in which to solve a medical problem quickly and accurately. The public knows it, and so does the doctor.*[18]

Judging from the response to publicity about the Alexandria group, emergency practice was on the minds of many others in the early 1960s. Mills was besieged with requests for information on his practice plan by physicians around the United States who were eager to start a similar type of practice. Many came to visit the Alexandria Hospital ED, both to see how the physicians worked and to see the ED physical set up. John McDade remembers, "…there must have been 60 or 70 visits. People coming in and saying, 'tell me what you are doing'."[7] One visit came from Robert Kennedy, of the American College of Surgeons, who was heading up a Hartford Foundation study on emergency care, but most visits were from physicians from nonacademic, community hospitals who had some level of responsibility for running the ED in their hospitals.

R. R. HANNAS: A GENERAL PRACTITIONER MOVES INTO THE WORLD OF ORGANIZED MEDICINE

One early visitor to Alexandria Hospital ED was Harris Graves, M.D., who was a GP from Nebraska, and a friend of R. R. Hannas. Graves was working part time in his local hospital ED, but was also active in the move to establish family practice as a specialty and knew Hannas from these activities. By 1965, R. R. Hannas had developed as an important medical figure in Oklahoma. He was a hard-working, highly respected GP, but had also assumed an important role in the Oklahoma State Medical Association, revitalizing their continuing medical education program. Hannas taught once a week at the University of Oklahoma Medical School. He would arise early to attend medical grand rounds, making the 125-mile drive from Sentinel to arrive at 8 AM. He developed a reputation as a good teacher in the medical clinics and was named the Oklahoma Chairman of the Council on Medical Education. In this role, he put on courses for GPs in towns around the state. Hannas was also on the board of directors for Blue Cross of Oklahoma and the Oklahoma Heart Association and was an active member of the American Academy of General Practice (AAGP).[19]

Although Hannas had prospered in Oklahoma, he was experiencing some stress from his busy practice and family discontent. Regarding rural Oklahoma and his patients, Hannas recalls, "My first wife hated it and they hated her and they should've, she was nasty to them….." His likable demeanor, excellent medical knowledge, and work ethic had made him a favorite physician for a whole region of the state. But this success left him almost no time for rest. He recalls,

> *You know my kids in Oklahoma, took them a long while to learn that this thing that you talk into, you know, when you dial—they didn't know it was just a telephone. They thought it was a fuckin' telephone, because every time it rang I'd say, "There goes that fuckin' telephone!"*[19]

The trials of this hectic lifestyle eventually persuaded Hannas to leave Sentinel, and in 1965, he moved his family to Kansas City, Missouri, where he took a full-time position with the AAGP. Hannas worked part time in a Planned Parenthood clinic and moonlighted in the ER of Research Hospital in Kansas City. This hospital had been called "German Hospital" until the World War made this name unsuitable in America, and the name had been changed to Research Hospital, even though it did not do research. Hannas enjoyed the ER work, but his focus was on helping the AAGP in their quest to have a specialty board in family practice. Hannas was secretary for the Commission on Education and the Commission on Hospitals for the AAGP. In 1967, he became the secretary for the Committee on Requirements for Certification. Sometime between 1965 and 1967, he met with Harris Graves, and they discussed the emergency practice plan that James Mills had created in Alexandria.[19]

The Pontiac Plan and Other Early Methods of Emergency Practice

The emergency care problem was seen throughout the United States in the 1950s, and just as James Mills would study the problem in Alexandria and develop a plan, others came up with their plans. This was the heyday of Hill-Burton hospital funding, and many new hospitals found upon opening their doors that they had underestimated their ED census and lacked coordinated physician coverage. In San Pablo, California, Brookside Hospital opened in 1954. The hospital's medical board developed a voluntary emergency service plan, and paid medical staff well—$10 an hour—to provide coverage. Initially 12 physicians volunteered, but by 1965, 40 physicians were working part time in the Brookside ED. As was typical with this type of staffing plan, many of the volunteers were young GPs who were building their practices and supplementing their incomes by working up to 80 hours a month in the ED.[9] The ED census for Brookside Hospital increased from 4000 patients per year in 1954 to over 22,000 by 1965, and the ED required major renovation and expansion.

This part-time, volunteer method of emergency practice was used in many nonacademic hospitals across the United States. Often a physician was designated the ED director and became responsible for securing enough physicians to staff the ED and addressing problems or concerns. Just down the road from Alexandria, Reinald Leidelmeyer, the Dutch immigrant physician who had trained at the University of Virginia, was in general practice in Fairfax from 1959 to 1961. When the new Fairfax Hospital opened in February of 1961, it did not have a plan for ED staffing. Leidelmeyer, who wanted to spend more time in the hospital setting, offered to help cover the ED. In the same month that Mills group began staffing the Alexandria ED, Leidelmeyer and another physician began working 12-hour daytime shifts on a part-time basis in the Fairfax ED, Leidelmeyer recalls,

> We had moonlighters for the night. We were busy when we had 30 patients—in a day. So when we started, there was no CPR [cardiopulmonary resuscitation]....There was nothing. I had two rooms each with two stretchers and one side room.[20]

Leidelmeyer was aware of Mills's group, and they met periodically over lunch to discuss how to best make a living in emergency practice. Billings, the financial interaction with the hospital, and controversies with community physicians were the usual topics of conversation. They had some awareness of what was happening in emergency care around the country, but during this time, they were focused on local issues.

In Pontiac, Michigan, Dr. Everette Gustafson, much like James Mills in Alexandria, was put in charge of doing a study on the problems in the Pontiac General Hospital emergency room in 1959. Pontiac was a blue-collar city, with a large concentration of autoworkers who had health insurance through the big auto companies. Pontiac General was a 381-bed, city-owned, teaching hospital. In 1961, the ED saw nearly 26,000 patients per year. Fifty-five percent of patients had prepaid health insurance.[21] Gustafson evaluated the situation by talking with ED patients,

> I talked to the people who came to the emergency room to find out what was happening. And I found out that most people came after 5 o'clock because most doctors closed their offices at that time. Another reason was that husbands come home from work at that time. Another reason was the often-long hours spent in doctor's offices. Another thing I found—and it was very sharp on their part—was that you could come to the emergency room and be seen, and Blue Cross would pay for that. One fellow told me, "I've been doing it for 7 years. My wife and kids have been getting all their care here. It's cheaper this way."[11,22]

Gustafson and Dr. Ralph Wigent came up with a plan for part-time, voluntary coverage of the Pontiac General Hospital ED. The basics of the plan were similar to what had been in place in Brookside Hospital and probably many other medium-sized community hospitals—a group of staff physicians who had full-time practices were hired to work part time in the ED. Coverage for the 8 AM to 4 PM shift was generally provided by moonlighting residents or other young physicians. The Pontiac Plan group initially provided coverage on evenings, nights, and weekends. The group comprised approximately 30 physicians from various medical specialties. Each worked from 16 to 32 hours a month, with a minimum requirement of 32 hours in a 3-month period. The difference between the Pontiac Plan and other part-time ED physician staffing methods of the early 1960s was how Gustafson, Wigent, and later Robert Leichtman, M.D., set up the business model. In 1961, the group of 29 doctors formed as association called the Professional Medical Service Group. They billed a minimum $4 fee for their services, but collections were handled by an accounting firm that charged 8% of gross fees. The physicians did not receive their fees directly, but were paid an hourly rate for each month's work by the Service Group.

After working with this arrangement for 5 years, the Pontiac Plan physicians formed a professional corporation. The reason was "the evident need for closer supervision of accounting practices."[21] Apparently, the physicians realized that they could make much more money in this type of arrangement. Gustafson and Leichtman chose a corporation rather than a general partnership to simplify the partnership agreements between such a large group of physicians and to make it easier for physicians to join and leave the partnership. It also gave control of the professional corporation to a small group of "resident agents," or incorporators, and the remaining partners were considered stockholders. The corporation elected five physicians to a Board of Managers, and this Board in turn elected a chairman, secretary, and treasurer.[22,23]

The Pontiac Plan Corporation hired a professional management consultant, Maria Maraveleas, who worked independently of Pontiac General Hospital to collect bills at a rate of $0.75 per patient. She also processed the insurance claims, disbursed money to the physicians, and handled all questions from patients about billing. Maraveleas would later play a brief role as an administrator for the early American College of Emergency Physicians. Physicians in the Service Group initially were able to charge individual fees on the emergency sheet, with no set fee schedule. However, due to variance in the fees charged, the professional corporation soon instituted a uniform fee schedule, which was based on the Blue Shield fee schedule. According to its leaders, the corporation distributed all monies equally at the end of the month on the basis of the number of hours worked by the individual physician member. Board members received a stipend for their administrative work. This early plan was "democratic" in nature and was an immediate financial success.[23] Blessed with a good payer mix, the practice management team was "...able to bill and collect physicians' fees so effectively that hourly income earned by physician members many times exceeds net earnings on an hourly basis in their private offices."[22]

By 1966, the corporation was paying physicians $16 per hour, compared with the previous rate of $10 per hour, and local physicians had formed a waiting list to get into the corporation.[21,23] The Pontiac Plan was also a clinical success. Despite an increase in ED patient volume from 26,000 in 1961 to 38,000 in 1965, the number of complaints about ED care and the number of incident reports filed in the ED decreased markedly.[23]

Just north of Pontiac in the Flint area of Michigan, Robert Rathburn, M.D., created a Pontiac-type emergency staffing plan that was even bigger than the original Pontiac Plan. Rathburn gave up private practice to work in EDs and administer a professional corporation of 60 physicians who provided emergency staffing for the McLaren and St. Joseph Hospitals. Many other ED staffing plans that were modeled on the Pontiac Plan were created in the mid-1960s but some did not involve incorporation of physicians, and thus were not true Pontiac Plans, but were more like the part-time voluntary staffing plans of the 1950s.

In the 1950s, most physicians who had been assigned, consigned, or otherwise coerced into staffing emergency rooms were not pleased with the work. By the 1960s, conditions in medicine had changed to cause a small cadre of physicians to actually choose to focus their work efforts in EDs. Other Alexandria-type plans, which used a group of doctors who committed to full-time emergency practice, emerged within 5 years of the Alexandria Plan. A group started in Binghamton, New York, and another at Ballard Hospital in Seattle, Washington, in 1966. In western Michigan, John Rupke, M.D., started a full-time group in 1966.

Most of the converts to emergency care were generalists or physicians who elected to drop out of their residency training—it was not common at this time for a specialist-trained physician to leave practice for emergency work. The movement of generalists to EDs was most likely a symptom of the ongoing decline of the status of GPs in America. GPs were increasingly finding themselves the second-class citizens of medicine. Whereas most specialists did full residencies, GPs typically had only internship training and were not as likely to be key players in hospital medical staffs. Their practices were also becoming more stressful. Part of this was the reduction in GPs so that fewer family doctors were seeing a greater number of patients. Another factor was the increasing complexity of medicine. New diagnostic and treatment options meant more in-depth workups, a higher percentage of patients requiring attention in the hospital, and vast new amounts of medical knowledge to learn and assimilate. GPs tried to meet clinical demand by increasing their numbers of appointments per day and hiring more staff. The product of these pressures was weary GPs who were wealthier than before, but who had little time to enjoy the fruits of their labors. It is not surprising that some, like James Mills, Jr., found that emergency practice might be a way to escape the rigors of private practice, while still providing an exciting and stimulating brand of medicine. Mills was the first to make the leap, but many other GPs in the 1960s were ready to jump after him.

Although some forward-thinking, enterprising physicians were beginning to develop plans for staffing EDs by the early 1960s, this did not mean that the rescue of emergency care was occurring on a large scale. Across the United States, especially in smaller hospitals, emergency care remained dreadful. Robert Kennedy, who was continuing his crusade as a surgeon wanting better care for injured patients, helped to produce a study on EDs for the American College of Surgeons and the Hartford Foundation. Over a 4-year period in the early 1960s, Kennedy and a hospital administrator, Lloyd Chadbourn, visited more than 325 hospital EDs in 34 states. They found no significant improvement in most EDs from the pre–World War II era—staffing by a single nurse, physicians not readily available, and a lack of equipment and facilities to handle emergencies. Many small EDs locked their doors at night.[9] It was only in the handful of U.S. hospitals where the "emergency problem" had been acknowledged, studied, and a plan developed with physician input that emergency care improved. In the academic world, the situation was also stagnant.

DAVID WAGNER, M.D.: THE SURGEON TAKES A PART-TIME JOB

David Wagner and his wife returned to Philadelphia from their work in the Indian Service Hospital in New Mexico in 1965 to put their children into Quaker schools in the Philadelphia area. The time spent in New Mexico serving the Native American population would turn out to be valuable training for Wagner's eventual work in emergency medicine. Wagner recalls the situation:

> Underserved, there was not a single specialist there. We had a little 28-bed hospital… We didn't even have an internist… It was unbelievable. It was such a privilege to be a part of, first of all, such an amazingly wonderful, truly American culture. Then to be let in their lives, but also to be able to have that experience of the diversity of conditions that one would see by a terribly underserved group of people…From an experience point of view, it was probably more useful than almost anything else.[24]

When he returned to Philadelphia, Wagner "just basically rang doorbells" to find a job as a surgeon. He was trained as a pediatric surgeon, but found a job at Women's Medical College where he signed on for a starting salary of $12,000 per year to do both general and pediatric surgery. Women's Medical College graduated 48 female physicians per year, and it was said that so few women graduated from U.S. medical schools at that time, if you were a woman in medicine, there was a 50% chance you had graduated from Women's Medical College in Philadelphia. Wagner was busy from the start, but his meager salary made it hard to support a family. A few months after he started at Women's, he encountered Bob Lambert, the medical director of the hospital in the hallway. Lambert looked flustered. Wagner recalls,

> I said, "Bob, what's going on? What's the problem?" He pointed his finger down there.
>
> He said, "Down there. We got these people. They keep coming to our emergency room. They keep coming—they are making us crazy. They are coming…and we've had to hire somebody down there at night because we just can't handle it with interns and residents doing it."
>
> I said, "Well, Bob, what's the deal?" He said, "We need somebody from 6 PM to 2 AM. After that we are shutting it down…we are going to pay $5.63 and hour—do you want it?"[24]

Wagner eagerly signed on and began his emergency medicine career working part time in the ED of Women's Hospital every other evening from 6 PM to 2 AM. He continued to do general and pediatric surgery. Because he was the only faculty member who had anything to do with the ED, he also became the *de facto* director of emergency care. Thus, Wagner caught wind of some of the happenings in community emergency medicine and, like a few others in the academic world, began to think about how someone might be trained for emergency practice.

JOHN WIEGENSTEIN, M.D.: TRAINING AT THE PINK PALACE AND EARLY YEARS AS A GENERAL PRACTITIONER

When John Wiegenstein was in his final year at the University of Michigan Medical School, he realized that he could not afford to do a full residency—with his growing family and lack of savings he would need to start a practice. He planned to do an internship at McLaren Hospital in Flint, where Robert Rathburn had started a Pontiac Plan–type emergency coverage. Wiegenstein was good friends with Robert Fisher, a charismatic student who was president of the class when Wiegenstein served as vice president. Wiegenstein recalls he and Fisher were having a beer in an Ann Arbor bar, celebrating their upcoming graduation,

> … and he was telling me about how he got his internship in Honolulu at Tripler General Hospital and I was going to that smoky town in Flint I said, "If I could go to Hawaii I would." He said, "Sure. They only take special people." So, it got me going and I got on the phone and called the Surgeon General and checked on their commitments, they had three openings still left and so I applied and, my wife didn't know about this, I was accepted. So while I was gone one day the wire—Western Union—people called my wife and said, "You have a wire can I read it to you?" And she said, "Go ahead." They said this was from the U.S. Army, congratulations you have been accepted in the internship in Honolulu and she said, "I think you have the wrong number obviously, because he is going to go to Flint in Michigan—he isn't going to Hawaii!" When I got home, she was not very happy—she was never going to leave the outskirts of Flint…we finally had it out and I called back and talked to the same Western Union person and I said, "Yes." He said, "Did you talk to your wife?"[25]

Wiegenstein's sense of adventure prevailed once again, and he prepared to go to the U.S. Army Tripler General Hospital, "the pink palace on the hill," for his internship. Getting there would prove to be a trying experience. John had a hectic last week of medical school. To pass pathology, he had to do seven more autopsies in that week. Perhaps his wife, Iris, had a premonition about the move—6 days before Wiegenstein was to graduate she and her children were involved in a serious car collision. Iris was brought unconscious to the hospital. One of Wiegenstein's daughters was thrown from the car and was "pretty banged up," but did not have serious injuries. Iris recovered but had a fractured arm that required surgery. She remained hospitalized, missing

John's graduation. After graduation, Wiegenstein loaded his three children into a Comet station wagon and made the drive from Michigan to California, where they would fly to Hawaii. He remembers padding the back seat with pillows so his bruised daughter could rest during the trip. Iris remained in the hospital with the plan that she would fly to California to join them once sufficiently recovered. When he was half way across the country, John called back to Michigan to find that Iris had developed an infection in the arm and was back in surgery. She was delayed a few more days, but was able to fly to California, where "black and blue, a cast on her forearm," she boarded a noisy plane with John and the three children and flew to Honolulu. Wiegenstein had to start his demanding internship at once and remembers the challenge,

> I had long hours, like in OB [obstetrics]—we had 36 hours on, 12 off during internship. Very active OB service. I had the record of eight deliveries in an hour. Two sets of twins in that hour. Anyway, we had lots of activity there. I'd go home and be exhausted…we got through that miserable year, internship.[25]

Wiegenstein finished his internship and as part of his commitment had to do two more years in a military setting and then had a requirement to do general practice in a rural community for 3 years. He was ordered to go to Port Louis in Washington, but his friend Fisher intervened. Fisher was to remain at Tripler for two more years and lobbied for Wiegenstein to also be assigned at Tripler. Wiegenstein received an assignment at Tripler for a 2-year program in the outpatient clinics. He took call and did rotations in anesthesiology; ear, nose, and throat (ENT); head and neck surgery; and pediatrics. He acquired broad-based knowledge and skills. He remembers liking surgery, but realizing that a few rotations did not constitute adequate training in the field,

> I decided I was not going to do surgery because the five appendectomies that I did, two of them were major problems. One was plastered up against the gallbladder and the other one had a tumor-obstructed appendix. I decided that if you open a belly you had better know what you are doing. Anybody can remove an appendix but not anybody can do a bowel resection or whatever else you might have to do. It taught me a good lesson not to do surgery.[25]

In 1963, Wiegenstein was released from his service commitment and he and his family headed back to Michigan where he found a rural practice in the small town of Holt, outside of Lansing, that would satisfy his federal loan repayment commitment. He joined another physician, but became concerned that this physician was practicing in a manner that would put Wiegenstein at risk. For example, he did a simple mastectomy in the office. Wiegenstein started his own practice and it became extremely busy.

> From 1965 to 1967, I just got overloaded with patients. I had more OB patients… I had a huge practice. I was never home. I was gone, a solo practice and it was just wearing me down. I got bored with baby checks, high blood pressure checks, and those kinds of things that just did not stimulate me at all. So, whenever they had an emergency—one of my patients would get in an automobile accident, I was right there. They would cancel all my appointments and I would go suture, and take care of this diabetic out of control, and whatever—I just went to the emergency department whatever chance I had, I loved that part…If they had one of my patients they knew I'd be there in about 20 minutes.[25]

St. Lawrence Hospital, the community hospital where Wiegenstein was on staff, experienced the same problems covering its busy ED that befell most hospitals at that time. St. Lawrence used itinerant physicians to cover the day shift and a rotation of all the medical staff to cover the nights. Wiegenstein recalls the situation,

> Day times they hired these people that come and go—mostly alcoholics you know. They moved from town to town. They really had a terrible situation because in the

daytime they couldn't get anybody to do it so they had to hire these people, vagabonds. At night time, the staff would cover it. I remember covering, they were hard up one day because one of these guys didn't show up because he was drunk or something, so I canceled my appointments and came and worked the day. That night the dermatologist came on board and I heard him say to the nurse, "You know, if there is a life-threatening rash, call me—I'm going to go upstairs." The nurse handled almost everything. If it was a surgical problem, she called a surgeon up, etc. If they didn't get there in time, the patients died. That's how bad it was. I was stimulated by that terrible situation and also the terrible situation in the ambulances....[25]

The "terrible situation" also stimulated St. Lawrence Hospital to study the problem, much as Alexandria Hospital had done 6 years earlier. The chairman of the committee to study the ED was a local family doctor, Eugene Nakfoor. Unlike James Mills, who had little to find when he researched ways to staff the ED, Nakfoor discovered a booklet, *Emergency Department: A Handbook for the Medical Staff*, that had just been printed in 1966 by the AMA's Department of Hospitals and Medical Facilities. The booklet included a detailed description of the Alexandria Plan, written by Mills, and the Pontiac Plan, written by Robert Leichtman. The handbook provided a wealth of other information on physician coverage, contracts, legal issues, and standards for emergency departments.[6] On the basis of his review of the handbook and other research, Nakfoor, despite being in Michigan where the Pontiac Plan had originated, decided to establish an Alexandria-type plan at St. Lawrence Hospital. He asked John Wiegenstein if he would join him, along with an industrial physician named T. D. Clark, who was friend of Wiegenstein. The three physicians staffed the ED, working 56 hours per week.[25]

Around the country, similar scenarios were playing out. In the Bay area of California, an enterprising young physician who was a Lieutenant Commander in the U.S. Coast Guard as part of the U.S. Public Health Service, was working in an emergency department part time, and thinking about the big picture of staffing EDs.

KARL MANGOLD, M.D.: "HOW DO THINGS WORK?"

Karl Mangold was born in 1938 in the blue-collar town of White Plains, New York, to German immigrant parents. Mangold, whose name would become synonymous with entrepreneurial emergency medicine, was a frenetic child—always busy and working a variety of jobs. As a large-framed boy at age 10, he told the local golf course owners that he was 14 and was hired as a caddy. He quickly moved up to manage a driving range and then the pro shop. He delivered newspapers, worked in a dining hall kitchen, and with each new job, he asked a basic question, "How does this work?" Later in medical school, his attention was on different things than most students,

> *...As a medical student you walk in an OR [operating room] and you're going to hold the "idiot stick." But what was going through my mind was how does all this equipment get here, who buys it, who pays for it, how is it maintained, how is it decided what equipment is here?...I looked at is as a systems approach—how do things work?*[26]

This fascination with systems was coupled with Mangold's sense that one person could make a difference in most endeavors. As a senior college student at Notre Dame in 1959, he was president of the Student President's Council. A team from Notre Dame won a television game show competition called the College Bowl, but Mangold knew that this accomplishment would not make much news at football-crazy Notre Dame. He had the idea that the school should make a strong show of support for this academic achievement that would rival the fuss that was made for victorious football teams when they returned home. He coerced a fellow student to gain access to a mimeograph machine. He and a couple of friends snuck out of their dorms after night check and stayed up all night printing thousands of flyers announcing the College Bowl victory, and encouraged students and faculty to come to the airport to greet the team. The next morning the dean of the College of Fine Arts found out about this initiative and invited Mangold to lunch. A few hours later, Karl was riding in a limousine with the mayor of South Bend to the airport to greet the students. Thousands of students lined the roads back to Notre Dame, banging on the car. Later *Television Age* and *Reader's Digest* magazines ran articles describing how the Notre Dame student body turned out to greet its academic winners.[27] That experience struck a chord with Mangold,

> The thing that really triggered in my mind was, like, "whoa!" I had an idea, one person has an idea, it just happened to me, I got it done, and I got it into (a national) magazine. It was really sort of a light bulb going on, like what one person could do… I was kind of astounded at where this idea went.[26]

Later in his emergency medicine career, Mangold would become famous and wealthy by taking ideas and running with them. Mangold had been raised as a Catholic and had been an altar boy. When he was making his postcollege career choice, he considered the two occupations his parents most admired—priesthood and medicine. He entered a Jesuit seminary for delayed vocations. Unlike John Wiegenstein, who had 6 years of seminary training, Mangold lasted only 6 weeks. Realizing he had made a wrong turn, he applied to medical school. He attended Cornell University Medical School in New York City where "they treated us like kings. They treated the residents like dirt but medical students were kings there."[26] Mangold remembers sitting in a lecture hall as a senior medical student in the 1963 school year as part of a public health/community medicine course and hearing that four physicians in Alexandria, Virginia, had left their practices to work full time in emergency practice. At the time "it just sort of went in and out." Mangold was most interested in the field of orthopedic surgery, but an internist faculty mentor encouraged Karl to do a year or more of internal medicine to provide a broader base in physiology before entering an orthopedic surgery residency. Mangold took this advice and started his internship in internal medicine at Presbyterian–St. Luke's Hospital in New York in 1964.

Then, like many in his generation, Mangold's path was affected by U.S. military involvement half a world away. As he completed his internship, Mangold could see that the Vietnam war was heating up, and his likelihood of being drafted was increasing. He took advantage of a program called the Berry Plan. Through this plan, graduating medical students could avoid the regular selective service draft by agreeing to be assigned to duty in military hospitals for 2 years. The Berry Plan helped to ensure an adequate number of physicians in the military medical services and gave physicians a chance to avoid combat duty. Provisions were available in the plan to do at least a portion of residency before or after the military assignment, but all physicians in the program had to complete their internship before their military commitment. Over the course of two decades, from 1954 to 1974, 23,000 young physicians participated in Berry Plan, including many of the early leaders of emergency medicine.[28]

Karl Mangold's wife Jan, who was trained as a nurse, but who also worked as a fashion model, needed to be in a big city, so when Mangold had the opportunity through the Berry Plan to be assigned to the Coast Guard in San Francisco as a flight surgeon, they jumped at the chance.

> …And so I was a flight surgeon and took care of the healthy recruits a couple of days and the Coast Guard inductees going through basic training 3 days. I was at the air station and did physical exams on pilots and nobody was sick, but I got a chance to do a lot of flying and got a chance to be lowered from helicopters down onto little dinghies and barges, and at the time that was a big rage because that's what James Bond was doing in the movies. Then my wife went back to work and my intention was to go back to New York but we really both liked California. We…got to thinking, well maybe we'll get a residency out here. I went over to UC and talked to a few people in orthopedics and…made the decision not to go back to New York or Chicago. Also, totally serendipitously—a guy in the Navy that I knew said let's make a little money, let's go moonlight in a couple of emergency departments before we go to

residency...and so we started to approach some hospitals and one of these hospitals basically said I've got 130 to 140 beds—I got 32 beds occupied...and we'll do anything. What do you propose? And we said, military docs, some residents, and we'll cover your emergency room nights and weekends. It surprised me out here, the only place that had emergency rooms as they were called then, were academic places and county places. Rarely was there a private hospital that had open emergency rooms. So, that's how we started. The first night I worked, then they said how much money do you want, how do you want to get paid? I had no idea...So the Administrator said we will you give you $7 per hour plus $25 a night shift and $5 a patient. So the first night I worked the door was locked. Literally locked, there was no publicity that we were starting and I saw two people. I have no idea why they came...That was the start.[26]

The typical patient load when Mangold first started covering the Memorial Hospital of San Leandro emergency department was less than 10 patients a night, but some real emergencies were in that mix.

I guess the single most harrowing moment I had in the emergency department all those years was in the middle of the night, about 3 AM, I got woken from sleep. Downstairs, a 17-year-old gal has belly pain. Well, I go down and pull the sheet back and there is a very pregnant abdomen, so I put her up in stirrups, there is a baby coming. No prenatal care, this gal had lived at home, the mother's outside, and what I see is a single cyanotic foot. I page anybody in the hospital—would have been dumb luck. Nobody is there, so I said put a call out for a couple OB/GYNs, and here I've got a single-footling breech coming my way with no prenatal care. I've never delivered a single footling breech—the only babies I delivered was in medical school in the OB rotation with a resident over my shoulder, never a breech and...all I could think of was the pelvis and the lectures that the OB guys would give, they put presentations up and they'd say now take this through the pelvis. All I remember was go slowly, and I thought at that moment, I said, "Poor baby, poor mother, and poor me." I felt so inadequate at that moment. Luckily, got a good baby out. I went out and told the mother and the mother had no idea, now you remember this was like maybe 1966. Totally different societal honesty about sexuality—a huge dishonesty in the society. The mother said, "Oh we didn't know she was pregnant!"[26]

Just a few weeks after Mangold and his friend started covering, the hospital administrator came to Mangold and said that he wanted to provide 24-hour physician coverage for the ED, and wondered if Mangold could do it. Since the military physicians had daytime commitments, they could not cover these hours. Mangold, sensing that a bigger role was possible, asked the administrator to let him find a daytime person.

He gave me two weekends to find somebody, because all I could think of...was— the person that is there during the day has all the power and control, he was running this little thing, and it's going to be out of our hands the minute you get somebody that's got some authority and respect of the medical staff.[26]

Mangold found a physician who was getting out of the military and was going to be an anesthesiologist to do the daytime ED shifts. Next, Mangold convinced another physician Herschel Fischer, who was leaving the Army to stay a year and work day shifts at San Leandro Hospital. Fischer had 2 years of internal medicine residency training before serving in the Army. He planned to return to Los Angeles to finish residency and go into practice. By late 1965, Mangold had managed to take control of staffing the Memorial Hospital of San Leandro ED while still working as a flight surgeon for the Coast Guard. Mangold explored orthopedic surgery residencies in the area, but then two things happened that would change his career path for good. Mangold recalls,

Medicare and Medicaid came in...There was such a stream of patients that were referred to us by the rest of the medical staff, because almost instantly they were

overwhelmed with all this deferred pathology. So, no surgeon wanted to get up and examine a belly any more. They had a full operating schedule the next day, so they sent them to us. The second thing that was sort of a defining moment…was at the 1966 Christmas party. They had a Christmas party, medical staff, in fact it was a medical staff and department head party—the Board of Directors, administration. And two women, wives of doctors, came up to me and literally hugged me and said you will never know what you have done for our marriage by being there in the emergency department. Then, I figured this cannot miss. This is going to sweep the country…We've got politics and economics called Medicare and Medicaid, and now we have hormones and marriages and women behind us.[26]

Mangold and Fischer began to talk with other Bay Area hospitals about staffing their EDs. This business became formalized when he and Fischer formed a corporation, Fischer Mangold, in 1966. Although he was listed as the second name in this partnership, Mangold was the driving force. From his initial instincts to take the lead role in recruiting physicians for the San Leandro ED, Mangold became a legendary physician recruiter and staffer of EDs. Fischer Mangold became the first multihospital, full-time emergency physician group in the country. By the time his service commitment was done in 1967, Mangold was in full swing, developing his business acumen, and Fischer Mangold was managing multiple EDs in the Bay area. Although he had originally done recruiting work for San Leandro for free, Mangold quickly learned some hard business lessons.

I gave about 300 free hours to one hospital designing their emergency department, setting up the whole thing from "didn't exist" to purchasing and resources and equipment and nursing staff, standards, and everything else and then that hospital at the last minute decided that they couldn't afford us and I had given away I figure about 300 hours. I learned to work with architects and city government, and on and on, but that taught me to never do anything for free. So, then the business side of me came in. These things have value; I'm never doing anything for free. The Fischer manual says docs never do anything for free. If you are making too much money, give it back to the hospital. If you give it back, they put your name in the lobby on a plaque. If you do it for free, they don't say thank you, they don't appreciate it, they take it for granted, they're exploitative—you never do anything for free. So…we would give the hospital donations as a group, or individuals, and get our name up there, all of a sudden we are philanthropists as opposed to flunkies doing whatever somebody said to do…A lot of people including everybody on the medical staff that wanted you to see their patients at night on the floor for nothing, resuscitate their patients, there is always people willing to turn you into a slave and we just wouldn't do it. I had that one bad experience and another light went on.[26]

Although Mangold was careful to not be exploited, he realized, as James Mills had in Alexandria, that good relations with the medical staff were essential to building a successful emergency group practice. He remembers how the interplay occurred,

I'd say, I've got a patient with a gallbladder here and…you have to teach me something before I give you this patient…you better teach me what you know because dead people don't pay. My job is to keep them alive until you, the real doctor, take them into surgery. Dead people don't pay…Look I'm an extension, I'm a free extension of your office. We're here nights and weekends and during the day. We don't steal your patient, we'll send them back to you so you have to teach me what you know so we can keep patients alive and happy and you can be efficient in your office, in the OR.[26]

WILLIAM HAECK, M.D.: STARTING EMERGENCY PRACTICE IN FLORIDA

Emergency practice was so wide open in 1966, that almost anyone with some initiative and an affinity for the ED could secure a working relationship or contract with a hospital to staff the ED. More physicians came to emergency practice by accident than by design. William Haeck, M.D., had a path that was typical for the early emergency practitioners. Haeck grew up in Grand Rapids, Michigan, the son of a prominent surgeon. He remembers as a child going to Butterworth Hospital where his father would make rounds,

> *He would park me in the emergency department waiting room. I would watch the ambulances come and go, and all the fast action there. Really kind of got fascinated by the whole thing and eventually became an orderly at the hospital and got assigned occasionally to the emergency room and that is where I really first got involved. Went to Northwestern, gravitated to Cook County Hospital for a lot of my rotations. Fell in love with the atmosphere there and interned there. At the hospital then the emergency department intern was king. Virtually 100% of the admissions to the hospital came through the emergency room.[29]*

Haeck did an internship and then through his Berry Plan arrangement was stationed at Hunter Air Force base in Savannah, Georgia. Then, like Karl Mangold had done in California, Haeck sought to make some extra money by moonlighting in local EDs,

> *I quickly discovered that most of the staff at the hospital there hated the emergency room and would actually pay you to take call there. I did a lot of it and at the same time discovered that a lot of little, rural, southeast Georgia community hospitals would pay somebody to spend the weekend in the emergency room. So I did a lot of that too and loved it. I thought you had to pick a specialty and I picked OB/GYN and got accepted in a residency program in Jacksonville, Florida. Got out of the service a couple of months early. Started in that residency program and I was really miserable. What I was not miserable doing was moonlighting. An obstetrician in Jacksonville Beach had a contract to staff the emergency room at Jacksonville Beach's hospital. His practice was busy enough by then that he really didn't want to continue to do that and asked me if I was interested. I quit the residency over my father's wishes, and over the residency director's objections. Their statements typically were, "That can't be a career, that's only something you'd do if you can't do anything else."[29]*

Haeck's "anything else" turned into a busy career. He started small, with the contract at the initial hospital in 1967, but his connection back to Michigan would soon have him in the thick of the national development of emergency medicine.

KROME, ROSEN, PODGORNY:
THE SURGEONS DEVELOP

While men like Mills, Wiegenstein, Mangold, and Haeck were beginning to figure out how to make a career in emergency practice, Ronald Krome, Peter Rosen, and George Podgorny—who would become three of the most influential figures in emergency medicine—were entrenched in their surgical residencies. Their counterpart, David Wagner, was a few years ahead of them and by 1967 was enjoying a hybrid career as a surgeon and emergency physician at Women's Medical Hospital.

Peter Rosen was leaving his surgical residency at Highland Hospital in Oakland, in 1965, just at the time that Karl Mangold was coming to the same area of California. Rosen, like Ron Krome, had chosen a surgical residency that did not have a strict pyramid system. He was married, had a child, and had another on the way. He knew that he would have to borrow money to supplement his $50 a month intern salary and wanted to make his surgical training as defined and brief as possible. Rosen developed some skills that he would use later in emergency medicine,

> *Highland influenced my career in emergency medicine although I didn't know it at the time, because at Highland the surgeons ran the emergency department. There were no medical residents in the ER except for one night shift a week that they would relieve the surgical house staff. We worked 12 on, 12 off, 6 days a week. That was considered an easy rotation. We took care of peds and internal medicine and surgical emergencies.*

So I ended up getting some training in nonsurgical emergencies that would come to play years later.[30]

Rosen then entered the Army and was stationed in Germany as part of the Army Medical Corps from 1965 to 1968. As a well-trained, brash young surgeon, Rosen started doing many operations in his first year, but then had some problems with his Army Colonel and was ordered to serve in a medical dispensary for a year,

My first year in the Army I was assigned to a 1,000-bed hospital that had one patient in it when I arrived because they had built another 1,000-bed hospital 50 km away. So, I started doing surgery because I had a pretty big population to care for in both troops and dependents and within a month, I had a waiting list of 6 months for elective surgery. Well, they noticed at the second major hospital that their workload was dropping because I was doing all the general surgery. He called me in and said that you can't do any more operations. I said, "Well, I was assigned as a surgeon what do you mean I can't?" He said, "It's not safe for you to do them there, we need to do them here. You have to refer them." I said, "What do I do for my occupation?" He said, "You might come up here and you could assist." I said, "You know, Colonel, that's ridiculous. It's 50 km, it's not too easy for people to visit, and these are the operations that I have been trained to do." He said, "Well I guess you are probably right. Go ahead and do them, but if you have any complications I'll cut your head off." Those were his exact words. Well, I did have a complication. I had a patient with an acute cholelithiasis who I actually referred up to that hospital because postop care was a little better and it was going to be a very hard case and I thought that two surgeons ought to be operating not just one. They sent him back. I sent him back. They sent him back again. The guy was dying so I operated on him and I nicked his common duct while I was trying to relieve his gallbladder abscess. The next day I got called up and this guy sends me to see the chief of General Surgery for Europe. The chief says I've given this guy the equivalent of a cancer. I said, "Colonel that's a little unfair. I didn't make the guy sick. I didn't reject him from surgery three times, and I had a complication which [sic] every surgeon has." He said well, "I don't think you're safe to operate I'm going to send you to dispensary for a year. If you behave yourself then we'll rethink it." I said "What's the logic of that Colonel? I'm not safe to operate, so if I don't operate for a year, I'll be safer?" That's precisely what happened and…it turned out to be an excellent experience because I didn't do surgery for a year…I had the very fortunate experience of discovering that it was possible to practice medicine without operating and still enjoy it.[30]

As his military duty came to an end in 1968, Rosen and his wife looked at the job possibilities back in the United States. The unrest in the big cities contributed to their decision to investigate practice opportunities in more rural areas, and Rosen accepted a position in the small town of Thermopolis, Wyoming. Rosen took call as a general surgeon for three towns, 30 miles apart, and also took call every fifth night in Thermopolis for all medical problems. He was the quintessential country surgeon, serving the community as needed. He even helped the local veterinarian with operations on dogs. As a surgical resident, Rosen had operated on dogs as part of laboratory research—he may have had more experience with dog surgery than the veterinarian. Rosen claims the distinction of operating on three dogs in Wyoming with stomach ulcers and operating on their owners for the same problem. Rosen began to become involved in nonsurgical areas of medicine,[30]

The Feds were trying to improve cardiac care and so they were giving money to establish coronary care units and I wanted an intensive care unit for my surgical patients. So to get the Fed money someone had to be named as Director of the Coronary Care Unit. I went and took a course in cardiac care management in Salt Lake City to apply for this grant. Got a grant for two of the three hospitals I worked in to set up a two-bed ICU/CCU [intensive care unit/coronary care unit] and became chief of cardiology at these two hospitals and within a year had more cardiac consultations than surgical consultations, which was funny. My very first paper was in cardioverting a patient with PAT and it was a postop patient. That was how that came about. So, actually my 3 years in Wyoming were extraordinarily useful years for emergency medicine because I did peds, OB, cardiology, as well as general surgery, orthopedics, and vascular surgery.[30]

Unfortunately, Rosen, who was only 34 years old, became a patient in the coronary care unit he had helped establish.

I had two heart attacks when I was in Wyoming...I had established a protocol where every patient in the CCU would have a central line and we used to put in peripheral centrals and the nurse wouldn't stick me, so I put in my own central line. If drug addicts could do it, I figured I could. Anyway, while I was lying in the CCU, I was thinking that maybe I should change specialties—that perhaps surgery was just too physically demanding, especially the way I was doing it, driving 200 miles a day. So, I wrote a letter to my surgical mentor at the University of Chicago, the guy who seduced me into surgery the first morning of my internship, and again by happenstance he had just died of a heart attack. His mail was being answered by a transplant surgeon who was in charge of the emergency department, but didn't want to be. They had decided to recruit a full-time director of emergency medicine and because I had gone to college there and interned there I was acceptable to them even though I certainly had no academic credentials at that time.[30]

Rosen negotiated well for this new job, and in 1971 became the first person to go from a position as a Wyoming country surgeon to a tenured associate professor of surgery at the University of Chicago. If Rosen thought that his heart would be less stressed in this new environment, he was gravely wrong.

Ron Krome graduated from medical school in 1961, just a year after Peter Rosen, and took a more direct path to emergency medicine than Rosen. After getting his military deferment, Krome did a rotating internship at Detroit Receiving Hospital, one of the busiest, inner city medical centers in the country. To serve his Berry Plan military commitment, he volunteered for the Public Health Service and was assigned from 1962 to 1964 at the Federal Narcotics Hospital, a minimum-security prison for narcotics addicts in Lexington, Kentucky. As part of that commitment, he served for 6 weeks on a Coast Guard cutter in the North Atlantic.

But I was okay, I took a suitcase filled with James Bond books, I really did...and I did things that you only dream of when you are a kid—went to the radar room....[31]

Working with chronic medicine patients at the Narcotics Hospital reinforced Krome's decision to go into surgery. He looked around the country for residencies at public hospitals, but decided that Detroit General Hospital had a good surgical residency that did not have a pyramid system, and he knew the environment. From 1965 to 1969, he was surgical resident at a place that was more like a war zone than a hospital, particularly in the ED. The ED at Detroit General (later to be called Detroit Receiving Hospital) was split in the traditional manner into medical and surgical areas, and residents from each of these services provided the staffing. Krome remembers, as a senior surgical resident, having the responsibility as "Pit Boss"—the person responsible for managing the ED.

...one of my chores as the Pit Boss was to make rounds in the morning. We had two shifts in trauma. There was a trauma straight days and trauma straight nights. On straight nights, the Pit Boss made rounds, I made rounds with the medical resident working nights, too. We'd make rounds in the morning. There were two doors to the ER, which convinced me that no ER should have two doors. Two entrances. We had the ambulance door and the walk-in up here, and the ER in the middle. So the drunks would come in the back doors and they would lie down on the stretchers and go to sleep...we served American cheese sandwiches, they would eat that, and they would go in the morning. There was no triage. I started triage there, and they would walk in, get on the stretcher, and have their sandwich, and in the morning we would wake them up and kick them out...and if you couldn't wake them up, get a neurosurgery consult!

That was an automatic, a head injury. It's true. You woke up, you were discharged; you woke up with the shakes, you were admitted to psychiatry. A simple triage mechanism.[31]

Krome was a surgical resident when riots struck Detroit in the summer of 1967. He remembers the National Guard was stationed at Detroit Receiving Hospital, and residents were not allowed to leave during the height of the violence. The riots were a temporary civil disorder that irrevocably changed Detroit, but inside Detroit Receiving Hospital ED, a constant disorder existed that periodically drew anger from the community. It was also not a good educational environment for the medical students from Wayne State Medical School. The chairman of surgery, Alexander Walt, who was a highly respected academic surgeon, was charged with cleaning up the mess. He would not do it personally—no senior level academic surgeon would get immersed in the ED. Instead, in 1968 he approached one of his bold, energetic, somewhat irascible chief surgical residents about the possibility of taking charge of the ED. Ron Krome, who liked trauma, was up to the challenge, and was also lured by the $25,000 annual salary that Walt promised. This was a higher salary than that made by most junior faculty—more in line with an associate professor salary. In 1969, Ron Krome began his great task. He had no faculty to staff the ED, just moonlighting residents who were paid $15 per hour. The local problems of emergency care in Detroit seemed insurmountable, but Krome and others would confront them head on and make a difference. Krome would then move to the national scene.

George Podgorny completed medical school a year after Ron Krome, and like Krome, initially chose a career in surgery. Podgorny, who had always been attracted to the ED as a medical student at Bowman Gray School of Medicine, was a fixture in the 1960s as a surgical resident at North Carolina Baptist Hospital, the primary teaching location of the medical school in Winston-Salem. Baptist Hospital at the time was still segregated, and black patients were seen at Reynolds Memorial Hospital. Podgorny started as a surgical intern in 1962 and did not finish his training until 1969. Along the way, he did a general surgery residency and served as chief resident, as well as a thoracic and cardiovascular surgery residency where he also served as chief resident. Podgorny was attentive to the ED as a surgical resident,

I was there a lot…every intern has to spend 3 months there, which was a harrowing experience. You were by yourself and of course, at that time no minor things came in. Nobody came in with a sore throat. Nobody came in for something minor and people either came with surgical trauma problems or came with massive medical emergencies, cardiac, pulmonary, endocrine, OB complications, botched abortions with a rip-roaring perforated uterus, peritonitis, shock, that type of a thing. There you were with a couple of nurses. The next one you could ask would be a first-year resident, who knew just a little bit more than you did. Faculty—almost never. I remember the first time I saw a faculty member in the emergency helping me was when the wife of the chief of pediatrics took an overdose. As soon as she arrived, some faculty internists arrived, being called by the husband to come and see what they could do, or if it was too late. So, I enjoyed the experiences because I enjoyed being able to do those things. Then, as I progressed in the line of surgical training, I became very adept and very comfortable at everything that had to deal with trauma and surgical issues. So, I made it known to interns under me that they would not have to hesitate to call me if there is a problem. So, eventually it got to a point that even the faculty and other people on other services knew I had a great deal of interest and knowledge in handling emergencies and they would call me for things I was not responsible for, officially, for them.[32]

Podgorny observed many changes during his tenure as a surgical resident. He served for several years as captain of Baptist Hospital's resuscitation team and saw the development of new methods of cardiopulmonary resuscitation (CPR). When he started, he would bring a scalpel to all cardiac arrests, open the chest, perform direct cardiac massage, and often would do a tracheostomy. By the later 1960s, the resuscitation team was doing closed CPR, assessing heart rhythms, defibrillating the heart, and using drugs like lidocaine. Podgorny also observed advances in the management of shock that had come out of the Korean and Vietnam Wars. But, he remained dismayed that interns were still staffing the ED and ambulances were still run by funeral directors.

> *I was talking to a faculty member who was officially in charge of the emergency room—he had never been there, never would go there. He made a schedule for interns, who eventually gave the schedule to me to make because he knew I was interested and he didn't want to bother with it. I tried to tell him that probably interns shouldn't be alone. Maybe a second-year resident also ought to be there. Of course, at that time, that was blasphemy. A second-year resident who is a "big man" at that time was a big position.*[32]

Podgorny never got his wish, but when he became a chief resident he made it a policy that interns must call a second-year resident whenever a patient with shock was seen in the ED. At the very end of his residency, Baptist hired a physician to provide some supervision of interns. By this time, Podgorny had read about the Alexandria group, but was not considering a career in emergency medicine. He shared his concerns about the ED with another person who had developed an interest in emergency care. Eben Alexander was the highly regarded chairman of neurosurgery at Baptist Hospital. Alexander had seen the ED patient census grow dramatically at Baptist Hospital, but was disappointed with the quality of care. He had the idea that training GPs in emergencies would be one way to improve the quality of care. Alexander submitted a proposal to the federal government for a training grant that would provide 6 months of training for GPs in emergency care. The proposal was considered but never funded.[32]

Forsyth Hospital, a large community hospital in Winston-Salem, was experiencing typical growing pains in terms of emergency care. As patient numbers increased, a rotation of the medical staff was attempted to cover the ED but was soon abandoned. By the end of 1968, three physicians had been hired to provide most of the staffing in the Forsyth Hospital ED. One of them, Dave Nelson, was a close friend of George Podgorny, and had been a year ahead of him in surgical residency. Nelson was waiting for his Berry Plan assignment, so he did not enter practice as a thoracic surgeon. He worked at Forsyth in the ED, but developed glaucoma, received an honorable discharge, and was free to stay at Forsyth, practicing emergency medicine instead of thoracic surgery. Podgorny was now finished with his long residency and was looking for jobs as a cardiothoracic surgeon. He was married, with four children, and none of the surgery jobs he explored was promising. His wife preferred to stay in Winston-Salem, but there were no cardiothoracic surgery jobs there for George. He began to work at the Forsyth Hospital ED with his friend, Nelson, and liked the work a great deal. The more time he spent in the ED, the less he thought about thoracic surgery. In addition, something was brewing on the national scene in emergency medicine that would prove intoxicating to George Podgorny and many other physicians who, for a variety of reasons, had found themselves practicing as emergency physicians.

3 "The Times They Are A-Changin'"

There's a battle outside
And it is ragin'.
It'll soon shake your windows
And rattle your walls
For the times they are a-changin'.

Bob Dylan,
The Times They Are A-Changin', 1963

The period from the advent of the full-time, Alexandria Plan emergency practice in 1961 to the beginnings of a national organization for emergency medicine in 1968 was one of the most active and trying times in U.S. political history. Hope, promise, and good will in the early sixties were gradually replaced by violence, civil unrest, and mistrust of the political system in the later years of the decade. The political movements of the sixties were not responsible for the birth of emergency medicine, but contributed to the development of the field from both a philosophical and practical standpoint. The major movements, including civil rights, the war on poverty, student activism, and the radicalism of the late sixties, influenced emergency medicine to varying degrees. More influential in changing the practice of emergency medicine were the two major governmental initiatives of the 1960s—Lyndon Johnson's Great Society programs, especially Medicare and Medicaid, and the Vietnam War.

President Johnson's Great Society Programs

As a new and vigorous president, John F. Kennedy created an atmosphere of change in the nation, but in the 3 years from his election in 1960 to his assassination in 1963, the Kennedy administration did not deliver any substantial changes in the health care system. The controversial concept of a federal medical care plan for the elderly was mired in Congress, and Kennedy did not have the support to push hard in this area. The stigma of socialized medicine was still attached to any federal effort to provide health care benefits to a large subset of the population. Hill-Burton funding continued to make hospitals and their administrators happy and tolerant of the inequities in health care delivery.

It was not until Kennedy's death that some of his social agenda began to move forward under the leadership of his successor, Lyndon Johnson. Johnson's relatively modest upbringing in Texas had brought him face to face with rural poverty, and he understood that health care for the poor and the elderly was abysmal or absent. Johnson was a pragmatist who liked to help people and who was fueled by the praise and adoration that came from helping. He did not advance strong ideologies beyond the belief that people were entitled to a job, a fair society, and a secure environment for their family. He said in his later years,

What the man in the streets wants is not a big debate on fundamental issues;
he wants a little medical care, a rug on the floor, a picture on the wall, a little music
in the house, and a place to take Molly and the grandchildren when he retires.[1]

At a time when much could be done in the area of civil rights and social programs, Johnson, a doer more than a thinker, was the right person to have in charge. His long career in Congress and powerful previous role as Senate majority leader gave him the knowledge and political capital to push legislation through that had been tied up in ideologic battles during the Kennedy administration. Both civil rights legislation and Medicare bills had been proposed during the Kennedy years, but were subject to opposition and compromises that prevented them from clearing Congress. After Johnson became president at the end of 1963, he realized that a big achievement in civil rights could propel him to victory in the 1964 presidential election. Utilizing all his political leverage, he helped the Civil Rights Bill through Congress and signed the Civil Rights Act in July 1964. The election in the fall of 1964 was a Democratic land-slide. The nation still had a lingering memory of Kennedy's hope for positive change. Now, with the momentum from his presidential election, with Democratic majorities in both halls of Congress, and a healthy economy, Johnson could hatch his Great Society programs.[1-3]

In his State of the Union message on January 4, 1965, President Johnson said, "A President does not shape a new and personal vision of America. He collects it from the scattered hopes of the American past."[1] Such was the case with Medicare and Medicaid. The "scattered hopes" that became Medicare had been batted around the U.S. political landscape since Roosevelt's 1935 Social Security Act. The program was successfully opposed for 30 years by conservatives in Congress and the American Medical Association (AMA). The Kennedy administration's original plan for Medicare in 1961 was squelched by Wilbur Mills, a conservative Democrat, and the powerful chairman of the House Ways and Means Committee. A combination of Republicans and Southern Democrats, with the financial lobbying of the AMA, led to the defeat of the Kennedy Medicare proposal. Following the 1964 Democratic election victory, Mills changed his position to support Medicare. The plan would provide reimburse-ment at competitive rates for care for the elderly, and consisted of two parts—payment for hospitals and physicians for inpatient care, and payment of physicians' outpatient fees. Mills understood that the second component would appease Republicans and the AMA. In a flurry of activity, Medicaid, a state-run health care program for the poor of all ages, was added as the third layer of federal medical insurance coverage. What had seemed a hopeless quest just a few years before emerged as Medicare and Medicaid in the summer of 1965.[1-4]

The impact of these programs on health care providers was felt almost immediately. Many elderly who had suffered with medical problems, but had not seen a physician for years, now were able to seek medical care. Although these visits did not usually represent emergencies, they affected emergency care. As general practitioners (GPs) and surgeons struggled to handle burgeoning patient loads in their offices, they were less available to come to see their patients who might end up in the emergency depart-ment (ED). They were also less likely to want to participate in a call system that might leave them up all night only to face a full schedule in the office the next day. This markedly decreased the availability of physicians for nonscheduled patients. It also made it untenable for hospitals to try to staff their EDs with a rotating schedule of the medical staff. The net effect of Medicare and Medicaid was the same as if the number of physicians per capita had been reduced. Karl Mangold remembers the effect in northern California,

> I can't underestimate what a boom Medicare/Medicaid was because doctors before that were very competitive for paying patients…They accused us of practicing… hospital medicine, which then was considered an absolute Communist conspiracy. But Medicare, Medicaid—turning them all busy into taking care of all that deferred pathology, really set the environment…for what happened.[5]

Some of the "deferred pathology" found its way to the emergency department when patients discovered that GPs and surgeons were overbooked or unavailable. The new patient burden seen in the mid 1960s may have pushed some GPs toward careers in emergency practice. This was certainly the case with John Wiegenstein, whose solo practice became so busy after Medicare/Medicaid was passed that he was overwhelmed and decided to enter emergency practice with Eugene Nakfoor.[6] In the rush to get Medicare and Medicaid passed, Congress and the Johnson administration had failed to fully consider access to care, particularly physician care. National efforts to increase the number of primary care physicians were just being implemented, and the effects of training more medical students and encouraging practice in underserved areas would not be felt until the early 1970s. David Wagner, who was just starting his surgical practice in Philadelphia, remembers the sharp increase in ED use by patients who had nowhere else to go:

> Family medicine was not really a formalized specialty...until [19]69 ...Physicians, graduates were all flocking into specialties. So there was nobody doing general medicine as it were and the offices were closing and institutions were bringing physicians together in sort of group practices associated with the hospital, but they were all specialists. It left the only place for people to go for their primary care was the emergency department. If you look back at the numbers in virtually every city of the country at that time they were just growing by leaps and bounds in terms of beating the door down to get some access to care...they couldn't find anyplace else. They were there because they couldn't find it anyplace else. They couldn't get access when they wanted it. It snowballed.[7]

ED patient visits had continued their progressive climb in the sixties, but Medicare/Medicaid accelerated the increase. From 1965 to 1970, ED visits in the United States rose from 29 million to 43 million per year.[8] But this increase was not just due to a lack of access to primary care (Table 3.1). By the mid 1960s the U.S. public, in particular the poor and elderly, viewed the hospital as the place where medical care was based. Hospitals had become little fiefdoms of health care in most communities, with outpatient clinics and private physician office buildings adjacent or annexed to the hospital building. For patients who were now entitled to care by way of having Medicare or Medicaid insurance, presenting to the ED at a hospital complex was the simplest and most convenient way to gain entry in to a system that could seem imposing and confusing from the outside. Patients understood that even if their problems were not very acute or severe, they would be seen and treated in the ED and referred to outpatient care in the same system. Even patients with a regular doctor used the ED in the evening and night hours when accessing their physician was becoming increasingly difficult. In the large cities of the Northeast and Midwest, the big urban hospitals, both municipal and private, became centers for care for a substantial portion of the nonaffluent population. For example, people who had moved from the Southern United States to Detroit to work in the expanding auto industry after World War II, when confronted with a medical problem would most likely be advised by friends and neighbors to go to the ED of Henry Ford Hospital or Detroit General Hospital rather than to a private doctor. By the late 1960s, the default

TABLE 3.1	Emergency Department Patient Visits to U.S. Hospitals
Year	**ED Visits U.S. Hospitals (millions)**
1954	9.4
1965	28.7
1970	42.7
1975	73.5
1980	82.0
1985	80.1
1990	92.1
1995	99.9
2000	106.9
2002	114.2

ED, emergency department.
From American Hospital Association Statistics, 1954–2002, and American College of Emergency Physicians.

point of contact for health care for millions of urban people had become the ED of the local municipal hospital.

The Medicare and Medicaid programs provided financial benefits that were most prominently felt by physicians who had previously treated the elderly and poor with minimal or no reimbursement. In emergency medicine, this played out in a number of ways. Many early emergency physician groups had contracts with a hospital, trading their physician fees for a stable salary from the hospital. Hospitals commonly did the billing, and charity care was a fact of life. The original Alexandria Hospital ED contract paid James Mills and colleagues a separate, fixed stipend for indigent care. Once Medicare and Medicaid were enacted, more incentive existed for emergency physicians to bill and collect their own fees. The Pontiac Plan physicians in Michigan realized this, and by 1966, had incorporated and used a professional management service for billing and collection. A large increase in physician salaries in the group was noted.[9,10] Other emergency physicians and groups took advantage of Medicare and Medicaid reimbursements to increase the size of their groups and develop larger, more corporate structures. The transformation of the ED from a money sink to a place where the hospital might make money, or at least break even, caused emergency care to be viewed in a different light in many hospitals. EDs, as the portals to the hospital system for many patients who were now more likely to be paying customers were enlarged and made more comfortable. Some hospitals hired hostesses or assistants to make ED visits easier on patients and families. Visitors to the Pontiac General Hospital ED in Michigan saw a sign in the registration area that said, "You have a friend in the Pontiac General Emergency Room. She is the Lady in the Light Blue Coat. Your patient representative." At nearby Beaumont Hospital hostesses, dressed in fashionable pantsuits, assisted ED patients.[11] Medicare and Medicaid made it possible for hospitals to begin to hire full-time emergency physicians or to expand coverage with more physicians. Whereas in the 1950s and early 1960s, hospitals could get away with hiring transient, poorly qualified physicians to staff their EDs, by the late 1960s, the increased potential to make money on emergency care and the competition for patients caused hospitals to recruit higher quality physicians for emergency coverage. Of course, in many inner-city municipal hospitals where not even Medicare and Medicaid could compensate for the burden of indigent care, the incentive to provide better emergency care was lacking, and the ED remained the domain of minimally trained, usually foreign house staff.

In the academic world, Medicare and Medicaid were the primary factors in shifting the focus of medical schools from biomedical research toward clinical care. Since the 1950s, medical schools had been ramping up their research infrastructures to be able to compete more effectively for federal research money from the National Institutes of Health (NIH). Clinical care was not considered a moneymaking venture, especially because many medical school hospitals and faculty members provided a large amount of charity care. Medicare and Medicaid, by converting a significant portion of poor, nonpaying patients to paying customers, made medical schools and teaching hospitals rethink where they should focus their efforts. In 1965, clinical service revenue accounted for only 6% of total revenues of U.S. medical schools. By 1975, this had tripled to 18%.[12] The new ability to generate revenue from clinical activities caused many medical schools to improve the infrastructure and clinical delivery systems of their teaching hospitals. Even grimy academic emergency departments were now viewed as potential revenue sources. Medical schools were for the first time in the strange position of having to compete with private hospitals for poor and elderly patients. Part of this competition was making their facilities more modern, spacious, and less "wardlike." Previously neglected areas were assigned administrators and more personnel. It is not coincidental that the practice of appointing a faculty member to be in charge of the medical school teaching hospital ED (usually a junior surgeon), came about in the late 1960s.[12,13] At the Medical College of Pennsylvania Hospital, David Wagner remembers being paid $4 per patient visit from Medicaid and notes that the hospital initially did not realize that ED physicians could bill for Medicaid patients. This money was eventually put into a separate institutional pot that Wagner was able to use to start the emergency medicine residency program at the Medical College of Pennsylvania.[7]

Medicare and Medicaid did not entirely solve the problem of health care for the poor. Millions of younger working adults who did not qualify for Medicaid still lacked health insurance. After the government programs were in place, some physicians were less inclined to provide charity care. John Rupke, an emergency medicine pioneer from Western Michigan who practiced before and after Medicare and Medicaid were enacted remembers,

> I started practice before they came in. At that time, everyone took care of the poor. When Medicare and Medicaid came in some of them said I'm not going to do that— let somebody else do that.[14]

The other major health initiative of the Johnson presidency that would affect emergency care came out of the Presidential Commission on Heart Disease, Cancer, and Stroke (Debakey Commission). This commission was strongly supported by wealthy liberals who wanted to see increased funding directed toward clinical advancement in cancer and cardiovascular diseases, as well as increased research funding in these areas.[2] Johnson, who suffered a serious myocardial infarction in 1955 that kept him in the hospital for 6 weeks, was sympathetic to this cause. Johnson's father also had heart disease and died at the age of 60 after a heart attack.[1] President Johnson addressed the commission at the White House on April 17, 1964:

> I have often been reminded myself of Shakespeare's line, "A good heart's worth gold." I am glad mine is good now and if the doctors and the Secret Service…will just permit me to get my exercise, I intend to keep it that way.[15]

Johnson spoke in grandiose, heroic terms of eradicating heart disease, cancer, and stroke.

> The point is, we must conquer heart disease, we must conquer cancer, we must conquer strokes. This Nation and the whole world cries [sic] out for this victory. I am firmly convinced that the accumulated brains and determination of this commission and the scientific community of the world will, before the end of this decade, come forward with some answers and cures that we need so very much…In my judgment, there is nothing that you will ever do that will keep your name glorified longer, and that will make your descendants prouder than this unselfish task that you have today undertaken to get rid of the causes of heart disease and cancer and stroke in this land and throughout the world.[15]

The commission's report recommended creating a network of centers, diagnostic and treatment "stations," and research units across the country for each of these diseases.[15] Part of the recommendation for "heart stations" was "immediate and emergency care for patients with acute cardiovascular emergencies."[15] The report also recommended huge increases in Public Health Service expenditures and grants for facilities, equipment, and training. Grants were created for the establishment of coronary care units in smaller hospitals. Peter Rosen secured one of these grants when he was in Wyoming to create a coronary care unit, where he eventually became a patient (see Chapter 2).

The Great Society programs of the Johnson Administration were the fruition of some of the hopes and dreams that John F. Kennedy had vaguely defined at the start of his presidency. Programs to ease poverty, improve education, and end racial discrimination passed through Congress rapidly. In most cases, the concepts were solid, but the implementation was less well planned and proved difficult. The expense of the programs was routinely underestimated. This was especially true with Medicare and Medicaid. Without a restrictive system for assigning fees, physicians and hospitals were allowed to bill federal and state programs at the going rates, with little control or standardization. Medicare soon became a cost monster for the federal government, and Medicaid program expenses stressed state budgets. Because of their overwhelming support from the populace, Medicare and Medicaid survived, but other Great Society programs did not.

While runaway costs were an issue, the downfall of the Great Society agenda came with the escalation of the Vietnam War. Lyndon Johnson did not have a great deal of foreign policy experience, and he viewed the world through the black-and-white goggles of his predecessors—communism was bad and must be curtailed. He was also loath to lose a fight, even if he was not originally a chief protagonist. As Johnson became more preoccupied with Vietnam, he had less time and energy to focus on his Great Society programs. A vicious cycle occurred—the more things went wrong in Vietnam, the more he became immersed in the details of the war, and his domestic agenda suffered. The war was hugely expensive and sucked up federal money that might have been directed toward domestic programs. The result was a gradual loss of steam for the Great Society programs at a crucial time. Many of the programs that attacked poverty in the inner cities might have had some effects on health care delivery. Community health centers were proposed, and many were started, but the size of the program was scaled back and it failed to have a large impact. The excitement of the president's commission about eradicating heart disease, cancer, and stroke was tempered by the shrinking availability of federal money for grant programs in these areas. What if the Great Society had been realized to its full potential? A case could be made that a reduction in poverty, additional resources for community health care in rural and urban areas, and increased funding of national service programs might have had a significant impact in shoring up primary care in the United States. This might have reduced ED utilization and the need for emergency physicians. However, it is unlikely that the Great Society—even if played out to its full scope—would have prevented the continuing boom in emergency services and the creation of the field of emergency medicine. The reality was that by the time a discouraged and weary Lyndon Johnson announced at the end of March 1968 that he would not seek reelection, emergency medicine was moving forward.[1,16] Months from then, a primitive organizational structure for emergency medicine would take hold.

THE TWO LITTLE BOOKLETS OF 1966

The old adage of not judging a book by its cover, if extended to include size, is very applicable to two 6 × 8.5-inch publications in the area of emergency services published in 1966: *Emergency Department: A Handbook for Medical Staff*, by the American Medical Association, Department of Hospitals and Medical Facilities, and *Accidental Death and Disability: The Neglected Disease of Modern Society*, by the National Academy of Sciences. These two booklets had a major impact on stimulating the birth of the field of emergency medicine and in guiding its early leaders.

The AMA, despite having as its primary focus the advancement and preservation of the private practice of medicine, was not a major opponent of emergency medicine. The constituency of the AMA included many private physicians who could testify to the poor quality of care in ED and who complained about the common practice by hospitals of consigning medical staff to work in the ED. The AMA became aware of the Alexandria and Pontiac Plans for ED staffing and followed the developments as more physicians elected to do emergency practice full time. The Hospitals and Medical Facilities Department of the AMA was charged with monitoring the developments in emergency care. The AMA watched carefully to see if emergency physicians were "stealing" patients away from community physicians, but this did not appear to occur. In fact, community physicians were increasingly happy to have emergency physicians on duty at night and weekends. They were also happy to have a place to refer complicated or very sick patients during the day. On the basis of the positive impressions of emergency practice in the medical community, the Hospitals and Medical Facilities Department of the AMA charged its Division of Socioeconomic Activities with researching how these plans developed. The AMA was receiving many more questions from its members about how emergency physicians practiced and how a group could be started. Before 1965, it appears that questions were referred to James Mills and the Alexandria group for those who wanted to do full-time practice and to the Pontiac emergency group for part-time work. Sometime in 1965, the AMA decided to develop a booklet that would provide inquiring physicians with the essentials of emergency practice. The project was headed by Richard Manegold, M.D., director of the AMA Division of Socioeconomic Activities. Detailed written descriptions were solicited from James Mills for the Alexandria Plan and Robert Leichtman for the Pontiac Plan, including samples of the original contracts. An emergency care plan at Chicago Wesley Hospital that used resident physicians with attending staff backup was provided in the booklet as a teaching hospital model. Other chapters focused on quality of care in the ED, medical education, and legal aspects of emergency care. The booklet did not advocate strongly for full-time, trained emergency physicians as a standard. Rather, it described the five ED physician-staffing patterns of the time: rotation of medical staff, intern or resident staffing, salaried physicians (full or part time), a medical group or partnership, and combinations of the previous four.[17] Hospitals and physicians were left to figure out the best staffing arrangement for their situation. One of the legacies of the AMA booklet was a small section called "terminology." Michael Silver, an AMA staff associate wrote about the use of the term "emergency room:"

> It is undeniable that the emergency service is at least as important as any other inpatient department in the hospital. For this reason, "emergency department" seems the most apropos and is used throughout this handbook. The recognition of the emergency service as a "department" of the hospital may be the first step in solving its problems.[17]

The AMA handbook had a significant impact. It was used as a "how to" manual for physicians who were looking to set up emergency practices. As noted previously, Eugene Nakfoor, the family physician who worked with John Wiegenstein to establish an Alexandria-type emergency-staffing plan at St. Lawrence Hospital in Lansing, Michigan, obtained the handbook and relied heavily on it when starting his group.[6] Many other community hospital physicians used the sample contracts, billing methods, and schedules suggested in the handbook. The handbook played a role in enabling enough ED groups with similar structures to come in to being, that by 1968, when one looked across the medical landscape of the United States, emergency physicians could be seen as a nascent but viable entity.

The second little booklet of 1966, *Accidental Death and Disability: The Neglected Disease of Modern Society*, was published by the National Academy of Sciences–National Research Council (NAS-NRC). The NAS, as an independent advisory body to the federal government and Congress on matters of importance to science and health, undertook this project to draw attention to the poor state of trauma care in the United States and to make specific recommendations on how to improve trauma care. Today, this function would be assumed by the Institute of Medicine, but this branch of the NAS was not created until 1970. The NAS Committee on Trauma, Shock, and Anesthesia, along with special task forces of the Division of Medical Sciences of the NAS-NRC studied the problem and reviewed the information and activities of many other organizations. Federal agencies—the U.S. Public Health Service, the National Institutes of Health, and the U.S. Army—were at the table, as were the AMA, the American Red Cross, and some representatives of the communication industry. The American College of Surgeons (ACS) Committee on Trauma, despite the fact that it led the effort to advance U.S. trauma care for over a decade, had a relatively small role in the proceedings. Robert Kennedy, the New York surgeon and ACS leader was consulted and provided some testimony for the NAS committee, but was not a primary author of the report. Although James Mills and his group had gained a certain amount of notoriety for their new emergency practice, and were in the shadow of Washington, they were nonentities when it came to the big picture of trauma care in the United States. No emergency physicians were included in the preparation of the report.

Most of the writing for the report was done internally by an ad hoc committee of the NAS Division of Medical Sciences. Alan P. Thal, M.D., a surgeon from Wayne State University School of Medicine was invited to be a committee member. He became the primary drafter of the "white paper" that would become the report. Thal was a well-connected academic surgeon who came to Wayne State as chair of surgery when Ron Krome was a first-year resident. Krome did not have much direct interaction with Thal, but remembers an annual summer party that the chair held. Residents were invited to attend but were required to wear suit and tie, even in the summer heat. Not all residents were invited. Krome notes, "That's how you knew if he didn't like you—you didn't get invited to his summer party."[18] Thal had a brief stay at Wayne State and moved to the University of Kansas before Ron Krome finished his residency.

The April 1966 NAS Committee on Trauma 2-day meeting to flesh out the white paper included an exhaustive, but disjointed agenda on trauma care in the United States. The meeting included general reports and testimony on disaster planning and the ED but digressed into specific areas like fluid resuscitation and a military film on wound ballistics. The participants debated whether to have the report include disaster management and decided to focus mainly on "standard" emergency medical services and trauma care. Ben Eiseman, the chairman of surgery at the University of Kentucky, who would later make life difficult for early academic emergency physicians, was a vocal participant during the meeting. Eiseman was valued for the experience he gained when he served as a civilian consultant to the Surgeon General in Vietnam from 1965 to 1966.

The meeting did not pay much attention to physician staffing in EDs, other than to note it was of poor quality. A brief discussion occurred about the U.S. Public Health Service grant submitted by Eben Alexander, the neurosurgeon who had discussed emergency care with George Podgorny at Bowman Gray School of Medicine in Winston-Salem, North Carolina. It was noted the grant proposal was to fund a 1-year training program for "postgraduate" physicians for "training in the requirements to become a director of an emergency department." One participant asked, "Did they get it?" Another responded, "Everything depends on appropriations."[19] The grant was never funded. Some of the participants had seen or read about the European approach to trauma care and emergency medical services (EMS). Belgium was mentioned as a model where physicians were part of the EMS ambulance response and delivered care at the scene.[19] Ignoring the impracticality of this approach when there were not even enough U.S. physicians to staff emergency departments, the final report made a recommendation for "pilot programs to determine the efficacy of providing physician-staffed ambulances for care at the site of injury and during transportation."[20]

The meeting participants were also very interested in the military approach to trauma care, and spent a good portion of the meeting discussing specifics of military injuries. Eiseman, full of himself at this meeting, said, "I am just writing up a paper here and I think maybe one quote would be in order." He then read the following from an article that, edited slightly, would appear in the *Journal of Trauma* in 1967,

> *Wounded in the remote jungle or rice paddy of Vietnam, an American citizen has a far better chance of quicker definitive surgical care by board certified specialists, surgeon, orthopedist, or anesthesiologist, than were he hurt on a highway near his hometown in the continental United States, and even if he were struck at the curb immediately outside the emergency room of most U.S. hospitals, including my own, would he be given such prompt, expert operative care as routinely is furnished from the site of combat wounding in Vietnam.*[19,21]

In the actual report, a less dramatic version of Eiseman's comments about the superiority of military to civilian trauma care was one of the most eye-opening concepts for American medicine and the public.[20]

The *Accidental Death and Disability* report defined the magnitude of the U.S. trauma problem, noting in 1965, that 107,000 American civilians were killed by accidental injuries, with 49,000 deaths due to motor vehicle crashes. In 2001, with 100 million more U.S. citizens than in 1965, and many million more miles traveled by automobile per year, only 43,000 motor vehicle crash fatalities were reported.[22] The 1966 NAS report describes the "epidemic" of trauma with inadequate attention at the public or federal levels. A key point was that trauma, as a medical problem, did not receive the same support as campaigns against cancer, heart disease, and "mental disease." The report pulled no punches in maligning the professional knowledge gap in managing traumatic injury. Chapters on accident prevention, ambulance services, communication, EDs, and research in trauma were included. The report noted that many emergency departments were unable to provide adequate care, and that physicians who staffed EDs were often the least trained in trauma care. Brief mention was made of "new patterns" of physician staffing of EDs, presumably referring to the Alexandria and Pontiac plans. The report concluded with more than 25 specific recommendations, many of which were taken up by Congress or private organizations to improve U.S. trauma care. Programs were recommended to pilot new delivery methods for ambulance service, helicopter programs, and training of emergency care providers. A system of categorizing and accrediting EDs was recommended. At the federal level, the report recommended the creation of an NIH institute for trauma research and a center for disaster management.[20]

The primary purpose of NAS-NRC reports was to influence legislators and governmental policy makers to create laws and programs to address public problems. By the end of 1966, more than 13,000 copies of the trauma report had been circulated to federal, state, and municipal agencies, medical organizations and to the media. Articles citing the major themes of the report appeared in the *New York Times* and *Boston Herald*. *Accidental Death and Disability*...had an almost immediate impact in stimulating the AMA to form a Commission on Emergency Medical Services.[23] The NAS-NRC acted internally to make sure emergency services did not fade from the Academy's attention by forming a separate Committee on Emergency Medical Services in 1967.

In the 5 years following the report, EMS benefited to some extent as the federal government allocated money for grant programs for ambulance service development and training of emergency medical technicians. Most of the funding came from Department of Transportation funding authorized by the Highway Safety Act of 1966. By the end of 1969, more than 300 state and local EMS projects had been provided $18 million. The federal government agency that should have been leading the charge in EMS development, the Department of Health, Education, and Welfare, and its public health service unit were slow to act on the NAS-NRC recommendations. In a 1972 follow-up report, the NAS-NRC Committee on Emergency Medical Services lamented, "Federal agencies have not kept pace with the efforts of professional and allied health organizations to upgrade emergency medical services...there are no federal focal points for overall planning, or for coordination of emergency medical services."[24] EDs received even less funding. Grants were available to hospitals for new models of emergency care, but the amount of funding was miniscule compared with the funding hospitals received through the Hill-Burton program. Disaster management was improved by the formation of federal agencies, but these were fragmented and the centralized Federal Emergency Management Agency (FEMA) was not formed until 1979. The American Trauma Society (ATS) was founded, but the NAS-NRC recommendation for a separate NIH institute for trauma was not realized.

Overall, the impact of *Accidental Death and Disability*...was greater than the programs and funding that emerged after its dissemination. For the first time, trauma was in the spotlight on a national level, with a collective concern from the public and the medical profession. Communities and health care providers were reminded that at a time when medicine was advancing rapidly and the space program was showing America's scientific promise, many trauma victims were being driven to the hospital in the back of hearses and cared for at poorly equipped facilities by medical professionals with almost no training in the diagnosis and management of traumatic injury.

The early emergency physicians had a keen awareness of the two little booklets of 1966, and how these publications might affect the field. The AMA handbook became a vital asset in establishing the practice infrastructure for emergency care. The NAS-NRC report demonstrated the gaps in trauma care, and in the recommendations of this report, early emergency physicians could see many opportunities for improving EMS and EDs. In 1961, the public charge to the medical profession was to provide physicians to deliver emergency care on a regular basis. By 1966, especially in the area of trauma, the charge was to improve the quality and organization of care. In reading between the lines of the NAC-NRC report, the missing component in trauma and emergency care was strong physician leadership. In the mid 1960s, that leadership was unlikely to come from surgeons or internists, most of who were busy enough with their booming post-Medicare practices and did not have the time or passion to move emergency medicine forward in a comprehensive way. Alternatively, the leaders would have to emerge from the "rag-tag" collection of emergency physicians, who in 1966 had little national presence and were viewed as a curiosity more than as a new physician movement.

The Sixties Surgeons, Trauma Care, and Emergency Medicine

The NAS-NRC report on accidental death and disability can be viewed as one of the crowning achievements of Robert H. Kennedy, M.D., and other surgeons who advocated for improved trauma care. Kennedy was not a primary author on the report, but provided important testimony and education to the government representatives who were responsible for compiling the report. Kennedy was the author of the 1955 "emergency room is the weakest link" maxim, and for the next decade worked very hard to improve ambulance and ED care for trauma victims.[25] The ACS created a Committee on Trauma in 1922, but it was not until 1960, when highway traffic injuries and fatalities were climbing dramatically, that it put a major emphasis on studying trauma care in the United States. In 1938, the American Association for the Surgery of Trauma (AAST) formed but remained a secondary organization to the ACS Committee on Trauma at least until 1961 when it began publishing the *Journal of Trauma.*

The ACS Committee on Trauma enlisted the help of the Hartford Foundation, an affiliate of the major insurer, the Hartford Company in the late 1950s. The Hartford Company had an obvious interest in reducing accidental death and disability. In 1960, the Hartford Foundation made the first of three major grants to the ACS, $150,000 over 3 years, for a Field Program of the Committee on Trauma. Robert Kennedy, who was then 71 years old, became the head of the field program. Kennedy, with the help of an assistant from the U.S. Public Health Service personally visited over 200 hospital EDs and surveyed 100 more. The summary of emergency care and the recommendations he developed from the field program resulted in two influential publications: *A Model of a Hospital Emergency Department*, published in 1961, and *Standards for Emergency Departments in Hospitals,* published in 1963. In the *Standards* the ACS Committee on Trauma calls for each hospital to have an ED director, but does not specify any standards for ED physician staffing other than stipulating that patients "will be seen by a physician within 15 minutes after arrival." The standards also call for EDs having departmental status in the hospital and state that "air conditioning in many parts of the country and good communications are essential."[26] By 1967, the ACS had distributed, on request, over 24,000 copies of these publications.[27] The ACS also used Hartford grant money to produce a film, *The Emergency Department: Organization and Operation* (1965). Copies of the film were loaned to hospitals and physicians on request. The influence of the ACS and other organizations in the federal government led to provisions in the 1966 National Highway Safety Act to improve emergency medical services through grants for training, communication, and equipment.

Buoyed by the success of its emergency department field program, the Committee on Trauma received a 3-year renewal of the Hartford grant for 1963 to 1966. Robert Kennedy turned his attention to the poor state of prehospital care for trauma victims. He and his staff visited more than 150 ambulance services in the United States and Canada to determine the best and worst practices of emergency medical services in the prehospital setting. Working with the American Red Cross, the National Safety Council, and the President's Committee on Traffic Safety, Kennedy developed *Standards for Emergency Ambulance Services* (1967). Kennedy also edited an important book in 1966, entitled *Emergency Care of the Sick and Injured.*[28] This pocket-sized, 128-page manual was aimed at EMS providers, law enforcement officials, fire department staff, and nurses. Kennedy was determined to make this book affordable, and arranged with W.B. Saunders Company to have the book sold for only $2 per copy. In its first 16 months, the book sold 25,000 copies. Kennedy also wrote a folksy monthly column in the *American College of Surgeons Bulletin* called, "What's New in Trauma in Your Area?" Exciting trauma and disaster situations, new EMS developments such as helicopter transport of trauma victims, and publication of courses on trauma were standard parts of the column. The column was not just about trauma, but included news about resuscitation techniques, including closed-chest cardiac massage, and new cardiac monitoring devices. The Hartford Foundation awarded a third generous grant of $275,000 to continue the ACS program in trauma from 1966 to 1969. In December 1967, the ACS honored Robert Kennedy's eightieth year at a dinner held at Kennedy's home base, Beekman–Downtown Hospital in New York City (see insert, Figure 3). Oscar Hampton, M.D., who served as the ACS Committee on Trauma chairman delivered a speech chronicling the huge amount of work and productivity achieved over 6 years in the field program by a man who might as easily have been retired. Hampton noted:

> His friends knew he had the expertise and experience to make it successful. He has, however, astounded everyone with his bulldog tenacity and indefatigability. Before 1960, he had become known as "Mr. Trauma." His continuing efforts have established him as the "King of Trauma." Long live the king![27]

About a year later, Robert Kennedy quietly resigned from the ACS staff at the age of 81. His contributions to the development of EMS and trauma care were greater than those of any other physician of his time. While Kennedy was a great proponent of proper training and standards for trauma care, his stance on trauma training for physicians other than surgeons, and his views on full-time emergency physician practice are harder to assess. In his earlier days, he had been very vocal about improving emergency physician qualifications as exemplified in his 1955 Oration on Trauma speech. Kennedy was certainly aware of the new emergency physician practices—he had visited James Mills at Alexandria Hospital as part of his Hartford field program study and had encountered many other nonsurgeons who were dedicated to emergency practice. But in his publications on ED facility development, trauma care, and EMS, Kennedy was quite mute on physician presence in EDs and chose to focus on educating paramedical personnel and nurses. Other surgeons adopted the same approach when dealing with emergency care. Rather than acknowledging that emergency physicians existed and might be helpful and useful in the early management of trauma patients, they sought to sequester or exclude trauma care from the rest of what was happening in the hospital EDs. Rudolph Noer, M.D., who developed a system at Louisville General Hospital to rapidly triage injured patients who were brought in by ambulance to a special area of the operating room, noted in 1963,

> Thus we see all too frequently a hybridizing of the emergency room which takes on, at one and the same time, the appearance of an outpatient clinic, a dispensary, a first aid station, and something halfway between the latter and the operating room suite or critical nursing area…(T)he critically injured patient belongs in the operating room or critical nursing area from the first; delay of these patients in the emergency room is likely to be detrimental to their most efficient and expeditious care, while at the same time placing undue burden upon the usually already overloaded emergency room.[29]

At the time, Louisville General Hospital ED was seeing an astounding 80,000 patients per year and was run by unsupervised house staff.[30] One of the advantages of bypassing the ED with critically ill trauma patients was that the patient would be seen sooner by an attending surgeon. Noer and other surgeons viewed this approach as an extension of military trauma care to the civilian world:

> The lesson learned by the Armed Forces should not be ignored: It is equally imperative in civil life that we separate promptly those needing resuscitative and operative treatment from those who can be treated on an outpatient basis.[29]

These surgeons cannot be faulted for their approach given that EDs of the time were generally unprepared from both an equipment and personnel standpoint to handle critical cases. However, in some cases their recommendations were remarkably short sighted. One editorial in 1965 notes that "Blood and plasma are being removed from accident rooms, for the patient requiring these will not be released…."[31]

The author seemed not to comprehend or acknowledge nontrauma emergency cases needing resuscitation with blood or plasma. Bypassing the ED, although possible in the larger teaching hospitals where surgery residents and operating room staff could immediately respond, was not possible in most nonteaching hospitals. In the days before trauma center classification, large community hospitals regularly received critical trauma cases. But, by the early 1960s, surgery was becoming increasingly specialized, and many surgeons did not want the increased burden of trauma care, especially when those patients were often uninsured or did not pay for services. It was also not practical to think that every ED could be staffed by a surgeon waiting for serious trauma victims to arrive. An editorial in the *Journal of Trauma* in 1961 lamented,

> *Why is trauma care unpopular? Either the injured patient intrudes on an already busy day or he demands care at night or on a weekend. He may or may not be an operative case and his convalescence may be prolonged. He does not come through the ordinary channels of referral but rather through assignment and while the patient may be grateful for his excellent care the surgeons will not therefrom build a practice. It would serve the surgeon better to treat, study and write in an elective field where his writings will attract patients from his colleagues.*[32]

Early trauma surgeons were similar to the early emergency physicians in that they were responding to a societal need and demand for improved emergency care. As they responded and defined themselves, both groups drifted outside of the mainstream of medicine. The small cadre of surgeons who were true believers in improving trauma care made important contributions in the 1960s. Surgeons, many of them from academic institutions, studied and published many papers and recommendations on emergency department design and organization, ambulance care, and injury prevention.[26,29,31–38] In contrast, the early emergency physicians, who were not in academics, developed their trade and wrote occasional articles on emergency care that appeared in less prominent medical journals or in the world of medical economics.

Robert Kennedy saw too few surgeons following his crusade for improved trauma care. Kennedy, as an elder surgeon, may have been tapped to be the head of the field program of the Committee on Trauma of the ACS because no one else was as passionate or able to devote time to the initiative as he. Although many surgeons wanted to provide definitive care for trauma victims, the field as a whole lacked the willpower or manpower to do so. In 1966, the AAST had 300 active fellows and about 150 senior fellows. This number could not even cover a majority of medical centers and large communities across the United States. But, the field of surgery was not ready to relinquish any aspects of the care of serious trauma patients to the upstart emergency physicians. The reasons Kennedy did not extend a hand to the committed emergency physicians he encountered in this travels lay in the gap between a trained surgeon and most early emergency physicians who had done only an internship.[39] The tone of his writings suggests that Kennedy believed full residency training was necessary for physicians who would provide emergency care. He wrote in a 1969 editorial, at the end of his career, that the hiring of physicians who had only completed an internship to staff emergency departments,

> *...may result in an inferior or second grade physician as regards the extent of his training. Those of us interested in the field of trauma need to aim particularly for completely trained emergency service coverage.*[40]

Surgeons like Wagner, Podgorny, Krome, and Rosen, with whom Kennedy might have formed a natural liaison, were still too early in their careers in the 1960s to have a chance to interact with the old "King of Trauma." It is not clear how Kennedy felt about emergency medicine as a separate specialty, but if a man's views can be partly discerned through his influence on colleagues, then it would appear that Kennedy was not supportive. Oscar P. Hampton, M.D., the chair of the Committee on Trauma of the ACS in the 1960s and 1970s noted in 1974, "Dr. Kennedy's friendship and advice have been of immense help to me for many years."[41] Hampton, like Kennedy, worked hard to advance trauma care, but was also a vigorous opponent of emergency medicine.

He later became the archenemy of people like John Wiegenstein, George Podgorny, R. R. Hannas, and James Mills in emergency medicine's battle for specialty status. Ironically, Hampton had served as James Mills's Sunday school teacher in St. Louis when Mills was a child.

The Vietnam War and Emergency Medicine

Military medicine continued to make impressive strides in the care of combat casualties in post–World War II conflicts. Korean War mortality rates for wounded U.S. soldiers who made it to field hospitals alive were reduced to 2%—in World War II the rate was around 4%. In Vietnam, the mortality rate went down even further to less than 2%.[42] A number of reasons are espoused for improved outcomes. The first is the system of triage, evacuation, and rapid medical care for casualties. Medics in Vietnam were better trained than their predecessors to provide resuscitation and care of serious wounds. Following initial battlefield care, the medic in Vietnam called in a helicopter for immediate evacuation of seriously injured soldiers. Helicopter ambulance units had been introduced in the Korean War, but were used to transport casualties who had been moved out of the field of battle. In Vietnam, helicopter transport from the battlefield became the modus operandi for evacuation of the wounded.[43,44] In 1969, at the peak of the war, 206,229 medical evacuation missions were carried out by helicopter crews in Vietnam.[44] The use of helicopters greatly decreased the transport time to deliver the injured soldier to definitive operative care. With an average flight time of only 35 minutes, Vietnam casualties requiring surgery were consistently undergoing definitive operative intervention in the field hospital within 1.5 to 2 hours after injury.[21,44,45] In addition to faster evacuation, resuscitation of casualties was improved in the Vietnam War. Physicians who served in Vietnam describe the liberal use of un–cross-matched blood in the early postinjury period. Kendall McNabney, M.D., a surgeon who would later start an emergency medicine residency in Kansas City says, "What I think improved trauma outcomes in Vietnam was the availability of O negative blood. It was everywhere—by the gallons."[43]

A 1966 study of 2,161 seriously wounded men who received blood over a 10-month period found a mean use of 6.6 units of blood per casualty.[45] Although blood was sometimes administered by medics at Vietnam battlefield aid stations, crystalloid solutions were more commonly used as the first line for treating volume depletion. Part of the rationale was that many soldiers became dehydrated in the hot, humid climate of Vietnam and needed salt and fluid replacement before blood administration.[21,45] This model of rapid field evaluation, administration of crystalloid solution and rapid transport for definitive trauma care was perfected in Vietnam and then became the goal for civilian trauma care.

Other advances in surgical techniques and care contributed to reduced morbidity and mortality in the Vietnam War. Specialist surgeons such as neurosurgeons and cardiac surgeons were more available. More vascular surgeons were available in Vietnam than in the Korean War, and arterial repair with synthetic grafts was introduced. The 1960s science boom figured greatly in supplying physicians with the infrastructure and devices to create a field hospital in Vietnam that was equal or superior to U.S. civilian hospitals. Inflatable (MUST) field hospitals were introduced in 1966. These hospitals could be flown to any location by a helicopter and included an air-conditioned operating room and enough space for a 20-bed ward. Battery-powered "suitcase" portable x-ray machines, a 46-lb laboratory, and plastic medical equipment were used in Vietnam. Heart-lung machines for cardiac bypass surgery and early dialysis machines were available on U.S. Navy ships off the Vietnam coast. Pharmacologic advances made far more drugs available in Vietnam than in Korea. Soldiers carried with them a minipharmacy kit containing antibiotics, antifungals, antihistamines, and analgesics.[21,46] Science figured heavily in every aspect of medical care in Vietnam, including well-developed research units that assessed the effects and outcomes of new medical therapies.[21,47]

For those who cared for the wounded and sick in Vietnam, the experience was life changing. The young surgeons who worked in the field hospitals operated more than they ever thought possible, returned to civilian practice or residencies with valuable experience, and were able to teach others what they learned in the military. Medics returned home with medical training and backgrounds far superior to what existed on the primitive civilian ambulance services of the 1960s. One medic who spent a year in Vietnam was Edward (Mel) Otten, who would later train as an emergency physician at the University of Cincinnati. Otten grew up in the middle class neighborhood of Price Hill in Cincinnati. When his football scholarship to Washington University in St. Louis fell through because the school dropped its football program, Otten had no way to go to college. He did what many of his friends did—volunteered for the Army. At age 17, Otten, a bright and motivated student who was pointing toward a career in medicine, went through the Army's medic program and pharmacy school. He remembers when he first set foot on Vietnamese soil: "It was September 26, 1967, at about 7:30 in the morning. The temperature was about 98, and it was light to moderate ground fire."[48]

Otten was stationed in the south of Vietnam, assigned to the 346 Medical Detachment. He was part of a medical civil action team that was assisting the South Vietnamese with medical care and care of the wounded. Otten traveled in to rural villages where he would identify diseases, prepare medicines, and provide care:

> *Everybody had a cough, everybody had worms, everybody had some kind of dermatitis. I would get things and mix them up according to Army regulations and the USP…and give these things out to the people and they were very grateful that they would get the things and we were supposed to be winning the hearts and minds of the people.*[48]

Unlike previous wars of the 20th century, Vietnam was primarily guerilla warfare, with a constant threat presented by a poorly defined and often invisible enemy. Otten recalls almost daily episodes of tragedy and terror:

> *I remember one day—we lived with the Vietnamese people, so I was going down to this place where I lived—and I heard this boom, it sounded like an explosion and I looked down the street and there was a Vietnamese Jeep that was burning and there was a whole crowd of people around there. I ran down and I look in the Jeep and it was a Vietnamese officer, his wife, and two children that were in this Jeep and somebody walked by and basically dropped a hand grenade in the Jeep and blew them up. The only one alive was a 4-year-old little girl. I pulled her out of the Jeep and I ran back to where our dispensary was, our medical dispensary, and tried to get her resuscitated but she—I cut her clothes off—I stuck an IV [intravenous] in her and she was gurgling blood and she had chest wounds and abdominal wounds and we lost her pulse and she died. That was a daily occurrence to see that kind of stuff. There was always the risk.*[48]

Otten remembers the impressive system for managing battlefield casualties. As a medic, he treated wounded soldiers in the field and attests to the important role of helicopter medical evacuation.

> *We could bring in a helicopter, which we called a "dust off"…As a medic I would try to stabilize the patient as best as I could, which mainly involved bleeding control. Most people die on the battlefield from bleeding. We would just put tourniquets on people; we put pressure dressings on people. Once in a while somebody might have an airway problem they might get their face blown away by a round or a piece of shrapnel in the neck or something like that, and then what we did we'd put in a couple of needles in their cricothyroid membrane to give them an airway. Mainly it was bleeding control. You give them morphine and you could put IVs in them and give them albumin, which was our main resuscitation that we used, and you'd also just use ringer's lactate. Most of it was just to control their bleeding. If they had abdominal injuries or chest injuries there wasn't a whole lot you could do. You could do a chest decompression.*

Some of the medics carried chest tubes. Some carried laryngoscopes and ET [endotracheal] tubes. Remember these guys had 10 weeks of training. The special forces medics were a lot better. They had about 50 weeks of training…(T)he Huey Helicopters—there wasn't much you could do inside of one. Because you put the stretchers in across the width of the helicopter so the patients' feet were kind of hanging out one end of the helicopter and his head was hanging out the other. Then you would put a couple of ambulatory patients, you would sit underneath the stretchers on the floor of the helicopter.[48]

The medics directed the helicopter pilot to take patients to the field hospital or to a larger hospital, depending on their injuries. Casualties who needed immediate resuscitation and surgery were taken to the field surgical hospitals where an assembly line–like approach to patients was used:

We used to say that getting shot in Vietnam was like getting shot on the steps of the hospital. You could actually be in surgery in 20 minutes in a lot of these places. Especially like at 3rd Surg. Hospital the helicopter would land right outside the door of the operating room or the preanesthesia area and they would take people out of the helicopter, they would put them on a stretcher and…they would just cut all his clothes off, and you still have your field gear, you still had your combat boots and your pistol belt and your canteen and hopefully they took your weapon away from you so you wouldn't accidentally shoot the pilot in the helicopter, or hand grenade going off inside the helicopter, but they would just cut all the stuff off of you. They had just a huge pile of all this equipment and uniforms they'd just throw it there. It just piled up, especially after big battles. You'd come by there there'd be a pile of field gear, piled twenty feet high…They would wheel you basically from the helicopter pad into the operating room and then start preparing your belly. Within five minutes of landing you'd be in the OR [operating room] getting your laparotomy. They'd give you blood, they could resuscitate you, they had a blood bank there, they could do vascular surgery at these places, it was amazing.[48]

The fact that the overall mortality rate in Vietnam was less than that in Korea is even more impressive given that many critically wounded soldiers who previously would not have made it alive to a field hospital were delivered in a highly critical state to the next level of medical providers in Vietnam. The paradigm of a well-trained initial responder, rapid transport, and definitive care by a physician in a well-equipped trauma hospital was one that was embraced and promoted by civilian surgeons in the 1960s. William Haeck, M.D., who was developing his ED group and was very involved in emergency medical services in Jacksonville, Florida remembers:

What was clearly evident in Vietnam was that you could organize trauma care and save lives by providing that care at the scene and then moving it upwards through an organized system…A lot of trauma surgeons came back, out of that experience, with that understanding and so it was easy for a lot of us who were organizing EMS systems to get support, particularly from the surgical community, for those systems. They were mixed in their support of emergency medicine.[49]

But duplicating a military-type EMS system in the decentralized, poorly regulated world of civilian medicine and prehospital care would prove to be a very challenging task. When Mel Otten returned home to the United States and started working for an ambulance company in Ohio around 1970, he found civilian emergency care to be very poor:

When I went to college I worked on an ambulance…as a fireman, on an ambulance responding to emergencies. I would go to emergency rooms and the doctors knew less about how to take care of these things than I did. We could get their airways under control, we were putting IVs in people, we were splinting people, we were putting people on backboards, and we were putting MAST trousers on them. We were doing lots of stuff that we had learned about in the Army but the civilians hadn't learned about it yet. Civilian emergency departments were still run by either people who didn't speak English or were bad doctors or people who were just doing their monthly rotation in the emergency room...The problem was between the guy who gets hit by the car in the street, gets splinted, gets resuscitated, gets an IV put in, by the time he gets to the emergency room the emergency room doctor doesn't know what to do and so they don't save him for the surgeon.[48]

As Kendall McNabney notes, military medicine is a single, highly regulated system, with no competition. Resources can be pooled and easily shifted between units. In a capitalistic system, with hospitals competing for patients, without a system for managing prehospital care or coordinating the flow of emergency patients, emergency care of the 1960s and 1970s could not begin to approach the efficiency of the military system.[43] Although Vietnam trained many fine surgeons, these surgeons did not come home to practice in civilian emergency departments. Since the Vietnam War concluded just as emergency medicine training programs were starting, far fewer emergency physicians than surgeons directly learned the lessons of wartime medicine and trauma care.

The first residency-trained emergency physicians were more likely to have opposed the Vietnam War than to have participated in the war. By 1968, the antiwar movement was in full swing and more than 400 medical students across the country had signed a pledge that they would not serve in Vietnam. The resistance movement was controversial, but some in established medicine were sympathetic to the students' cause.[50]

Civil Rights and Violence in the Cities

The civil rights movement was the model for the social movements of the sixties. Parallels can be drawn between what was happening in civil rights, and what was happening in emergency care. A fundamental premise of emergency medicine was that emergency physicians would take care of anyone, with any emergent problem, at any time of the day or night. James Mills and colleagues had expressed these tenets in their original Alexandria Plan rules in 1961.[17] This approach to the sick and injured was congruent with the ideals of civil rights and racial equality. Morgan describes the feeling of participating in this movement:

More than anything else, the civil rights movement galvanized the phenomenon known as "the Sixties." The heightened sense of moral awareness, the loneliness of breaking from one's social roots, the exhilaration of being part of history, the bonds of kinship reinforced by music and communal work, and the courage gained from collective effort, all became characteristics of the activist "Sixties generation" as it broadened its assault on American society.[51]

The aura of the civil rights movement can be seen in some of the features of the sixties emergency physicians—the "heightened sense" of providing care to the down-cast in society, the loneliness (and fear) of breaking away from traditional medicine, and later, the exhilaration of forming a new specialty. The discrimination faced by early emergency physicians from the rest of the medical world was not as harsh or violent as the discrimination faced by blacks in the sixties, but like racial discrimination, it was a constant, subverting influence. The kinship of fighting for the cause of emergency medicine echoed the feel of the civil rights movement as emergency physicians moved in to the seventies.

LEWIS GOLDFRANK—A YOUNG ACTIVIST IN THE WORLD OF MEDICINE

Lewis Goldfrank was born in 1941 in Pleasantville, New York, to parents who had been very active in the 1930s in civil rights, the fight for workers' unions, and helping to organize Nazi resistance in Europe. They were for a period of time active in the

American Communist party. Goldfrank's mother, who was an author of children's books, was investigated by the McCarthy Committee. Goldfrank remembers,

> ...she had no political activity at that time at all but the book they questioned her on was a book called Apple Pie for Lewis. She had written children's books, and my favorite apples, when my grandmother gave me apples, were the red apples as opposed to the green apples. That was at least one of the questions they raised.[52]

Goldfrank's home was filled with the big thinkers of the day—scientists, artists, writers, and philosophers, and young Lewis read extensively and became interested in the interface of politics and medicine. He attended Clark University in Massachusetts, which he found to be "a very progressive and interesting school," and then set his sights on medical school. As a bright student with a strong science background, he was accepted to many medical schools, but chose Johns Hopkins University because the school encouraged students to be involved in research and because "it was in the South and I thought I could carry on the civil rights activities that I worked on before." Goldfrank started as a first-year medical student in the fall of 1963, and one of his classmates was the first black student to be admitted to the Johns Hopkins medical school.

Things did not go well for Goldfrank at Hopkins. Although he did well in class and received good grades, he could not tolerate the attitudes and traditions of the South. He saw this the first day when he was taken on a tour by a senior medical student and was shown the "white" entrance and the "colored" entrance to the emergency room. The tour guide then said, "See that old black drunk in the corner? Who wants to sew him up?" When classes started, Goldfrank observed behaviors toward the single black student that he found appalling. He remembers,

> ...this young black guy, every time there was a class he was called to the front, we'd all get called to the blackboard to point out things and he'd be brought up and harassed and abused and so a couple of us would get up and say, we'd come up, and say you can't do that. There was tremendous racial hostility. A lot of these guys from the deep South had never met or worked with a black guy. The goal was clear to flunk this guy out. Several other guys and myself were trying to protect him, and then we had been there in school for 3 months when Kennedy was killed and there were parties in the dormitory.[52]

Goldfrank tried to engage faculty members in discussions about how socialized medicine might help be "the solution for all these poor people waiting in the emergency department." He went to nearby Cambridge, Maryland, to participate in demonstrations and rallies for civil rights and against poverty. He refused to wear the tie that was required attire for medical students; he engaged the dean in heated philosophical arguments about segregation. Finally, the dean of the medical school had enough of the young idealist and activist. Goldfrank remembers,

> I really didn't accept this higher structure of how you are supposed to behave to the dean, ...I wasn't going to succeed and at the end of the year by the time I got home... a few weeks later I got a letter that you have been terminated and you not a member, you do not need appear at class next year.[52]

After exploring the possibilities at other U.S. medical schools, and not receiving much encouragement, Goldfrank had a chance encounter. He recalls,

> I met a Professor from Brussels, Professor of Philosophy, who was an organizer of the...Jewish underground, in Brussels during the second World War. He said, "We and the faculty in Brussels, when the Nazis came in they told us to teach in Dutch. The people in Brussels spoke French. Our faculty said we are French speaking, we will teach in French and for the next 7 days, they took one faculty member out in the courtyard and hanged them. He said that's why we are called 'Free Spirit, Free Examination, Free Thought.' Who cares what you believe? If you are a good student

you'll pass, so come to Brussels and you'll enter in the school. Anybody can enter, depends on whether you can do the work, whether you succeed or not." My wife and I got on a boat.[52]

Lewis Goldfrank thrived at the University of Brussels Medical School from 1964 to 1970, and he and his family "were really looked after immensely well." He found a diverse student body, with African students from the Congo and the Sudan. The national health care system in Belgium was a sharp contrast from what he had observed in the United States, and Goldfrank marveled how "everyone was taken care of." Meanwhile, back in the United States, involvement in the Vietnam War was expanding, and Goldfrank notes, "it became more and more of a problem for me personally, so it was just as well to be there."[52] Goldfrank was a conscientious objector for the U.S. draft, and if he returned to the United States, he "was afraid I was going to get drafted." As Goldfrank was finishing medical school and contemplating his future, he had contact with a person who was in Europe recruiting for resident physicians for a new residency program that was affiliated with the University of Connecticut at Mt. Sinai Hospital. With some reluctance, Goldfrank and his family returned to the United States, and he did his internship at Mt. Sinai Hospital. He had a good internship year in Connecticut, but found that the hospital "was just too slow for me." After proving that he could function well as a physician in the United States, Goldfrank wanted to be in a setting where public health issues and the state of humanity would be a bigger challenge. He ended up in the Bronx, New York, at Montefiore Hospital where he did a 2-year residency from 1971 to 1973. Goldfrank would make New York his base, his public health pulpit, and a battleground for the development of emergency medicine.[52]

EDs were on the front lines of many of the urban riots of the mid 1960s. Despite the passage of the Civil Rights Act in 1964, and the limited success of the war on poverty, the tinder for unrest lay in cities where de facto segregation and racism were common and unemployment was high in minority communities. In almost all cases, an incident of alleged police unfairness or brutality, combined with a summer heat wave, ignited the riot.[53] The first cities to experience "race" riots were Harlem and Rochester, New York, and north Philadelphia in 1964. In 1965, a major riot erupted in the Watts ghetto in Los Angeles. Six days of violence resulted in 35 deaths, the burning of whole sections of Watts, and 4,000 arrests.[16] Gail Anderson, M.D., who in the early 1970s became the first chairman of emergency medicine in the United States at Los Angeles County, University of Southern California, was an obstetrics and gynecology faculty member at that time, and remembers:

…the Watts Riots added fuel to the flame because of sudden awareness that there had to be more focus on the training of emergency people…We got quite a few patients from the riots but…the riots added to the idea that there had to be training and training programs for physicians in emergency medicine…I think there was a national recognition of a serious problem.[54]

The summer of 1966 brought riots in 16 U.S. cities, but the largest and most deadly of the sixties riots occurred in the summer of 1967 in Detroit. The auto industry had attracted many blacks from the South to relocate in Detroit in the 1930s and 1940s, and the city prospered with largely segregated black and white neighborhoods. In the post–World War II period, the auto industry lost lucrative defense contracts, began to decentralize, and moved more operations to the suburbs or out of state. This resulted in increased unemployment for Detroit laborers. In the 1950s, the black population in Detroit climbed to nearly 30%, and the city lost nearly a quarter of its white population. The black population of Detroit had a 1959 median income 40% lower than whites and had far poorer health, as measured by rates of tuberculosis, infant mortality, and death.[53] Poor blacks in Detroit usually lacked health insurance and relied on municipal hospitals like Detroit General Hospital for their care.

The city was cognizant of the disparity in income and quality of life between white and black citizens, and by 1967, Detroit was praised for its state and federally supported antipoverty programs. This did not prevent the riot that was triggered in

July 1967 when police made a fairly routine bust of an after-hours drinking establishment in a black neighborhood of Detroit. An angry crowd gathered in the hot, muggy, early-morning hours to protest the arrests, and a few people incited a violent rampage that would become 20th-century America's "worst civil disorder."[53] More than 2,500 businesses were looted, burned, or destroyed; nearly 1,200 people were injured; and 43 people were killed over 4 days. The hospitals of Detroit, primarily Detroit General, received the seriously injured. Detroit General enacted its disaster plan soon after the riot broke out, and by the end of the first day, it "looked like a military field hospital…with state police and National Guardsmen stationed at every entrance."[53] Resident and staff physicians were called in, or not allowed to leave, and four times as many doctors were in the hospital as normal. Ron Krome, then a senior surgery resident, was on duty during the riots and worked 12 hours on, 12 hours off during the 4-day stretch.[13] The spectrum of injuries included gunshot wounds, stab wounds, and burns. Critical cases were taken to the operating room or intensive care units, but the hallways were lined with rioters who had less severe injuries. Some of them lay on the floor in leg irons. Physicians and hospital personnel struggled with feelings of anger and resentment at the injured rioters. Many injuries resulted from police beating rioters, with frequent allegations of police brutality. Newspaper reporters witnessed a bloody black rioter brought to the Detroit General Hospital by police. When the man called out to ED staff for help, the policeman kicked him in the groin and shouted racial slurs at him.[53]

Urban riots continued into 1968. In Kansas City, where Kendall McNabney worked as an attending surgeon at Kansas City General Hospital, riots broke out in April after the assassination of Martin Luther King, Jr. In this case, "overzealous" police action—spraying a crowd of high school marchers with tear gas—led to more violence and property destruction. McNabney stayed in the hospital for 4 days to treat injured patients and because the hospital was in the vicinity of the riots and it would not have been safe to commute home. McNabney remembers that the number of cases presenting to the ED during the riots was actually less than normal, as many nonriot patients were fearful of venturing to the hospital. National Guard troops were placed on top of the hospital and patrolled outside with bayonets drawn. ED personnel were particularly disturbed when one of their co-workers, a black orderly, was brought in as a gunshot victim and died in the ED.[43]

Urban municipal EDs were at the epicenter of civil unrest in the 1960s, but poor health care was not often cited as one of the main reasons for the riots. The leading factors, according to surveys conducted after the riots, were police brutality, substandard housing, crowded living conditions, poverty, and anger at local business people.[53] Ron Krome remembers that even if it was not a factor in the riots, people had cause to be upset with emergency care, especially prehospital care in the greater Detroit area. Krome recalls the case of a head-injured child that demonstrated the deficits in emergency care and transport in Detroit:

> [A] young kid fell out of a tree at a public park. There was no EMS—the police picked her up took her to the hospital and there were only interns on. The interns couldn't speak English, so they put her back in the station wagon. She was seizing, they couldn't start the station wagon, they called for a second station wagon. By the time they got here, she was inoperable. That provoked a lot of public pressure on the mayor to shake up EMS, the categorization of hospitals as far as their ability to respond.[13]

The forgiving attitude of the urban public toward hospitals and EDs in the 1960s, despite the tremendous inadequacies in most of these institutions, stems from the fact that the EDs were always open; did not openly discriminate on the basis of race, ethnicity, or ability to pay; and would care for acute and nonacute problems. In a society that was rife with segregation, discrimination, and inequality, EDs were in some sense little bastions of egalitarianism. This did not mean that the care was good—the urban poor were more resigned to than content with their emergency care. Long waits to be seen and poorly trained or inexperienced physicians in the EDs made an emergency visit a frustrating and risky event. In Cincinnati, Ohio, dissatisfaction with hospital and emergency care at the Cincinnati General Hospital was one of the factors in urban riots in the late 1960s. The riots helped to stimulate the formation of the first training program in emergency medicine.

The civil unrest of the sixties sometimes alerted city governments and the public to the poor state of emergency care. The riots also highlighted the important role played by hospitals and EDs during a disaster. However, the riots, assassinations, and violence of the sixties did not greatly affect the course of the early practitioners of emergency medicine. Men like Mills, Hannas, Wiegenstein, Leidelmeyer, and Podgorny were not working in areas of major unrest and went about their business, developing their skills in emergency medicine, and thinking about how the field might evolve.

SEX, DRUGS, ROCK AND ROLL—AND EMERGENCY PHYSICIANS?

By the mid 1960s, much of the hope, optimism, and good will that had characterized the early part of the decade had evaporated. Politics became more personal and radical. As sixties' scholar Edward Morgan noted, "The process of radicalization began with three crucial ingredients—belief in community-based, egalitarian democracy; a sharp personal awareness of social ills; and a feeling of confidence that something could be done."[51] As more young people took a direct participatory or observational role in helping the oppressed or suffering in society, they developed "a heady sense of empowerment," described by participants as a "combination of fear and ecstasy resulting from taking risks to change one's environment—Out of this profound personal engagement came the distinctive personal politics of the sixties."[51]

The first emergency physicians were not part of the "sex, drugs, rock and roll" culture of the sixties. They were middle-aged, white, male professionals, some of whom had served their country in wars. Most, like Mills, Hannas, Wiegenstein, and Wagner, had practiced medicine in the traditional way before making the leap to emergency medicine. They were educated and well to do by most standards. John Wiegenstein, with his prematurely gray–white hair; R. R. Hannas with his military-style crew cut; and George Podgorny with his early-1900s–style handlebar mustache would have been viewed by the younger activists of the sixties as part of the "Establishment," even though they were still early in their careers. However, these emergency pioneers were not part of the medical establishment. They were viewed as an oddity by most in medicine. In their migration to a new type of medical practice, they were exhibiting somewhat radical behavior. When asked if the events of the sixties helped to fuel the emergency medicine movement, most of the emergency medicine founding fathers deny a clear association. However, as George Podgorny notes of the young radicals of the sixties:

> They probably philosophically contributed to people understanding that there is such a thing as change. The only thing that is constant is change…Maybe it kind of vaccinated people, that, you know, there can be significant change…I don't think that in itself it gave an impetus. I think there is probably a coincidence that of course emergency physicians by far were very young people. So, maybe there was a parallel as the young hippies were rebelling in the society, young emergency docs were rebelling in house of medicine.[55]

Ideas of participatory democracy, individual freedoms, and interest in alternative lifestyles were concordant with the new field. Emergency medicine was clearly a new way to practice medicine, and for some, it became a less radical way to express their individualism. The early face of emergency medicine resident education was partly shaped by some of the free-spirited products of the sixties. Three men who would have a prominent role in the first emergency medicine residency training program—Bruce Janiak, Richard Levy, and Phillip Buttaravoli—grew up during the sixties. They were not radicals, but all three felt, and were moved to act, by the mood of the times.

BRUCE JANIAK, M.D.: AN ORDINARY KID FROM OHIO

Bruce Janiak was born in Cleveland, Ohio, in 1943. Janiak's father, Len, had been a Navy man, but his biggest talent was football. He was a professional football player for the Cleveland Rams and then became a high school football coach. Bruce attended high school in Brecksville, Ohio, and had a typical suburban upbringing. He washed dishes at a YMCA camp during the summers and enjoyed hunting and fishing. He followed his girlfriend to Marietta College in Ohio in 1961. As for football, Janiak notes that although he played high school and 1 year of college football, "I just never inherited my dad's skills in that regard." Janiak liked the sciences and biology, but was not especially passionate or confident as he considered medical school. He remembers thinking,

> …I'll try medical school but I don't care if it works or not, because I'll be a detective—I thought police work would be fun. I was rejected by several medical schools and finally got on the waiting list at Cincinnati. I was accepted by the Chicago College of Osteopathy and had interviewed there and was going to go there when I got accepted by Cincinnati and it was quite a chore to decide where to go, because I thought osteopathy, it sounded kind of interesting to me. I guess I fell back on my conservative instincts—I guess if I roll the dice an M.D. would be, at the time now, a little more valuable than a D.O. and that probably was the last time that I was willing to take the same path everyone else did… [B]ut I went to medical school with…an incredible apprehension—surrounded by people I knew were brilliant and knew everything, and I was a dunce who knew nothing.[56]

Janiak calls medical school "the best years of my life." For the first time, he learned how to study and despite his apprehension was able to keep up with his peers. He does recall skipping out on biochemistry lab to play pick-up basketball with some of his classmates, but overall he was a diligent student. Like John Wiegenstein at Michigan, Janiak became aware of an opportunity to make some extra money during his senior year of medical school. A hospital in Northern Kentucky hired medical students to cover its emergency room.

> It was just over the river. It was one of those really ancient hospitals…Actually, advertised for medical students to be the emergency doctor at night and on weekends. I was called in by the dean who got word of what I was thinking of doing who warned me that I could destroy my career and of course being a jerk, I said "Ah, I'm going to do it!" Well, I took my little Lilly doctor's bag and drove to this little hospital, parked my car, and walked in the back door when a rather anxious, semicorpulent nurse in her white uniform and cap ran out the door and said, "I'm glad you are here—there is a cardiac arrest upstairs!" Honest to God, you'd think I would make this stuff up!… [W]hen I went in and I watched the nurses push on this body, it's when I decided that either I am going to never do this again or I'm going to learn to do it right. That was the watershed thing that made me go back and say, "Where can I get training in emergency medicine?" So…what I remember about the resuscitation is a nurse giving a drug called Coramen, which I'm sure most people won't remember, basically it's caffeine IV to stimulate the heart. Of course, the patient didn't live. I, of course, had to change my underwear after that and I went and worked in the emergency department. I did a bunch of shifts over the next year, it was $45 for a 24-hour shift—reading most of the time, because there were only three or four patients a day, it was very, very quiet. It was an emergency department with what truly were "wet readings." Most people don't know what wet reading is. This was the x-ray hand-developed and still dripping when they handed it to you. It was really interesting, I watched them develop and it was fascinating.[56]

As a medical student, Janiak was not aware of the Alexandria group or other practicing emergency physicians. When he was on a senior rotation at Jewish Hospital, across the street from the Cincinnati General Hospital, he asked one of the teaching faculty if he knew anything about training in emergency care. The faculty member did not, but said that he had heard that a couple of the Cincinnati medical school faculty members were talking about training in emergency medicine. Janiak was referred to Herbert Flessa, M.D., a hematologist who had been put in charge of the ED by the chair of internal medicine. Janiak knew Flessa as a young faculty member who wasn't afraid to mix it up with the students,

> Herb was a great clinician but also an incredible defensive back on our touch foot-ball team. He hit you and you knew you were hit. He had fun with us and we as students really appreciated the fact that he did that.[56]

Flessa, who quickly appreciated the overwhelming task of bringing control to the busy Cincinnati General ED, was thinking about developing an emergency medicine training program. The ensuing discussions between he and Janiak would lead to Janiak becoming the first emergency medicine resident.

RICHARD LEVY, M.D.: FROM THE "HOLLERS" OF KENTUCKY TO THE HALLS OF HARVARD

Richard Levy, who became the leader of the prominent academic emergency medicine program at the University of Cincinnati in the 1970s, was born in 1947 and raised in Irvine, a hamlet in southeastern Kentucky. How a rebellious Jewish boy from this background came to be a leader in emergency medicine can be partly understood by exploring the immigration and assimilation of Jews in to American society in the 1900s. Levy's great-grandfather had left Lithuania for America to avoid being "fodder for the czars." Jews were conscripted into the czar's armies and "they were put up front."[57] Levy's grandfather came to the Midwest and peddled dry goods before he settled in Irvine, Kentucky, and opened a dry-goods store that his son, Levy's father would inherit. As Levy recounts, this area of Kentucky,

> ...had been over 100 years systematically raped of all of its resources, all the way from its coal to its oil to its timber, but what was left when I grew up was a little bitty town that had a railroad that went through it that connected the southeast part of the state with the rest of the world and had a tiny bit of farming and...commercial activities. It was a town of 3,000, so it was pretty small. I was there because my parents, specifically my father, moved there as part of the submigratory pattern of Eastern European Jews who were second generation or first generation, you saw them through-out the south and throughout the small midwestern towns of the country. They were there as merchants because there were wholesalers in larger communities like Cincinnati that gave them favorable terms and so it made sense for them to go into these smaller communities and set up dry-goods stores. My father had a small depart-ment store kind of thing. Very typical, in looking back, every town had one, as a Jewish merchant. Typically there was only one or two per community, in our instance we were the only Jews in a small town.[57]

"The Right Way Store" provided a good living for the family, and the people of Irvine accepted but did not embrace their lone Jewish family.

> My father was well respected as an individual, however we were the Jews. If you went into the back roads of our area, there were hollers, the people—stereotypes make fun of them—those people really did exist. They would have called my father's little department store "the Jew Store." They would do it not in a verbally anti-Semitic way, but in a descriptive sense, that we were different.[57]

The Levys' religious and cultural base was in Lexington, Kentucky, about a 2-hour drive through the mountains from Irvine. Levy's parents drove him to the synagogue in Lexington three times a week for Hebrew school. Levy viewed Irvine "as the place where I grew up and had a good time...but also viewed it as—I was going somewhere else." As a restless student who sometimes caused trouble, Levy had an accelerated exit from Irvine.

> *...when you talk to some of the early people in emergency medicine, [some] of us were misfits in certain ways, either conventional or nonconventional. I don't have a high school degree. I was rebellious; I think you could classically describe me as the smart troublemaker. Junior year, I got in a lot of trouble and high school really was sort of tolerating me. I made okay grades, but they were tolerating me. Through a suggestion of my principal, I went to a program at UK [University of Kentucky] for students going into their senior year of high school and he was fairly...explicit...that if I stayed at the University of Kentucky he'd be real pleased he wouldn't have to deal with me as a senior. So, I went into the dean, this is only back then, these kind of things I don't think happen any more, but I went and saw a dean and said well I guess I had ought to go to college, and he said well if you make two "A's" this summer you can go to college. I just went, no degree...I'm the only professor that you probably know that doesn't have a high school degree....[57]*

Actually, Peter Rosen was another rambunctious young man who became an emergency medicine leader and does not have a high school degree. Levy started college in 1964. Influences that moved him toward medicine were the favorable view of medicine in the Jewish community—"my son the doctor"—and his memories of two GPs, a man and a woman in Irvine who were role models:

> *...they were semi-God–like figures growing up...[T]hey were very well respected and well thought of. They worked real hard, but they economically were well off compared to everybody else... [T]he best and the brightest at that time no matter what your ethnic group went into medicine...[I]t was before the explosion of medical schools and was right at the point where Medicare and Medicaid were on the cusp of exploding and science was progressing very rapidly at that point in time. So, being a doctor was like a very cool thing to do but also very competitive.[57]*

Levy stayed in state to attend the University of Louisville Medical School. There he met an interesting faculty member who introduced Levy to emergency medicine. Don Thomas was an anesthesiologist by training who had developed a keen interest in EMS. Red-haired and loud, he had a persona like a Wild West sheriff. Thomas was always on the move; he had an EMS radio in his office and a white station wagon with a siren on it parked outside the hospital. He often packed a gun. Thomas also ran the Louisville General Hospital ED when Richard Levy was a student preparing to suture a patient:

> *I'll never forget my first exposure to emergency medicine. He ran into the suture area at the time and he handed me forceps and he even put the needle on and he said; "You make sure, Levy, that you get the white stuff to the white stuff and the red stuff to the red stuff and holler if you need any more help." I taught many people how to suture based on that principle because it wasn't a bad one. That was Don Thomas....[57]*

As noted previously, the Louisville General Hospital was considered to have an advanced trauma program and ED, but Levy remembers it as being chaotic, disorganized, almost surreal,

> *There was a guy there who was also from anesthesiology but I think he may have been a resident. God I can't remember his name except he was really a strange, strange guy. I mean entertaining but he carried a gun—carried a gun in a holster at that. He told great funny, funny stories but I remember one time he came in, he was dressed as the Grim Reaper and another time he came in and he had a priest outfit on, and he would go from patient to patient. It just was a time when, that was a charity hospital, and there weren't any controls, and so there were a lot of free spirits that could do crazy stuff because no one said you couldn't do crazy stuff unless you were so far out that maybe you came to the attention of a higher up, but that was unlikely.[57]*

Levy was influenced by and became a participant in the movements of the sixties. One of the Great Society initiatives was the development of neighborhood or community health clinics to provide health care access to the underserved. As a medical student, Levy cofounded a network of student-run health clinics called the Greater Louisville Organization for Health (GLOH), because "health care really sucked back then when it came to poor people."[57] As Levy notes, for a college student of the sixties,

> [T]here were two things going on that were both significant crosscurrents. One was the Vietnam period and I was a medical student active in the antiwar movement, as a matter of fact I am absolutely sure, only because I can still see those guys snapping pictures of me—I'm sure I'm in the FBI [Federal Bureau of Investigation] files somewhere from that activity way back when. So there was that and the very real concern that if I did do internship right after medical school there was a possibility that I would end up over in Vietnam. I really didn't want to do that. A deferment by way of more of graduate education wasn't a bad idea in and of itself. The other thing…there was a strong cultural directive of healing the world, fixing what's wrong, doing something good for mankind, and these all may sound kind of silly and self righteous but it was the time…So, I was pretty idealistic. Another factor was I really did have this feeling of how can I make a big impact on the world. For whatever reason something was starting to click in me that I wanted to do more than just be a doctor. I can't tell you why or what, but something was starting to foment inside… I wanted to try to do something, so I went off to public health school.[57]

After graduating from medical school in 1972, Levy went to Harvard and earned a Masters in Public Health. When he entered the world of emergency medicine, he became one of the first leaders who was a product of the movements of the sixties. Levy notes:

> …my college and medical school years were very interesting times in America— drugs, sex, rock and roll; times were changing rapidly, and many of my generation were caught up in the spirit of creating a better tomorrow.[58]

Phillip Buttaravoli, M.D.: An Observant Student in the Sixties

Phil Buttaravoli grew up on Long Island in New York. As a 20-year-old premed student at the University of Vermont, he was hired as a summer orderly in the ED of Meadowbrook Hospital on Long Island (now Nassau County Medical Center) in 1965. Buttaravoli remembers the experience:

> I just found it absolutely thrilling, fascinating—action, drama, all the things. I can recall at the time asking the nurses there, "Does anybody ever do this full time? Do doctors practice this full time?" The response that I recall very vividly was, "Not in this country!"[59]

Although he knew little about medicine at the time, Buttaravoli, in the summer of 1965, could see that conditions were not optimal at Meadowbrook:

> I also remember being quite struck by the lack of quality in medical care that was provided to the patients. It seemed like, my goodness, even as a layman it didn't seem like the patients were getting cared for with the same quality that I thought was going on in the rest of the hospital. There were interns basically that were running the emergency department and didn't know anything. I would see patients deteriorate and die without much intervention; there seemed to be a lot of confusion. It seemed to me that, wow, if you could provide a service for these patients, of quality, they sure would appreciate it. It seemed like patients were needing somebody, it was a crisis, my goodness, no one seemed to be coming to their rescue. Wouldn't it be nice if somebody could rescue them? The doctors who were staffing the emergency department were interns,

foreign medical graduate interns for the most part, that I could recall. They just didn't seem to have much on the ball…I didn't have much on the ball when I was an intern either. You needed supervision.[59]

Buttaravoli filed these memories of poor ED care away and began medical school at the University of Vermont. He eagerly looked forward to his ED experience in medical school, assuming that a university medical center would have vastly better emergency care than he had seen back home at his county hospital. He was wrong. He found interns staffing the department, with a nurse in charge. Buttaravoli also noticed that emergency patients did not have access to the same resources he knew existed for patients elsewhere in the medical center. He became somewhat incredulous at what he was seeing, and decided to make the study of emergency care his "project,"

As I became so enthralled by this discovery of an area wanting a specialist… I ended up doing some papers. These were not expected of me, I just did it because I needed to do it. I did a critical evaluation entitled, "Medical Center Hospital of Vermont, Emergency Department a Critical Self-Evaluation" and then…I basically interviewed the staff and looked at all the various aspects of the emergency department and then I published student recommendations for the Medical Center Hospital of Vermont, based on the findings of my study….[59]

Presumptuous as it was, Buttaravoli's assessment of emergency care at Medical Center Hospital of Vermont was painfully on target. He did not interview attending physicians and wrote, "because I felt that with the limited amount of time that is spent by them in the emergency unit they could not be truly and intimately familiar with the actual problems as they exist there."[60] Buttaravoli's report identified problems in emergency unit staffing, triage, care of critically ill patients, equipment, communication, and teaching. He noted that during the night, the only respirator available to the emergency unit was kept locked in a room. If the respirator was needed, someone had to go to the main hospital operator to get the key to the room. In citing the poor documentation in the ED, he described how a new technology, instant Polaroid photos, could be used to document physical finding in emergency patients, and then used for teaching purposes and inclusion in the medical record. He wrote an article on this new use of instant photographs to enhance the medical record that was published in the *New England Journal of Medicine* in 1970.[61]

Buttaravoli cited the meager but important literature of the 1960s on emergency care in his report. He knew about practicing emergency physicians and called for the Medical Center Hospital of Vermont to appoint an emergency director and hire full-time physicians to staff the emergency unit. Buttaravoli's prescient parting message to the Medical Center of Vermont came in his article, "The University Hospital Emergency Department Unwittingly Exploited: A Possible Solution." The conclusion to his treatise reads,

The scope of emergency practice lies beyond the simple sum of the acute care aspect of the other specialties. It encompasses communications, transportation of the ill and injured, the design, staffing, and equipping of emergency facilities, disaster planning, community wide coordination of all emergency related services. The present basic non-system of emergency care has been proven to be grossly inadequate and the public is tiring of impersonal sub-standard treatment. Emergency departments will remain at the lowest end of the health care system though, no matter what the community needs are, until responsible leadership takes over and treats this aspect of medical care with the same respect as any other specialized division. Training and utilization of emergency specialists must be actively encouraged by all of today's health care personnel. A university hospital should have a model emergency department along with its other superior services. Eventually, under a system with full-time, adequately staffed emergency physicians the emergency service would have the means to provide care equal to if not higher than the quality provided by the other departments. Computerization, helicopter service, specialized emergency technicians, etc., should be supplied to give the public the highest quality of emergency care that modern medical science and technology has to offer.[60]

Phil Buttaravoli was not around to see if any of his recommendations came to fruition in Vermont. After an internship in Santa Clara Valley Medical Center in San Jose, California, he joined the second class of residents in emergency medicine at the University of Cincinnati in 1971.

THE SIXTIES WIND DOWN AND UNRAVEL

The importance of Phillip Buttaravoli's work as a medical student goes beyond his exposure of the inadequacies in emergency care in his own medical center—most teaching hospitals were in a similar, sad state. A key point is that a young man who had no national exposure was independently able to see the problems in emergency care and make recommendations that were on par with what was being promoted by the early leaders in the field. Other young medical minds of the sixties were doubtlessly seeing the same problems and a few realized that through emergency practice they might be part of the solution.

The sixties were a defining period in American medicine. For the first time, government assumed a prominent role in health care through the Medicare and Medicaid programs, and through the Johnson administration's community health initiatives and federal grants for diagnosis and treatment of specific diseases. Government also fueled the rapid pace of biomedical discovery through NIH support of research at medical schools. The advances in military medicine in the Vietnam war demonstrated the potential for improved civilian trauma care, and the government responded to some degree to stimulate trauma programs and EMS. The net effect of these government programs was to bring more attention to emergency care and to demonstrate that it was an area desperately in need of progress.

Outside of the government, the themes of the social movements of the sixties were in synchrony with the development of emergency medicine. Many of the people, like Janiak, Buttaravoli, and Levy, who would become the first residents to train in emergency medicine, were college students in the sixties. They would bring to the field a different set of values and ideals and the dress, music, and culture of the sixties. Both the civil rights movement and student activism on college campuses pitted young idealists who believed they had a moral calling against institutions that were prepared to defend the status quo.[51] In a similar manner, the early practitioners and trainees in emergency medicine found their "calling" opposed by the medical establishment. The feel of the sixties permeated the groundswell that would become emergency medicine. The emphasis on social programs, the attention to the needy in society, and the new possibilities in medicine were all part of an atmosphere of change that propelled emergency medicine toward full-fledged medical specialty status.

The latter years of the sixties became increasingly violent, sour, and radical. Instead of moving peacefully toward social change, young people were increasingly "dropping out" to alternative lifestyles or using confrontation and violence to make their points. The student activists of the sixties, many of whom seemed to be living the American dream by attending prestigious universities, rejected the American dream, rebelling against the capitalist and commercial themes of their world, looking for a less oppressive and more inclusive and fair society. Analogous to this, the early emergency physicians rejected the idea of traditional medicine—they did not want to see patients in an office-based practice, follow them over time, or limit themselves to a specialty area of medicine. While these physicians did not leave an oppressive medical world to practice emergency medicine, they faced strong opposition once they were identified as a real entity in the world of medicine. Societal cynicism and outrage with the government was made even more intense with shocking events like the National Guard shootings of Kent State antiwar students in 1970 and the Watergate scandal. The students who experienced this radicalism were less likely to trust authority and more likely to value independence. Their mark would later be felt in emergency medicine.

The year 1968 has been called "The Hard Year."[62] The United States was hopelessly mired in Vietnam. In January, the Vietcong launched the Tet offensive in to South Vietnam, killing more than 1,100 U.S. soldiers in 30 days. In February in South Carolina, students attempting to desegregate a bowling alley were fired upon by state police, and three students were killed. At the end of March, Lyndon Johnson, with a lowly approval rating of 36%, announced that he would not seek reelection. On April 4, Martin Luther King, Jr., was assassinated in Memphis, and many cities rioted in response, with nearly 50 deaths. Later in April, 1,000 students at Columbia University took over several campus buildings in protest of the University's policies on the war and toward poor neighbors. On June 6, Robert F. Kennedy was assassinated after winning the California Democratic primary election. The August Democratic presidential convention was marred by violent protests and police brutality. In the last few months of 1968, an emotionally worn-out nation saw peace talks initiated with the Vietcong and the victory of Richard Nixon over Hubert Humphrey in the November presidential election. This marked an abrupt end to the big government, Great Society mindset of the Kennedy and Johnson era. The economy was also about to experience a downturn that would have major ramifications for health care funding.[3,4,16,51,62]

The frequency and intensity of tragic and unsettling events in 1968 shocked and then numbed the nation. But, in the midst of all this, average Americans went about their work and raised their families. Among them were the early emergency physicians who were aware of, but not visibly affected, by the tumultuous proceedings. Some of the pioneers of emergency practice, bridled with hope and energy, were starting to look beyond their own situations. Although it was a "hard year" for the nation, 1968 would become a momentous year for the organization of emergency medicine.

4 Emergency Medicine Gets Organized

By the late 1960s, American medicine was relatively fixed in its professional structure. There were internists, pediatricians, surgeons, and subspecialties in these domains, along with hospital-based specialties such as anesthesiology and radiology. Decades before, these fields had been organized and established certifying boards. The two major areas of practice in medicine that had not formally organized were general practice and emergency medicine. General practice had a longer history than any of the other specialties, but finally took the step to expand its training beyond an internship and to establish a certifying board in family practice in 1969. Family practice was not a new threat to the medical establishment, and with the shortage of primary care doctors, many were glad to see family practice as a new "specialty." The organization of emergency medicine would not proceed as smoothly. Practicing in the emergency department carried a negative stigma, and seemed to violate the traditional concept of a doctor caring for his patient over time, rather than in an isolated episode. Emergency medicine was also perceived as a direct threat to the autonomy and pocketbooks of traditional medical specialties. The resistance to this new medical entity, along with the ephemeral nature of some emergency practitioners, would make it challenging to organize emergency medicine.

The Seminal Ideas

John Wiegenstein and Eugene Nakfoor established their Alexandria-type group at St. Lawrence Hospital in 1967. Before the group was established, Wiegenstein was encouraged by the administrators at St. Lawrence to talk with John Rupke, M.D., the young director of an emergency department (ED) in Grand Rapids. Rupke had an interesting road to emergency care. He had been in a preseminary program at Calvin College, but like Wiegenstein, did not pursue a career as a clergyman. He was drawn to medicine while in college.

> I was working the emergency department as an orderly for 5 years and in the summer I would go up to Alaska and there are no doctors or nurses up there in Pacific-American Fishery Canneries and then I would be the "8 Man," so called. I learned how to pull teeth and deliver babies and so forth. I was an orderly. Up there in Alaska, you practice as much medicine as you are able. You give full disclosure, hey I'm no doctor, this is what they do in the emergency department.[1]

Rupke went to medical school at the University of Maryland. He was a year behind Ron Krome, and like Krome decided on a surgical career. Rupke came to Butterworth Hospital in Grand Rapids, Michigan, and did an internship and 2 years of a surgical residency. He was familiar with emergency care from his previous work, and when nearby St. Mary's Hospital announced in 1965 that it was looking to hire a full-time physician to run its ED, Rupke was interested, but had some stipulations. He remembers, "I went down there as head of the emergency department on one condition that I had learned enough as an orderly. I will hire and fire all of the help down there." Rupke dropped out of his surgical residency, became the ED director at St. Mary's Hospital, and hired three other physicians to form an Alexandria-type emergency group called Emergency Physicians, Inc. At the time, his was one of six or seven similar groups in the country.[1]

St. Mary's was one of a large network of Mercy hospitals of Michigan, and it was therefore natural for the administrator at St. Lawrence, another Mercy hospital, to suggest in 1966 that Eugene Nakfoor and John Wiegenstein visit Rupke to find out more about ED management. Both Nakfoor and Wiegenstein were still in general practice and expressed doubts to Rupke on whether emergency medicine was going to progress. Rupke remembers telling them, "General practice isn't going to go anywhere." But he told them that emergency medicine was "…going to go all over the United States because this is a mess all over the United States."[1] Nakfoor and Wiegenstein went back to Lansing and started their group in 1967, and Rupke and Wiegenstein saw each other several times in the next couple of years at medical meetings. Both were seeking education in trauma and other medical emergencies to improve their clinical practice. Rupke and Wiegenstein also attended a presentation by Irvin (Chief) Henderson, the head of the new American Medical Association (AMA) Commission on Emergency Medical Services in San Francisco in January of 1968. Wiegenstein and Rupke developed a relationship others would call "The Two Johns."[2]

One of the main issues the men discussed was the financial viability of the groups. Wiegenstein learned that Rupke used the Maraveleas's company, Medical Ancillary Services, to bill for his group. In the first year of his group's operation, Rupke had allowed the hospital to bill for ED physician services, but they did such an "atrocious job" that Rupke was forced to look elsewhere. He found Medical Ancillary, the same management and billing company used by the Pontiac Plan groups in eastern Michigan. The Maraveleas husband-and-wife accountant team had been enterprising enough to expand their service across the state by 1966. Wiegenstein decided also to use Medical Ancillary Services for his ED billing at St. Lawrence.

Wiegenstein was struck and bothered by the utter lack of knowledge and training possessed by those who delivered emergency care—including his own deficiencies. He was not sure where to turn for training. He signed up for courses offered by other medical fields. He went on a cruise to take a course on emergency orthopedics. When he showed up at 9 AM for the first lecture, he was the only attendee. The lecturer seemed annoyed that he would have to provide the lecture to a single person, but Wiegenstein, thirsty for knowledge, insisted they proceed. Early in his ED work, Wiegenstein had also observed that prehospital care was nonexistent or dreadful.[3]

> I noticed that the ambulance people didn't get trained at all. They would bring in a real sick patient and both of them would be sitting in the front seat, they'd have oxygen on the guy in the back. I remember one time they brought this patient who was dead at the door. "Well, he must have died on us!" That's the kind of service we got…I knew about the programs that were being offered in Akron, Ohio, by the orthopedists, so I went down there feeling certain I would be the only doctor to attend the course, it was for EMTs [emergency medicine technicians]. I became an EMT because I finished the course. I got my badge and all the stuff.[3]

Orthopedic surgeons along with general surgeons had played a leading role in trying to improve the prehospital management of trauma and ambulance training. In the 1940s and 1950s, the American Orthopedic Association pushed for proper emergency splinting and management of fractures. The American College of Surgeons (ACS) and American Orthopedic Association worked together to develop guidelines. By the late 1960s, the orthopedists had in some ways supplanted trauma surgeons to become the leading proponents of ambulance technician training. In 1964, the Committee on Injuries of the American Academy of Orthopaedic Surgeons (AAOS) began offering 3-day courses for emergency medical personnel. Federal grants for emergency medical services (EMS) training that were stimulated by the National Academy of Sciences–National Research Council (NAS-NRC) Accidental Death and Disability Report of 1966 became available from the Public Health Service and Department of Transportation as early as 1967. Around this time the Committee on Injuries of the AAOS, headed by Walter Hoyt, Jr., M.D., began to produce a comprehensive training manual for emergency medical personnel. Assistance and support was garnered from the ACS, AMA, American Red Cross, the U.S. Public Health Service, the NAS-NRC, the U.S. Army, and the Department of Transportation. The project took 4 years to complete, but the famous "Orange Book," titled *Emergency Care and Transportation of the Sick and Injured*, published by the AAOS in 1971, became the authoritative work for EMS training in the 1970s.[4] Thousands of EMTs and paramedics who were trained in community college or other programs viewed the Orange Book as the bedrock of their education.

The course that Wiegenstein attended in 1967 was run by Walter Hoyt at his home base in Akron. Hoyt, who thought it a bit strange that a physician was taking his EMT course, invited Wiegenstein for cocktails that night. Also attending was Joseph Owen, who was at the course representing the U.S. Public Health Service's Division of Accident Prevention. The three men discussed emergency care and Wiegenstein talked about his desire to see an organization that could help train emergency physicians. He asked whether Hoyt or Owen knew of any national organizations for emergency physicians. Both responded that they knew of no such organization. Owen said he would check with his colleagues in Washington. After Wiegenstein returned to Lansing, he received separate letters from Hoyt and Owen informing him that their inquiries had revealed no national organizations for emergency doctors. Both encouraged Wiegenstein to form one.[3] Wiegenstein mulled over the idea and sought input from John Rupke. His idea for a national organization stemmed mainly from his desire for better education in the developing field. Rupke was receptive to this, but approached the concept more from a business standpoint. A few months later Wiegenstein invited Rupke to Lansing. They met at a bar in the Lansing airport, and "over a brew or two," Wiegenstein recalled:[5]

> I invited him to talk about this and so he came down and we talked about it and he said, "I really think we ought to start a business, multihospital." I said, "What do you think we need the most? Do we need to make money or do we need to learn what we are doing first?" He had to admit that was probably more important, getting training programs.[3]

When he was referring to training programs, Wiegenstein did not mean residency programs—that concept was not prominent in his mind and would be left for others to pursue. He was referring to training in emergency care for physicians who entered the field. This is now known as continuing medical education, but in the case of the early emergency physicians, there was nothing to continue. Most had minimal to no training in emergency care and needed to improve their knowledge base and skills to match their enthusiasm for the field. Wiegenstein decided to push forward with plans for an association. He did not know the other emergency physicians in Michigan very well, but did know that many of them used Medical Ancillary Services to bill. Wiegenstein contacted the billing company.

> I said I want the leader of each group. I want the person who's the go-getter in each group that he billed for. He gave me those names of the people. So that is how I brought them in. First of all, I had to come up with a by-laws and constitution, so I collected all the by-laws and constitutions of the Academy of General Practice, Radiology, Internal Medicine, Surgery, and a few others and looked at all of them. I kind of put pieces and parts together that I thought were good and then made a list of purposes of ACEP [American College of Emergency Physicians] and then had my LPN [licensed practical nurse] type it for me and then I took that document with me to our first meeting on August the 16th.[3]

A College of Eight

Wiegenstein used the list from Medical Ancillary Services to telephone the other key members in each emergency group in Michigan. Because many of the physicians practicing emergency medicine were part timers as part of Pontiac Plan–type practices, only a few people could be identified who were full-time emergency practitioners.

Eight were invited to a meeting at 1:30 PM at the Holiday Inn in Lansing on August 16, 1968: Wiegenstein and his partner, Eugene Nakfoor; Rupke; John Rogers, who was an obstetrician/surgeon by training; Robert Rathburn, the mastermind of the huge Pontiac Plan–type practice in Flint; Richard Lingenfelter; Robert Leichtman; and George Fink. Rathburn, who understood business and legal aspects of how organizations were formed, came with an attorney so that the group could incorporate that first day. Maria Maravelas functioned as the secretary to the meeting. The main points of discussion were the principles and purpose of a national association, membership status, how the association would be funded, what to call it, and the legal identity.[6]

The discussion about a name was dominated by Dr. Rogers. As an obstetrician/surgeon, he did not have a favorable view of general practice organizations or training. Because Wiegenstein drew heavily on the constitution and by-laws of the American Academy of Family Practice for his initial drafting of the constitution and by-laws of the new organization, he turned to the term "academy" when thinking of a name. However, when Wiegenstein suggested this, Rogers strongly objected, saying that the association would be viewed like general practice—a weak player on the national medical scene. Rogers favored the use of the word "college" to describe the association, like the American College of Surgeons. The eight physicians unanimously, and somewhat presumptuously, voted to call themselves the American College of Emergency Physicians. Lingenfelter, who practiced at Beyer Hospital in Ypsilanti, where a decade earlier Wiegenstein had worked as a medical student, objected to the inclusion of osteopathic physicians in the College. Many osteopathic physicians practiced in the state of Michigan, including several who worked as emergency physicians. In a new organization desperate for members, it did not seem reasonable to Wiegenstein to exclude anyone. After a tense discussion, the group voted to allow osteopathic physicians in the college. Active membership was "limited to those physicians who voluntarily devote a significant portion of their medical practice to emergency medicine and surgery."[5,6] Lingenfelter was so displeased by this that he never attended another meeting. George Fink, who was present in place of an invited physician from Ann Arbor who had suffered a heart attack, felt strongly about maintaining the private practice of emergency medicine. Presumably his feelings centered on billing and the ability of emergency physicians to have a fee-for-service practice. His influence could be seen in the stated purpose of the college—"to promote and maintain the ethical standards of private practice in emergency medicine and surgery."[3,6] The inclusion of the word "surgery" would come back to haunt this young college. Surgeons who caught wind of the new organization and its purposes assumed that emergency physicians wanted to see patients in the ED and then take them to the operating room to perform surgical procedures, although none of the original eight did this. Since many general practitioners (GPs) performed surgery in the 1960s, and some of the original college members (like Wiegenstein) were GPs, it was a plausible threat to surgeons that emergency doctors might siphon off some surgical procedures. Just as James Mills had to confront concerns from local physicians about "patient stealing" when he started the Alexandria group, the founders of the ACEP faced early resistance from surgeons and others who were threatened by this growing new practice.

The organizational meeting concluded with the election of Wiegenstein as chairman of the ACEP, Rogers as the treasurer, and Maria Maraveleas of Medical Ancillary Services as the executive director. The physicians apparently did not perceive a conflict of interest in naming as executive director of their new organization the person who was doing the billing for their private emergency practices.[6]

The motivation for forming a national organization had two main components. First was the altruistic desire, best expressed by Wiegenstein, who noted:

> *Actually it was fueled by my desire to have training programs. I had to train myself, selfishly. I wanted to…have an association where we invite people in from surgery, internal medicine, and say what do we do the first hour? I'm tired of going to courses that tell us about how you handle an emergency in the operating room. I want to know [for] that first hour what needs to be done. You come and tell us that. I wanted somebody to come in and sort of outline for us what we need to know in order to be good emergency physicians.[3]*

It is interesting to note how, at this stage, Wiegenstein's ideas about what emergency medicine encompassed and what it might become were so undeveloped that he looked to established medicine to tell him "what we need to know."

The educational component was clearly a necessity for the early emergency physicians. Many who were practicing by 1968 had only 1 year of internship. Because it was believed from the start that the best emergency physicians were "generalists," the standard had become, by default, 1 year of postgraduate training.[7] This was reinforced by the hiring practices of the early leaders. By 1968, many of the early emergency physician groups were enticing interns, even those who may have planned further residency training, to join their groups. By offering attractive annual salaries of $25,000 or more, the groups were able to lure many interns away from additional residency training to become, at least temporarily, emergency physicians.[8] Expectations were also starting to change in what an emergency physician could offer. No longer were EDs primarily the domain of drunks and itinerant physicians. As physicians and the public came to understand that in some communities a group of physicians was now "specializing" in emergency care, these physicians were expected to have advanced knowledge like a specialist. Unfortunately, the great majority did not have the residency training of specialists, and most were not inclined to go back to the harrowing work hours of residency to obtain further training. Even if they had the inclination, the existing residency programs in other fields like internal medicine or surgery were not geared toward emergency care and would leave gaps in training. The early emergency physicians soon learned that internship training alone did not necessarily prepare one well to deliver quality emergency care. In addition, the rapid pace of medical advances in areas like cardiac care, resuscitation, and pharmacology in the mid 1960s was making what they learned in medical school and internship obsolete. Physicians such as Wiegenstein developed a healthy sense of awe and fear about what needed to be learned to function well in the emergency department. Desperate for that education, Wiegenstein envisioned a national organization that would provide courses in emergency care to boost the inferior knowledge base of those in emergency practice.

In spite of the emphasis placed by Wiegenstein on education, the stated purpose of the original ACEP did not include any mention of education or training of physicians. This is most likely due to the dominance of the second motivating factor for the formation of a national organization by the Michigan physicians—finances. The decision to become an emergency physician in the 1960s was as much about lifestyle and income as it was about practice content or the science of the field. Both for those physicians who left their practices to become emergency physicians and for interns who were deciding if they wanted to join emergency groups, a fundamental question was, can I make the same or better money as an emergency physician as I would in other fields? Whether the answer was in the affirmative depended on the business setup of the group and reimbursement for services. Blue Cross and Blue Shield ("the Blues," or BC/BS) was an important part of the private health insurance marketplace in the state. Physician fee schedules were stratified, with specialists receiving higher reimbursements for patient care than generalists. Procedures received higher reimbursement than nonprocedural care. Emergency physicians were a new entity, and insurance companies did not have separate billing categories for emergency physician work. Because most emergency physicians were not specialists, reimbursements were at the level of a GP. R. R. Hannas, who was a strong proponent of education and specialty development, nonetheless realized the importance of finances, noting, "You must remember…that like a lot of specialties we started basically for an economic reason."[9] The economic reason in this case was explained by John Wiegenstein in a 1969 article in *Medical Economics*:

> Essentially…our economic goals stem from an experience Michigan E.R. physicians had in the summer of 1967, when Blue Shield began cutting the fees it paid for emergency room services. We protested and won. But we recognized the fact that emergency room M.D.s ought to be able to make their weight felt with third parties, and we incorporated that idea when we formed an organization….[10]

Wiegenstein recalled that BC/BS, with no explanation, cut emergency physician payments from $15 to $7.50 per visit. While Wiegenstein was upset, he knew that the perfect warrior for this battle was John Rupke. Rupke's conservative, Calvinist upbringing made him suspicious of bureaucracy, government, and big business. He was a champion of individual freedom, especially when it came to physician autonomy in practice. In Western Michigan, where BC/BS did not have as much of the insurance market, Rupke became infuriated by the arbitrary nature of BC/BS reimbursements for emergency physician services. The Blues had set a "usual and customary fee" for emergency physician care that he felt was unreasonably low. He and his group stopped participating in BC/BS insurance and informed patients that their emergency physician fees would have to be paid directly. Rupke recalls,

> We did not participate with them. I'll tell you why and that's because they think that all the other health insurance companies are going to subsidize their subscribers. That is crooked and we will have nothing to do with that. No reason you should have your health coverage subsidized by the subscribers to other companies.[1]

This began a long, acrimonious battle between Rupke's group, and other allied emergency physician groups, and Blue Cross and Blue Shield.

Wiegenstein, Rupke, and colleagues understood that the first step to being recognized, both professionally and as a distinct economic entity as emergency specialists, was to form an organization or association. Once they had a name, members, and a purpose, they could claim that a specialty group existed. The added benefit to greater financial clout was the educational programs and services a national organization might offer to members. Wiegenstein and colleagues at this point did not conceptualize emergency medicine as a new specialty in the traditional sense of residency training programs and a certifying specialty board. They were more focused on getting existing practitioners together to determine how they could function better in the ED and maintain a financially successful and viable practice. Thoughts of residencies and a Board would come only once they made their fledgling organization truly "national." Technically, the group had become more national by the fall of 1968. William Haeck, who had started an emergency practice in Jacksonville, Florida, heard from his father back in Grand Rapids that John Rupke and some colleagues were forming an organization of emergency physicians. Haeck flew up to Michigan to attend one of the first ACEP Board meetings.[11]

The First Contact—Michigan Emergency Physicians Meet Reinald Leidelmeyer

It was shortly after the August 16, 1968, seminal meeting to incorporate ACEP when John Wiegenstein became aware of an article in *Medical World News* featuring Reinauld Leidelmeyer entitled "Does it Take a Specialist to Run Emergency Room?" The article begins with this bold statement:

> *Physicians who practice regularly in hospital emergency rooms need a national organization of their own. And one of the principal aims of such an organization should be recognition of ER work as a full-fledged medical specialty. So argues Dr. Reinald Leidelmeyer, co-chairman of the ER department at Fairfax Hospital in Falls Church, VA.[12]*

The article quotes Leidelmeyer on the benefits of a national organization relating to hospital contracts with emergency physicians.

> *…every time such a contract is worked out, the same problems arise. There are problems of compensation, of relations with the staff physicians, of administration, of liability. It is a terrible waste of time and money and effort for each hospital to go through the same growing pains when these problems have already been solved by others. A national organization of ER doctors could pool the experience of its members and help hospitals and physicians starting out along this path.[12]*

Leidelmeyer did not just focus on the business side of the field. Like Wiegenstein, he believed that training was essential, but his ideas may have been more advanced than the Michigan emergency physicians. After describing the great variety of medical conditions and procedures an emergency physician deals with, he noted,

> No average doctor knows how to handle all these things. That is why specialized training is necessary for ER work and why such work must be, and I believe soon will be, recognized as a specialty.[12]

Reinald Leidelmeyer, in 1968, was emerging from the shadows of his more famous neighbors in the Alexandria group. Leidelmeyer had initially practiced part time in the Fairfax ED, while still holding onto his general practice. By 1965, he was working full time in the ED. He became very interested in EMS and training of ambulance personnel. His contact with James Mills and the other Alexandria group physicians was minimal—they had occasional luncheons to discuss issues, but did not otherwise meet or socialize. As noted previously, Mills and his group had received a great deal of national attention and commonly received visits from physicians who were starting emergency practice in other parts of the country. Leidelmeyer, who started emergency practice at the same time as Mills, did not receive as much attention. An example of his spreading the word about emergency medicine was a visit to talk before the Pulaski County Medical Society in Little Rock, Arkansas, in April 1966.[13] Leidelmeyer authored an article entitled, "The Emergency Room: How to Cope with This New Challenge," which was published in *Virginia Medical Monthly* in 1966. The article, which can be viewed as an expansion of James Mills 1963 article on the Alexandria plan in the same journal, described many of the problematic issues facing emergency rooms and provided pragmatic solutions.[14] An intensely competitive man, Leidelmeyer also seemed to look forward and at the big picture more than the Alexandria emergency physicians. John McDade, one of the original Alexandria four, notes that before Leidelmeyer's initiative, "We never had an idea of forming a medical specialty."[15] One of their surgeon colleagues at Alexandria Hospital had suggested to James Mills that the group should think about forming a national emergency medicine organization. According to McDade, "He didn't want it. He wasn't interested in it."[15] The 1968 article in *Medical World News* put Leidelmeyer on the national scene in emergency medicine. He was contacted by numerous emergency physicians who supported a national organization, and Leidelmeyer subsequently developed plans for a national organizing meeting in Virginia in November 1968. Upon hearing about Leidelmeyer's meeting, McDade remembers Mills saying, "Oh God, who needs that?"[15]

John Wiegenstein was one of those who phoned Leidelmeyer, but unlike the others, he had already created a "national" organization. Wiegenstein described the newly formed ACEP, and invited Leidelmeyer to attend the next ACEP Board meeting. After their formative meeting in August, Wiegenstein had been busy creating a humble infrastructure for the new organization. He secured some space—a storage room in the basement of the Michigan State Medical Society (MSMS), where Herbert Auer, the executive director, was sympathetic to their cause. It was in this space that Leidelmeyer, who flew up from Virginia, observed the ACEP board meeting in the fall of 1968. Using an overturned box as a table and card table chairs, the Michigan physicians described their nascent organization. As Wiegenstein notes, Leidelmeyer, "just wasn't impressed"[3] (see insert, Figure 4). Leidelmeyer stated that his primary objection to ACEP was the large number of part-time emergency physicians in the developing organization. Although he too had been a part-time emergency physician for the first few years he worked in the Fairfax Hospital ED, Leidelmeyer did not like the Pontiac Plan–type practice and believed a national organization should have full-time practitioners as members. Based on his later writings, he also did not understand that many of the Michigan emergency physicians like Wiegenstein, Nakfoor, and Rupke were practicing full time in their EDs.[16] Sensing that things were not especially collegial, Wiegenstein sought a way to warm up Leidelmeyer. He knew that Leidelmeyer was Dutch, and figured that a visit to Holland, Michigan, a scenic and heavily Dutch community on the Lake Michigan shore, would improve Leidelmeyer's feelings toward the Michigan group. Wiegenstein took Leidelmeyer on a 2-hour trip to tour Holland, Michigan, but Leidelmeyer, again, was not very impressed. During a high-speed drive back to the airport, Leidelmeyer told Wiegenstein that he was still going to have the November meeting and that he did not consider ACEP to be a true national organization for emergency physicians.[3,5,17]

After being rejected and somewhat scorned by Leidelmeyer, Wiegenstein realized ACEP needed to look more professional and official if they were to impress others. He developed a plan to make ACEP appear like a national organization before the November meeting. First, he had to come up with some money. Dues for members had been set at $50 per year, but with only eight original members, this did not constitute much of a budget. Wiegenstein telephoned Bob Rathburn asking for help. Rathburn had 60 part-time physicians in his Flint group. He decided to make ACEP membership mandatory for his group, and collected $50 from each. The ACEP budget was now up to around $3000. Wiegenstein also needed a brochure and official membership cards. He also needed a logo, and asked Herbert Auer to help him design one. Wiegenstein said, "I don't want any snakes. I want something really professional, real sharp looking."[3,5] Auer had a son, Art, who was in his twenties and had some experience with design. He enlisted his help to work on the logo. Art Auer created a square made up of 56 smaller squares. All were dark except a "missing" white square in the middle of the third row. This represented ACEP—what was missing in American medicine. The missing square was then turned 90 degrees to become a diamond, which dotted the "i" in "American" on the logo.[18] Herbert Auer presented the design to Wiegenstein who liked it very much.[3,5] Later, Herb confessed to Wiegenstein that his son had done the logo. Within 2 years, Art Auer would become the executive director of ACEP. Wiegenstein also had a brochure, membership cards, and copies of the ACEP constitution and by-laws smartly bound in a red cover. This type of preparation would become the hall-mark of Wiegenstein's work in the world of organized medicine. Loaded with boxes of his materials, with "the ink still drying on the pages," five of the original Michigan eight—Wiegenstein, Rupke, Nakfoor, Rogers, and Leichtman—made the trip to Arlington, Virginia, for Leidelmeyer's national emergency medicine meeting. Rupke, who did not like to fly, drove and the others traveled by plane.[3,5]

The First National Meeting of Emergency Physicians

The meeting began on Saturday morning, November 16, 1968, at the Marriott Twin Bridges Motel in Arlington, just across the Potomac River from Washington, D.C. Three of the Alexandria four drove the few miles from Alexandria to Arlington. James Mills was staffing the ED that morning and had an agreement with John McDade that Mills would come to the meeting at noon, and then McDade would cover the Alexandria ED that afternoon. R. R. Hannas and Harris Graves had made the trip from the Midwest. William Haeck had flown up from Florida. The remaining physicians at the meeting were emergency practitioners from 12 different states. No physicians from the West coast, Northwest, or Texas attended. Twenty-nine emergency physicians were in the room. Other guests included Alan MacIntosh, M.D., from the American Academy of General Practice (AAGP), E. B. Struxness, M.D., from the U.S. Department of Health Education and Welfare, and Jim Reynolds from the magazine *Medical Economics*. Maria and Peter Maraveleas were there and assisted with minutes and distribution of the ACEP materials. Eugene Ford, who represented Detroit Bank and Trust and was called a "financial advisor," made the trip from Detroit to attend the meeting.[19]

Reinald Leidelmeyer, who referred to the gathering as "my meeting," welcomed the guests and opened with a presentation detailing the "evolution, growth, and utilization" of emergency departments in Fairfax County. He also discussed the need for better ambulance services and training.[19] Leidelmeyer then introduced Wiegenstein.

Although John Wiegenstein hated public speaking, his nervousness was not appar-ent, and he willed himself through his speeches. Those in attendance would have noticed a marked contrast between Leidelmeyer and Wiegenstein. Leidelmeyer was a short man, balding, with large, dark, horn-rimmed glasses. With his Dutch accent, brusque mannerisms, and umbrageous personality, he was not the type of man behind whom others would naturally rally. Wiegenstein had a presence about him. Tall, slender, with his prematurely gray–white hair coifed in a neat swirl over his forehead, Wiegenstein cut a commanding figure. Even at the age of 38, he had the air of a statesman or experienced politician (see insert, Figure 5). As the ACEP brochure and red, bound constitution and by-laws were distributed to the attendees, Wiegenstein described what had been accomplished in Michigan. He was low key and did not make a big sales pitch for ACEP at that moment, but did make note of the newly printed membership applications.

The next person to be introduced by Leidelmeyer was Alan MacIntosh, M.D., of Vienna, Virginia. MacIntosh was representing the AAGP and presumably became aware of the meeting from Hannas and Graves, who were active in that organization. The AAGP was less than a year from becoming the American Academy of Family Practice and was eager to absorb the emergency physicians as a subsidiary of their group. MacIntosh made his pitch, but it met a tepid response. After this, following an illogical agenda, Maria Maravelas was introduced. She stated that Medical Ancillary Services, Inc., had "offered its organizational assistance and facilities to the American College of Emergency Physicians for as long as its board and its members felt that a need for such assistance existed."[19] Leidelmeyer thought that this arrangement was inappropriate, and later expressed his dissatisfaction to Wiegenstein in private.

A formal discussion of the merits of joining the AAGP then occurred, and consensus was reached that the emergency physicians should not be a subsidiary of the AAGP. Ironically, the next presenter was R. R. Hannas, who at the time was working for the AAGP on its move toward official specialty recognition by the American Board of Medical Specialties. Hannas was secretary of the Exam Committee, charged with developing the board certification exam. Hannas had learned a great deal about what it takes to become a medical specialty from his work with the AAGP. While at the AAGP, Hannas met Ward Darley, M.D., who was a giant figure in medicine in the 1950s and 1960s. Darley was from Colorado and was trained as an internist. He was dean of the Colorado Medical School and then became president of the University of Colorado. Darley was very active in the American Association of Medical Colleges (AAMC) and helped develop the National Intern Matching Program. He served as AAMC President in 1953.[20] While working for the AAGP in the 1960s, Darley did research on the evolution of medical specialties, and he referred Hannas to literature in this area. Hannas also relied upon Lynn Carmichael, M.D., a family practice leader from Florida who was a key leader in organizing the family practice movement toward medical specialty board approval. When Hannas went to the Arlington meeting of emergency physicians, he still viewed himself as someone who was moonlighting in EDs, but through Harris Graves, he was becoming more interested in the field. Unlike Wiegenstein, Hannas had no problem getting up in front of others and expressing his views. Having traveled the same road with general practice, he believed that he knew the basic elements of how to become a specialty. Hannas recalls:

> I said the first thing you guys have to do, I told them about the evolution of specialties…I said you have to first define your content and I said, here we got a start. I had a long sheet of paper, they all called it the toilet paper, but I had the things that they could do and how they should do it, outlined even the content itself.[9]

When Hannas got up to speak at the initial meeting he presented concepts that were somewhat dizzying to most of those in the audience. Neither the Alexandria group or Wiegenstein's primitive ACEP organization were at that time thinking of a new specialty of medicine—they were trying to bring emergency physicians together for advantages in the business side of the field and to develop educational programs.[3,15] Hannas was looking a few more years down the line; he was promoting the idea of a new specialty. Perhaps this seemed like the logical way to proceed because he had been immersed in this process with the GPs. Going to the blackboard, he drew a circle of components that could lead to a new specialty of emergency medicine, enumerating the importance of each, and noting how a circle of activity and achievements would lead back to the start of the circle (see insert, Figure 6). The first component was definition of the content of the field. Next was the development of graduate training programs and departments of emergency medicine in medical schools. The development of a specialty board with a certifying exam was next. Continuing education to maintain standards and the development of research were the final components that would feed back to continually redefine the content of the specialty.[18] Hannas drew a specialty organization as a catalyst in the center of the circle, promoting each step toward specialty development. Those in attendance were impressed with Hannas's knowledge in this area. John McDade remembers, "I thought geez, we got this, this guy is going to be useful!" Hannas would give this same presentation repeatedly in the next few years, showing the simple but essential steps. He closed his presentation by making a strong pitch to adopt ACEP as the national specialty organization for emergency medicine, saying, "We came here to set up a national organization, but the Michigan guys have already done it, lets just join their group and make it national!"[3,5]

After some brief discussion, a motion was made to install ACEP as the national organization of emergency medicine, with the retention of its board and officers until a congress of delegates was convened to elect a national board. Wiegenstein humbly acknowledged the approval of the group and directed it for its first task. Nine regional representatives were selected from those physicians attending to assist with recruiting on a national level. The morning session then adjourned. James Mills had arrived late and was very quiet during the discussion. Reinald Leidelmeyer may have been somewhat miffed by the adoption of ACEP as the national organization, but he did not offer any formal resistance. Lunch was held in a dining room at Fairfax Hospital. Leidelmeyer had arranged for a photographer to take some pictures as the doctors dined (see insert, Figure 7).

The meeting reconvened at 3 PM and as a result of some lunchtime discussion and negotiations to "de-Michiganize" ACEP, Leidelmeyer and Mills were elected to the board of directors. Over the next few hours, the group discussed committees and who would serve in what roles, but a final decision on committee memberships was left to the board. The meeting adjourned at 5:30 PM, and John Rupke volunteered to drive some of the physicians to dinner. Many of the men wanted a drink or two to celebrate the events of the day, but Fairfax County did not sell alcohol—it was a "dry" county. Rupke, who had previously lived in Washington for several years during medical school and his Army service, offered to take the men "across the creek" to Washington to a bar. However, the ebullient Rupke decided the group should first have a tour of embassy row. As the tired and hungry men in the back seat moaned, Rupke motored up and down the streets, giving historical details of the sites and buildings.[5] Later, over dinner, the men were full of excitement at what had been hatched that day. But, they were also cognizant of the amount of work that lay ahead.

The following day, Sunday morning, the new ACEP met again for a few hours to recapitulate how they would further organize, expand, and communicate. Probably with Leidelmeyer in mind, Wiegenstein emphasized that "all communications to members applicants and news media must emanate from the American College of Emergency Physicians headquarters, following board action and approval."[19] Leidelmeyer would soon violate this understanding by sending out his own version of the minutes of the meeting to all who attended, as well as a letter. In the letter, he seemed to still be smarting from the transfer of power from him to Wiegenstein. He commended the participants, and then had these observations:

> So often these charter–organizational meetings degenerate and or deteriorate from the start in to power plays or grabs by ambitious individuals or groups, and I do hope your wisdom to leave the provisional structure and board in the hands of those who so obviously wanted and deserved it, will prove to be another and maybe the most important accomplishment of this meeting for the future, the unity, and the long range plans for the organization.[21]

Despite his conciliatory remarks, Leidelmeyer received a stern rebuke from Wiegenstein for sending out communications without getting approval from the full Board.[3]

The struggle between Leidelmeyer and the Michigan group was an undercurrent in the meeting, but the overall tone was one of excitement. The attendees left inspired, invigorated, and feeling as if they had brethren in their new practice. William Haeck remembers,

> The meetings were pretty intense...because of the amount of work that got done, and the amount of work that needed to be done that tumbled out at the end of the meeting. There needed to be strategies for membership. The organization needed support, dollar wise. Some direction needed to be given to dealing with the AMA, the American College of Surgeons. There needed to be a strategy for the members to be effective in their local communities, in their county medical societies, in their state medical societies—to get grass root support going for emergency medicine.[11]

Before the meeting ended, Wiegenstein told all the participants that he would have membership cards made for them with their names typed in. One of the attendees, Robert Ersek, M.D., did not want to wait for a typed card. He implored Wiegenstein to become a member immediately, handed him a completed application form, and pulled out the $50 membership fee. Wiegenstein shrugged, and thought, "Why not?" He hand-wrote Ersek's name on the membership card, and Ersek, a research fellow and surgery resident from Minnesota who had been moonlighting in emergency departments, became the first card-carrying member of the new national ACEP. Ersek was active in ACEP for a few years, but then went on to become a prominent plastic and reconstructive surgeon in Texas whose antiaging medical and surgical techniques have received national media exposure.[22]

Wiegenstein and his colleagues returned home delighted with the outcome of the meeting, but knowing they would have to ramp up their organization in a hurry. The other participants, except perhaps for Leidelmeyer, were enthused and filled with a new sense of purpose, but few of them would become active in ACEP. Six attendees of the original meeting, including Wiegenstein (1968–1971) would go on to become presidents of ACEP in the next decade—Mills (1971–1973), Hannas (1973–1974), Haeck (1974–1975), Graves (1975–1976), and McDade (1979–1980). The stance of James Mills at the end of the November 1968 meeting might be described as watchful waiting. Mills and his colleagues had not promoted emergency medicine as a medical specialty. As this emerged as a goal for the new organization, Mills was reticent at first. Within a few years, he would become a leader and a strong voice for the establishment of emergency medicine as a medical specialty. But, in 1968, the man who had started it all in 1961 was more of a passive participant than a prime mover in the national organizing process in emergency medicine.

Growing Up As a National Organization

The formation of ACEP was a classic case of "if you build it, they will come." Word of the November national organizing meeting was picked up in the national medical newspapers. In the December 13 issue of *Medical World News* a boxed article in "News of the Week" entitled "Emergency Room MDs Form National Group" described the organizing meeting and requirements for membership. Wiegenstein also remembers an article in a national medical newspaper that stated the purpose of ACEP was "to get a better deal from hospitals."[5] Although Wiegenstein was appalled to have this message broadcast as the reason for ACEP's existence, he admits that it greatly boosted membership. The national publicity came before ACEP was ready to handle an onslaught of new members. Hundreds of emergency physicians contacted Wiegenstein, sending letters and telephoning him, expressing their appreciation for his work and the existence of a national organization. They also were looking for help. Wiegenstein remembered that many of the letters had the tone,

> "Thank God! We finally have somebody to send all these problems to solve." I sent back a note saying we are a young organization. We will have those answers in the future, but right now I'm afraid we are all in the same boat, but continue your interest and we'll find out how to answer your questions and problems.[3]

Wiegenstein remembers being flooded with requests for membership. He was also getting requests by hospitals and emergency groups who were seeking to hire emergency physicians. Young physicians and medical students wrote to find out if residency programs existed in this new field.[23] Federal agencies, state departments of health, Boeing Corporation, emergency department directors, and hospital administrators all sent letters to ask questions, request assistance, or show their support.[24] Wiegenstein tried to phone or write back to many of these inquiries, but he had no support staff,

> No one was working for us. All these applications were received, and I kept them in my briefcase. I'd say a couple of hundred. I just couldn't handle it myself and so I went to the Medical Society and said can you give us some part time help? Can we share a secretary or something? They said sure so they introduced us to Jackie and we paid one third of her salary and took up seven eighths of her time.[3]

The Michigan State Medical Society again helped ACEP by offering the secretarial services of Jackie Van Deventer. After a few weeks of organizing and informal communications, board meetings were held in Lansing every 2 to 4 weeks through June of 1969. Naturally, the out-of-state board members, Leidelmeyer, Mills, Hannas, and Graves were unable to attend most meetings. In the February meeting, it was announced that John Rogers, one of the original eight Michigan ACEP members, had assumed the role of acting executive director because the Maraveleas' had resigned from the position due to "the possibility of a question of conflict of interest."[25] Leidelmeyer's concerns about this conflict had apparently been heard by Wiegenstein and the rest of the board, resulting in the Maraveleas's exit. They did not go quietly and soon sent a bill to ACEP for several thousand dollars for the services they had provided. This debt would become an albatross around the neck the ACEP budget for at least 2 years. Other key business during this meeting was the installation of William Haeck of Florida as the Membership Chairman, replacing Robert Leichtman, who had resigned. Leichtman resurfaced a few years later as a "psychic physician" and faith healer.[26] During the February 1969 meeting, Wiegenstein also announced the appointment of John Van de Leuv, M.D., as the chairman of the Commission of Publication. Van de Leuv replaced George Fink, M.D., who had written the first ACEP Quarterly Report. Fink's first editorial in the Quarterly Report was a bit too saucy for Wiegenstein's taste,

> He said don't let anyone "shit on your statue" or something like that. He used language that I didn't think was appropriate for our first report.[3]

Fink was angry when Wiegenstein told him to tone down the editorials. He vindictively told Wiegenstein that he was aware that Wiegenstein had a medical school loan from the Washtenaw County Medical Society. Fink told Wiegenstein that it was "real poor taste for a national organization leader to have a debt to the Medical Society."[3] According to Wiegenstein, Fink offered to pay the loan off and said that if Wiegenstein could not pay it, he should resign. Wiegenstein decided to bring the matter up to the board. In a closed-door session, with Wiegenstein out of the room, the ACEP board debated and sided with Wiegenstein. Shortly after, Fink quit the organization. This left only Wiegenstein, Rupke, Rogers, Van de Leuv, Nakfoor, and Robert Rathburn to do the work. Whether by design, or circumstances, ACEP resembled a regional organization more than a national organization for the first 8 months of its existence. Leidelmeyer sent frequent letters addressing board business and complained about being left out of the loop. After about 6 months, Wiegenstein agreed to hold board meetings at the Detroit Metropolitan Airport to make it easier for out-of-state board members to attend. It was only after this change that the Board meetings truly had national representation.

ACEP was on shaky footing at this point. It had reserves of around $6000, but the Maraveleas's debt had to be paid. Also, there were problems with the landlord. Upon learning that ACEP was now a national organization, the MSMS was in the strange situation of being a state medical organization with a national specialty organization headquartered in its basement. Although the MSMS agreed to house ACEP offices for another year, it was clear that the ACEP could not reside in the MSMS long term.[27] Despite these local problems, ACEP forged ahead with a national focus.

Wiegenstein realized he needed help with his plans for a national organization. The American Medical Association was a logical place to turn, and R. R. Hannas had mentioned in his talk on specialty formation that it was essential to work with the powers that be in the AMA. The AMA had not been opposed to emergency medicine. In fact, it had published the well-known booklet on emergency departments in 1966 and shortly after that had formed the Commission on Emergency Medical Services. Wiegenstein decided he would go to the AMA headquarters in Chicago. As a neophyte to medical politics, he did not realize that a prescheduled appointment might be a good idea. Instead, he called up John Rupke, picked him up in Grand Rapids, and they drove the 3 hours to Chicago. They walked in to the AMA offices and asked to speak with Leo Brown, the executive vice president. Amazingly, they were ushered in to meet Brown, and they presented to him their dilemma. Wiegenstein recalled,

> We told him, we have this organization, we've got memberships galore, and don't really know what to do with them. And, they're asking questions, very important questions like, how do we manage an emergency department? These were the things I wanted to know![5]

Brown was understanding and helpful. As Wiegenstein remembered,

> …he sort of was amused by it all and I think it was kind of refreshing—that we wanted to do this. He said, "I'll help you out. Do you want to have a meeting here in Chicago? We can help you here." I said, "That would be fine. Where would we have it?" "At the Palmer House," he said, "You need a brochure?" I said, "Can you help us with that?" He said, "Yeah, we'll print your brochure for you."[3]

John Rupke remembers that Brown was supportive when they told him that they wanted their new organization to be "under the umbrella of the AMA." Brown, who would work for the AMA for 25 years said, according to Rupke, "This is one of the most exciting things I have heard in the period of time I have been here."[5] Rupke notes that Brown was probably having visions of many new AMA members pulled from the ranks of ACEP.[1]

An AMA-prepared brochure was sent out, with the ACEP logo on the front. The AMA also invited, and in some cases paid for, outside speakers to attend. About 50 ACEP members came to Chicago for the February 7–8, 1969, meeting. One of the main purposes was to shore up the regional, state-wide system for membership. The original plan was to have states form chapters, which would be granted charters by the national ACEP. The problem was a lack of resources and experience on the part of those who were trying to form the state organizations. William Haeck, who was the Membership Committee chair, had done a laudable job in Florida. Very much like a traveling salesman, he traversed the state soliciting for members of the Florida chapter. He recalls that he,

> Went to the Florida Hospital Association and got addresses for all the hospitals in Florida and mailed out those packages to the emergency rooms in all the hospitals in Florida. When I had 3 and 4 days off together, I took that list and divided the state into four or five areas and just got in my car, had a leased old Buick convertible, and I just drove to the section I had outlined and just walked blind into the hospital emergency room. Probably in most of the hospitals in the state of Florida. If a doc was there, I talked with them, if there was no doc there I left material all over the emergency department lounge, talked to the nurses, tried to get names and addresses of docs… I just went cold turkey into the emergency room and discovered what was going on. That's all I was really looking for—I was looking for members. By 1970 I had identified, I'm guessing, 100 and got 100 to sign up. That was the big trip, getting them to pay a little bit of dues money and sign up.[11]

Other states were far behind Florida. Given that the national office had only around $5000 in its coffers, it could not provide financial support for state ACEP offices. In the days before inexpensive copiers and electronic communication, it was not only more difficult, but far more expensive to copy notices and publications of interest to members and to mail them out. One of the early priorities for ACEP was to get tax-exempt status from the government to get a better rate on mailings and purchases.

The national meeting at the Palmer House in February 1969 was attended by about 70 emergency physicians from 16 states.[28] The meeting allowed members from various practice settings to compare strategies and devise solutions to common problems. The meeting was also a chance for ACEP members to see how big an impact their organization might have on the national medical scene. Jack Hall, M.D., the vice president and director of medical education of the AMA, spoke to the group. Irvin "Chief" Henderson, who was the chairman of the AMA Commission on Emergency Medical Services spoke about how the AMA was promoting emergency medical education and EMS.[5,25] Next was Herbert Flessa, the Cincinnati internist who was the director of outpatient services at Cincinnati General Hospital. Flessa became aware of ACEP and came from Cincinnati to present his plans for starting a residency program. Flessa had approached the AMA with his idea and presumably found out about the ACEP meeting through his contacts at the AMA. At this point, Flessa had no residents. Bruce Janiak, who was a few months from finishing medical school, had committed to doing a rotating internship and would begin the emergency medicine residency in July 1970. Flessa presented his tenuous vision for training emergency medicine residents to the new, tenuous national emergency medicine organization.

On the following day, more prominent guests gave presentations to the small ACEP board. R. R. Hannas spoke about becoming a specialty. Joseph Owen, from the U.S. Public Health Service, who Wiegenstein had first met a few years earlier at the Akron EMT course, talked about community emergency services. Sam Seeley, M.D., from the National Academy of Sciences (NAS)/National Research Council, and one of the principles in the "Accidental Death and Disability..." report talked about the role of the NAS in emergency care services. Clearly, ACEP, with barely 200 members in 1969, was important to those in government and medicine who had been working in emergency services. The government officials probably saw the inexperienced but eager emergency physicians as potential worker bees for their lofty goals of improved emergency department, EMS, and trauma care in the United States. ACEP members, most of whom, like Wiegenstein, felt like amateurs in the professional world of medical politics, were surprised at the stature their young organization had achieved. Even before ACEP had proved itself as a legitimate organization, it was attracting attention far beyond its years.

The final speaker at the ACEP organizational meeting in February 1969 was Robert H. Kennedy, M.D., the surgeon who had pioneered trauma care improvements, who had coined the term "weakest link" for emergency departments and who had personally visited and surveyed hundreds of emergency departments in the early 1960s. Kennedy spoke about the role of the American College of Surgeons in emergency care. While it may not have been fully appreciated by those in attendance that day, the address by the 82-year-old Kennedy to the new group of nonsurgeon emergency practitioners, who were on average less than half his age, was an important passing of the torch for the field of emergency medicine.[25]

Wiegenstein and the other ACEP leaders returned from the Palmer House meeting feeling both energized and overwhelmed. The spring and summer of 1969 were spent processing new member applications, dealing with the bleak financial picture, and planning the first educational meeting for members in the fall. John Rupke was now able to use the national presence of ACEP in his campaign against medical insurance companies. He conducted a survey of ACEP members to see how Blue Cross and Blue Shield were perceived by emergency physicians in Oklahoma and Michigan. Rupke presented a statement for inclusion in the May 1969 ACEP board of directors meeting minutes that questioned,

> ...the ever increasing stature of third party intervention in the provision of medical services...Regional representatives are advised to endeavor to determine what amount

of money is being expended yearly to support prepaid insurance plans and what percentage of these monies are never paid to the subscriber, the hospital or physician. The cost of the third party in medicine is never published in the public media, but constitutes a very significant portion of the medical services dollar.[29]

Rupke relished his role as the back room, man in black, getting his hands dirty with the finances and hidden politics of emergency medicine while Wiegenstein and others were the up-front diplomats of the organization. When asked why he came to fill this role, Rupke says,

Because we needed an activist role, and I'm ugly. I'm dead serious. I'm meaner than any of those guys. I've been around. I've seen what had been going on in the hospitals all the time and the way the hospitals operate and the way the health insurance companies operated, and I already had enough experience with them and knew it was going to be bad.[1]

One idea that Rupke, Wiegenstein, and John Rogers had explored from the start of ACEP in Michigan was an arrangement for profit sharing and pooled insurance for ACEP members. Although it was not widely spoken of, or recorded in the minutes of the initial meetings, this was probably the reason why a Detroit banker, Eugene Ford, made the trip to Arlington for the first national ACEP meeting in 1968. From its early months, ACEP had an Insurance Committee, headed by Rogers, which explored financial benefits for ACEP members. The profit-sharing scheme was initially proposed as "a master agreement by which a bank would manage profit-sharing money generated by incorporated ER groups."[10] The plan was explored with various financial companies and banks but had died out by the middle of 1970 when non-Michigan ACEP board members such as R. R. Hannas were not enthusiastic about a profit-sharing service for ACEP members. In retrospect, it was ironic that ACEP leaders spent time and energy trying to secure financial advantages for individual members while the organization was on such tenuous financial footing. Rogers and others looked to foundations as possible sources of money for ACEP, including the nearby Kellogg Foundation in Michigan, but no significant outside funding was forthcoming in the early years. ACEP also explored a group life insurance plan for members, but a survey of members did not reveal much interest, and this was also tabled by late 1970.[30] Around this time malpractice and liability insurance was beginning to become a problem, and by early 1971, ACEP was exploring a college-sponsored professional liability program.[31]

Changes were made to the constitution and by-laws in the first year of ACEP's existence to reflect the broader mission. William Weaver, who was an original Alexandria group member, was put in charge of revising the Wiegenstein version of the constitution and by-laws. Revisions adopted in June 1969 included deleting the word "surgery" from any mention of emergency medicine practice and adding to the purposes and objectives statements about promoting research and providing representation in organized and academic medicine. The board debated whether ACEP members should be full-time practitioners of emergency medicine. The purists believed that the future of emergency medicine depended on well-trained, full-time emergency physicians. The pragmatists in the organization realized that in 1969, not many full-time emergency physicians existed and that building ACEP membership numbers and revenues would require including part-time emergency physicians. The result was the requirement for an ACEP member to devote "a significant portion of his medical practice to emergency care." Except for dropping the word "surgery" at the end, this was no different from the description in Wiegenstein's original ACEP constitution. The constitution and by-laws also allowed for up to three of nine members of the board of directors to be "not exclusively engaged in the practice of emergency medicine."[32] The organization worked with this constitution and by-laws until 1972, when Harris Graves directed a major revision of the document.

The next major thrust was for ACEP to put on a credible educational meeting for members. R. R. Hannas, as the chair of the Education Committee was charged with this task. In typical presumptuous manner, the group called this meeting the First

Scientific Assembly of the American College of Emergency Physicians. R. R. Hannas wanted to hold the meeting at Estes Park, Colorado, where he had spoken before on emergency medicine topics at an annual medical meeting. Hannas received a commitment from the Estes Park organizers to allow ACEP to hold the meeting in November, but they then reneged. Hannas remembers:

> Flat-ass turned me down. Made my shit list, of course. But, I got in a phone booth the day he turned me down...I called John. I said, "Colorado won't sponsor us so let's do it on our own." He said, "Can we do it?" I said, "Yeah." So we did. We did it on our own.[9]

They made arrangements with the Hilton Hotel in Denver, Colorado, and the first national educational meeting for emergency physicians, developed by emergency physicians, was booked, but far from ready to go. Speakers had to be secured, and Hannas relied on his many friends and colleagues from other fields to serve as presenters. The presenters were asked to cover the emergency aspects of their topic. At the bottom of the brochure announcing the meeting was an indication of how early ACEP was an all-male organization: "Bring your wife along with you. And don't forget your skiis [sic]. The skiing is great in Denver." Wiegenstein remembered that a few months before the meeting, they still did not have a final program,

> I was really worried because R. R. kept procrastinating. I said please send me a list of speakers, we have people coming to this thing! And so he finally sent me this hand-written, scribbled program, laid out, and he said I'm going to leave it up to you to get the psychiatric speaker. I couldn't find anybody locally. So I went to the membership roster and called on this guy named Abraham Twerski, and he was a psychiatrist from Pittsburgh...He came. John Rogers of course was the treasurer—he and I were the whole staff at that time. We had a little cart standing outside the door getting walk-ins and things of that nature, and we paid him money to drive. We were kind of waiting, he hadn't shown up. His talk was going to come up in an hour and we haven't seen the guy, what would we do? And this guy walks in with full black robe on to the floor and a rabbi hat on. He walks up and he says, "Is this the American College of Emergency Physicians meeting?" And I said, "Yes." I said, "Who are you?" He said, "I'm Dr. Twerski." John and I looked at each other and said, "Oh my God!" I said, I'm very happy you got here and so forth and then he said, "By the way can my brother watch my lecture?" We said, "Sure." "Do we have to pay anything?" "No, he can just show up." I said, "How will we recognize him?" He said, "He looks just like me. He's a rabbi too!" They both went in. He gave a talk. The guys were rolling in the aisles laughing. It was the funniest, funniest psychiatric lecture. They really enjoyed it. I remember one thing, he said, "There's a psychiatric condition—we're trying to determine what's real, what's organic, and what's psychiatric. This psychiatric condition is very classical. They tell you they've got this terrible headache, like a spike driven right in their head." Then he shows some x-rays. "Sometimes you can take an x-ray." And this guy's got this spike right through his head! That was our meeting at Denver...."[3]

The first ACEP Scientific Assembly had 130 attendees. This was about 20% of ACEP's 650 members at the time. More might have attended, but to save money, the brochures for the Scientific Assembly were sent by third-class mail and took over 5 weeks to reach members.[33] The program was a hodgepodge of lectures on emergency topics given by nonemergency physicians, including a cardiologist, ophthalmologist, trauma surgeon, thoracic surgeon, and plastic surgeon. The other presentations focused on emergency practice and were given by Hannas, Nakfoor, Mills, Graves, and Rathbun. Wiegenstein, who at this stage was too podium-shy to deliver a presentation, deferred to the others and had no official role in the program. But, despite the slapped-together nature of the meeting, the emergency physicians who attended were very pleased. Wiegenstein remembered, "You could just feel the enthusiasm in the hallway. They were just vibrant."[3]

The board of directors met in the evening with dinner. For the first time, some of the wives of ACEP members attended the meeting and were even present for the board meeting. Friendships were started among the wives and couples that would go on to span four decades. Although the first scientific assembly was not the most professionally produced educational meeting, its impact on the early emergency physicians was considerable. William Haeck, who attended the meeting, remembers how difficult it was to become educated as an emergency physician:

> You have to realize that all of us came from different backgrounds and none of us had been particularly trained across the broad spectrum of what we were seeing. Just as an example for me, I was reading all the x-rays after hours and sometimes during the day and had no training beyond internship in doing that. My own solution was to, through a friendship with a radiologist at the hospital, arrange that I would spend 2 hours in the radiology department behind his back as he read films for the first 2 hours in the morning after I was coming off the night shift. I recall going to an American College of Surgeons meeting in San Francisco, very early on. Picked topics that I wanted to listen to, and getting about 2 or 3 or maybe 5 minutes worth of good stuff out of there. It was really clear that we needed education that we designed and at those very early times of scientific assemblies it was really a joy because you were spending time at a lecture where you got the stuff that you needed and we really had to repeat over and over again to speakers that we weren't interested in how to do an appendectomy, we were interested in the diagnosis and that was about it. Had to coach the speakers…The other joy of those early meetings was to discover that there were people all over the United States who had the same experience you had had, and were doing the same thing that you were doing.[11]

The first scientific assembly was also successful in that it did not lose money. With a balance of $4006 on December 15, 1969, treasurer John Rogers was happy to report that the scientific assembly had expenses of $9900, but had made a little over $10,000.

The ACEP leaders had little time to reflect on their first successful "scientific" meeting. They were now planning another national meeting for February 1970 (see insert, Figure 8). As Wiegenstein noted in his chairman's comments in the January 1970 Quarterly Report, the purpose of this meeting, was "to set goals for 1970, within the limitations of our budget. In other words this will actually be a *workshop* for committee action."[33] The meeting was held in the Downtowner Motel in New Orleans, just off the French Quarter. Ninety members attended, many with their wives, and the committee structure was shored up, with many new members assigned to committees and given tasks to carry out.

A couple of the new faces who showed up in New Orleans were George Podgorny, the extensively trained surgeon from Winston-Salem, North Carolina, and Karl Mangold, who had started his northern California emergency group about 3 years before. Podgorny found out about ACEP in 1969, and with a colleague applied for membership and a charter for a state chapter in North Carolina. He remembers his first experience with ACEP:

> We all met in one room and after, decided that there is no way we can deal with everything as a group, decided to break into four original committees. One was called Hospital Committee, one was called Finance Committee, one was called Education Committee, and one was called Publications Committee. Then since we had only one room, we moved the chairs and gathered them in the four corners. It was very noisy because everybody was talking and we said that we got to get organized. So a decision was that if we were going to progress we would need to do four things and that is why the four committees. (a) We got to have some money, got to have dues and/or something; (b) We got to deal with hospitals, we are not in office practice. We are totally dependent on hospitals… (c) We will need to have an Education Committee, because we need to educate ourselves. In order to do that we need to have—(d) Publications and meetings. It was decided that as soon as we could gather some money we're going to get full-time staff.[34]

Wiegenstein and the board were delighted to have people like Podgorny and Mangold in the organization. Sharing the workload was an absolute necessity.

Wiegenstein and the other original leaders were struggling with the enormity of their responsibilities. Membership was approaching 1,000, and the only hired staff was part timer, Jackie Vandeventer. Wiegenstein's clinical emergency department work at St. Lawrence Hospital called for 56 hours per week. When he was out of town on ACEP business, his partners Eugene Nakfoor or Gaius Clark had to fill in his shifts. Wiegenstein was concerned about unduly burdening his partners. None of the ACEP leaders received reimbursement for travel, or any other compensation for their organizational work—the early budget did not allow it. Wiegenstein estimates that in the early years he spent almost a quarter of his salary each year conducting ACEP-related business.[3] At the New Orleans meeting, the ACEP board decided to reduce the frequency of meetings to a maximum of four per year. Reinald Leidelmeyer, perhaps wary that the Michigan ACEP leaders were trying to ramrod items through during board meetings, asked that board meetings be scheduled for longer periods of time to allow "the proper time for many important decisions."[35]

The burgeoning membership now provided enough dues money for Wiegenstein to hire a full-time executive director. He did not have to look far. Art Auer, the young man who had covertly designed the ACEP logo at the request of his father, Herbert Auer, the executive director of the MSMS, was bright, energetic, and readily available. Herb Auer's generosity in providing physical space in the MSMS basement for ACEP to grow may have figured in Wiegenstein's employing his son. Hired in the summer of 1970, Art Auer had an exciting start. One of his first tasks was to travel to Las Vegas and the Hotel Sahara for a planning committee meeting for the upcoming second Scientific Assembly. Auer prepared an outrageously detailed, five-page account of his trip for Wiegenstein, including the fact that he was "treated to the midnight show starring Jack Benny at the Hotel."[36]

The ACEP board realized that part of what R. R. Hannas had described as "content" for a developing field was having a credible journal. The ACEP Quarterly Reports were an extremely valuable source of information for members, but provided only bits of medical practice or scientific education. A journal called *Emergency Medicine* already existed and by 1971 was widely circulated. This was a "throw away"–type journal, published out of New York City. ACEP had approached the editor, Irving Cohen, about advertising for the ACEP Scientific Assembly in *Emergency Medicine*. A few months later, Cohen made an offer to provide ACEP with two to four pages of his journal per month for ACEP related news or articles. The ACEP Publication Committee discussed the advantages in publicity that *Emergency Medicine* might provide, but rejected this offer. George Podgorny, a member of the Publications Committee led the opposition. Podgorny was the most "academic" of the early ACEP members. He was a member of the American College of Surgeons and the Association for Academic Surgeons, which had just created its own journal. Podgorny had already published in surgical journals. He notes, "I understood the importance of it…I was attuned to it and couldn't understand why anybody would want a new group to have a captive journal."[34] The Publications Committee decided that ACEP would produce its own journal by early 1971, with John van de Leuv as the editor.[37] Since the name "Emergency Medicine" was already being used, and Cohen claimed sole rights to the name, ACEP could not use those words in the name of their journal. They settled for the bland but accurate name, *Journal of the American College of Emergency Physicians* (JACEP). It took van de Leuv about a year to get the journal up and running. The first bimonthly volume of the JACEP was published in January of 1972. There were no true scientific articles or original research contributions. The articles were reviews of topic areas of interest to emergency physicians. The back portion of the journal was reserved for a section on ACEP news and was printed in a light blue. These "blue pages" served as the chief source of information on ACEP and the drive for specialty status for emergency physicians.

ACEP continued to develop "socioeconomic" policies relating to contracts between emergency physicians and hospitals with the primary intent to "assure the allocation of the professional fee to the emergency physician." The organization also seemed to be acquiring more of a social consciousness as it became larger and more national in scope. The Socioeconomic Committee of ACEP modified its purposes in 1971 to include actions to "promote and maintain the highest quality of emergency care to the entire social spectrum of the population" and to reinforce that delivery of emergency service is "primary and independent of the ability of the patient to pay for these services." However, ACEP was not advocating that emergency physicians work for free. John Rupke's hand can be seen in the next section of the principles: "To promote the policy that it is the community's obligation to responsibly bear the cost of these and other health services for those unable to pay for their medical care."[38]

The second scientific assembly at the Sahara Hotel in Las Vegas in the fall of 1970, and the concurrent "General Assembly" meeting of ACEP is viewed by many early leaders as the point when ACEP and emergency medicine truly became a national entity. This meeting was attended by over 650 emergency physicians—representing about half of the ACEP membership. The ACEP organizers had expected no more than 400 attendees, and the assembly halls overflowed. The name of ACEP was flashing in neon on the hotel sign. Surveying this, John Wiegenstein remarked to A. L. Jenkins, an early ACEP leader from Tennessee, "A. L., now I believe ACEP will really go."[28] The educational sessions at the second scientific assembly had a more professional feel to go along with the larger audience. Commercial exhibitors from the pharmaceutical and medical supply industry were present. This meeting was not simply a group of early leaders brainstorming about how to keep their organization afloat. It was now a real business meeting, with an agenda, committee reports, matters brought to vote, and the use of Robert's Rules of Order to govern the proceedings. The entire board of directors attended. Elections were held, and John Wiegenstein was re-elected as chairman of the board. R. R. Hannas was elected vice chairman, and William Haeck was elected treasurer. Money was now flowing in—$118,000 in dues in 1970 to 1971 and $46,000 in registration fees for the Las Vegas meeting. As ACEP grew, its physical space at the Michigan State Medical Society became prohibitively small, and in April of 1971, the college moved to the nearby 241 Building in Lansing. Accommodations were better, but still not spacious or well appointed. New staff were hired and by 1975, ACEP employed more than 40 personnel.

As emergency medicine became more of national entity, the ACEP board of directors had to consider broader issues and interact with other organizations. ACEP was viewed as a focal point for every issue in emergency medicine and was often put in the position of having to react to proposals and initiatives from other organizations. For example, the Emergency Department Nurses Association formed in 1970 and immediately asked to form a strong working relationship with ACEP. These demands consumed the leaders' time and hindered ACEP in attending to its own internal needs as a rapidly growing organization. Nonetheless, in its first 4 years of existence, ACEP directed several key initiatives to move emergency medicine forward in the realm of practice, toward recognition as a medical specialty, and in the development of residency training programs.

The early leaders were beginning to find their niches in the organization and were able to use their talents accordingly. Many became good friends. The meetings themselves were more informal than today. One popular session at the early scientific assemblies in the early 1970s was called "Think and Drink." These were seminars, held from 1 to 6 PM, where "round-table discussions...provided an exchange of practical and useful information"[39] (see insert, Figure 9). The image of physicians at an official medical conference sitting around a table, some drinking alcohol and smoking cigarettes as they learned and discussed their trade seems unusual today, but was fairly standard for the early 1970s. The relationships were further developed, as would be expected in a small, new organization, not in the official meetings of the board and committees, but in the late night, informal gatherings over dinner, at a bar, or at poolside. Ideas and policies for the new organization were as likely to arise after a few drinks as they were at a board meeting. More than once, thoughts sketched on a napkin or tablet in a bar or hotel room later were formulated into proposals or policy.

R. R. Hannas played a key role in the education realm. He was the chair of the ACEP Commission on Education in the early years. Hannas appears to have favored the term "commission" over committee on the basis of his previous work with the AMA, where the former term was popular. Commonly described as "a real character," by the other early leaders, Hannas was full of energy, irreverent, fun loving, and always ready to have a beer or two and socialize after a busy day's work (see insert, Figure 10). R. R. was an excellent tennis player and would encourage other ACEP leaders and their wives to play. One of the things that colleagues of Hannas remark about is that he always wore red socks. The reason for the red socks dates back to his days in Oklahoma, and a general store that was probably very similar to the one Richard Levy's parents had owned in Kentucky,

> We were living in Sentinel, Oklahoma, I was in the rural general practice there. My number-two boy, Jake, was probably 5 or 6 years old. All those little towns there had their Dixie Store. You know most of them were run by a Hebrew family and this was. This was Joe Levine's store... (I)t was Father's Day and Jake goes down to the Dixie Store and sees Joe. Of course, everybody knows everybody in those little towns. He says, "Joe, what am I gonna get my Dad for Father's Day?" Joe says, "Jake, I got just the thing." He reaches up on the shelf. He's got a stack of three red socks that he probably has had for decades. He hadn't been able to sell them, you know. He said, "Jake, your Dad will love these." Jake said, "Fine, wrap them up." So Jake brings me these three red socks for Father's Day that year. I wore them, I loved them, I haven't worn another color since except when I'm playing tennis and I'm wearing white socks. But, it saves decisions.[9]

Hannas was responsible for the annual scientific assembly, continuing medical education, and ACEP's efforts to promote residency programs in emergency medicine. In 1971, his commission recommended that all ACEP members be required to complete 150 hours of approved postgraduate study every 3 years. This added a layer of complexity and more work for the ACEP office in verifying member's CME, but was rapidly adopted as policy by the board.

The other key area for Hannas's Commission on Education was developing some general guidelines or requirements for emergency medicine residency training. One of the requirements for recognition of emergency medicine as a specialty was the approval of emergency medicine as a separate section on emergency medicine in the council of the AMA. One of the best ways to show that emergency medicine was a separate specialty, and deserved its own section, was to establish viable residency training programs in emergency medicine, and a system for reviewing and approving those residencies. Since the Cincinnati residency had only started 7 months before, and the Cincinnati organizers were not involved in ACEP, none of the members of the original, 1971 ACEP Subcommittee on Graduate Education had any experience with emergency medicine residencies. Some, like Karl Mangold, had never completed a residency. This did not stop them from developing Proposed Essentials for a Residency Training Program for Emergency Physicians.

The chairman of the subcommittee was Ron Krome, the young surgeon from Detroit, who, just out of his residency, had been placed in charge of the Detroit General Hospital Emergency Department in 1969. By 1970, Krome had heard about the plans for the Cincinnati residency, and was thinking about forming a residency in emergency medicine at Detroit General. Krome also discovered ACEP in 1969 and applied to become a member through the Michigan chapter. He encountered some difficulty. Krome and a surgical colleague had surveyed Michigan hospitals on their emergency capabilities and rated hospitals with a point system. According to Krome, at least one early Michigan ACEP leader worked at one of the hospitals that received a low score, and held a grudge. Krome believes he was "blackballed" from becoming an ACEP member for about a year.[40] Once he was granted membership, Krome was recognized as a residency-trained academician, and he became very involved in the development of residency guidelines. Along with Hal Jayne, who was also working in the ED of Detroit General Hospital, Krome revised the original guidelines that were sent to him by Hannas. Then, at the Sarasota ACEP Winter Workshop in 1971 they were finalized, approved by the board of directors and sent to the AMA Council on Medical Education. The AMA Council refused to approve the ACEP's Proposed Essentials for a Residency Training Program for Emergency Physicians, and was not cordial in its response. At the same time, in the fall of 1971, ACEP put forth its first request for section status to the AMA. The AMA, not quite sure of what to do with this new aggressive, yet unsubstantiated group of physicians, sent the request to each of its existing sections to get their input and approval. The petition for Section status would languish for a few more years.

Hannas's good friend Harris Graves was an active member of the ACEP Board in the first four years (see insert, Figure 11). His two main accomplishments for ACEP were editing and doing much of the writing for ACEP's first published work, *The Emergency Department Management Guide*, and supervising the rewriting of the ACEP constitution and by-laws in 1971 and 1972. *The Emergency Department Management Guide* was a 19-page booklet that came out of ACEP's Commission on Hospitals, which was chaired by Graves. The booklet provided the basics of how to organize, staff, and run an ED. It was provided to all ACEP members and was sold to hospitals and other interested parties for $1 per copy.[18] One of Harris Graves most important contributions to ACEP was the revision of the constitution and by-laws. Wiegenstein's original constitution and by-laws had required several amendments and modifications in the 3 years of ACEP's existence, and it became apparent that ACEP was constrained by the system of representation and management outlined in the original constitution and by-laws. The original called for a House of Delegates that met once a year and developed policy resolutions and referendums, which the Board was obligated to carry out. The system had never been fully enacted, and early ACEP was clearly run by the board of directors, but as the organization grew to over a 1,000 members, Wiegenstein and the other founders came to realize that very little would be accomplished if an active House of Delegates began to flex its muscles or became at odds with the board of directors. This type of arrangement had periodically paralyzed the AMA for years. An Ad hoc Committee on Revising the Constitution and By-laws was appointed in 1971, with Graves as chairman, and plans were made for a Constitutional Convention in November 1972.

The ad hoc committee met on the Lake Michigan shore in Holland, Michigan, in summer 1971. George Podgorny was an important contributor to the discussion. As the committee considered different models for organizational structure and representation, Podgorny described how the American College of Surgeons was run, with a powerful physician executive director, a board of governors and a board of regents. As Podgorny remembers, the committee was "leery" about putting too much power in the hands of a physician executive director,

> We decided we were going to have a strong board of directors...have a president who changes every year...have a nonphysician management-type executive director who doesn't understand the medical issues, but will just run the mechanics of the College, and that's how we prepared the constitution and by-laws.[34]

The new constitution and by-laws created a council for ACEP, consisting of one elected councilor from each chartered chapter, and one additional councilor for each 100 members in that chapter. The ACEP Council was advisory to the board of directors, but aside from resolutions that could be submitted to the board for "consideration," it had no way of directly controlling the board. This later became important during the contentious negotiations for specialty status. The revised constitution and by-laws called for the officers, including the ACEP president, to be elected by the board of directors. The executive director was considered an employee of the board of directors. At the time the new constitution and by-laws were written, John Wiegenstein had served as chairman (president) for over 3 years. In the revised constitution and by-laws, the president was restricted to a 1-year term, after serving on the board of directors for a year as president-elect. Wiegenstein, sensing that a 1-year term was too short to understand the workings of the organization, tried to have the president's term increased to 2 years, but this motion was defeated by the board of directors.[41] In terms of members, the new constitution and by-laws mandated that active members be physicians who devote a significant portion of their endeavors to emergency medicine and who fulfilled the requirements for postgraduate education (the 150 hours of CME over 3 years).[42]

The by-laws also included ACEP's Principles of Ethical Practice. One of these principles addressed the practice of one emergency physician group covertly stealing a contract from another group: "The emergency physician shall not negotiate for a position as emergency physician in a hospital without first notifying the incumbent emergency physician concerning the proffered position and his interest in it."[42] There was no monitoring or enforcement of this principle, and it would come to be violated many times as large emergency medicine group practices and corporate groups competed for hospital contracts. Another ethical principle was "An emergency physician shall not associate himself in any fashion with any institution which permits medical practice by other than a physician." This presumably addressed the use of physician assistants or unsupervised medical students by some hospitals to provide emergency service.[42]

The new constitution and by-laws had to be approved by the ACEP House of Delegates, and a "Constitutional Convention" was held in November of 1972. Delegates objected to the new proposal for a council that had no power over the board of directors and introduced revisions to modify the arrangement. However, the existing rules called for any proposed revisions to be submitted in advance. In a narrow 32 to 28 vote, the House of Delegates voted to abide by the ruling of the chair, and then voted to adopt the new constitution and by-laws, thereby extinguishing its own existence. But, as soon as the new council attendance was called, new debates on who should be allowed to be an active member and a proposal to reinstitute the associate member status sprang up. With the new structure of ACEP, this debate was shunted to the Resolutions Committee of the Council.[43] The constitution and by-laws that Graves and his committee prepared was less egalitarian, but allowed for a more streamlined, responsive organization. The 1972 version stood the test of time and had only minor modifications over the next 25 years.

The years from ACEP's eight-person start in 1968 to the end of 1972 were a period of growth for the founders as well as the organization. By the end of 1972, ACEP was a credible national organization. The world of organized medicine and the government were very aware of ACEP, and looked first to ACEP on matters relating to emergency medicine. Where before, surgeons were viewed as the spokesmen for emergency care, it was now emergency physicians, led by ACEP. The academic world of emergency services was still confused and detached, but by 1972, it showed signs of joining the dialog. In its first 4 years, ACEP grew from its original eight to around 3,000 members. Younger emergency physicians were joining the organization. Early ACEP was run exclusively by men, but by 1971, ACEP had women members. Meeting rosters show that Isabelle Ackles, M.D., from Pittsburgh and Carol Hurley, M.D., from Lombard, Illinois, attended the ACEP Winter Workshop in Sarasota in February 1971, and Marjorie L. Smith, M.D, attended the ACEP board of directors meeting in Atlantic City in June 1971.

ACEP was no longer run out of a briefcase, on a shoe-string budget. From a budget of a few thousand dollars in its first year, ACEP grew to a budget of $340,000 by the end of 1972. The organization was financially solvent, but its only sources of revenue were member dues and meeting profits. William Haeck, the treasurer in 1972 noted that he had to sound a "recurring theme…That's a great idea but we don't have the finances."[43] John Wiegenstein served as chairman of ACEP from its inception until 1972, when James Mills was elected to replace Wiegenstein just before the new constitution and by-laws were adopted. Wiegenstein had developed dramatically as a leader in those few years. In the beginning he had been reserved, self-deprecating, often looking to others for the answers. By the end of his service as chairman, he was viewed by those within ACEP and outside as a master politician, and he was on a mission, determined to see that emergency medicine became a recognized medical specialty. R. R. Hannas, who like Wiegenstein came to the new field in a serendipitous way, remembers,

> John, was a natural leader and he knew instinctively the diplomatic way to go, whereas I would have probably run over them.[9]

Karl Mangold echoes Hannas's remarks with his assessment:

> Wiegenstein could have been Secretary of State of the United States of America. He is so diplomatic…an understated, awesomely competent, wonderfully diplomatic, great human being, kind of presence. I really believe he could have done Colin Powell's job and done it well.[44]

James Mills, Jr., who had been somewhat tepid in his initial enthusiasm for ACEP, particularly the idea of a new specialty, had been converted by his forward-looking, energetic colleagues. As the new ACEP president in 1972, he was ready to move aggressively forward toward specialty recognition. Like Wiegenstein, Mills was viewed as an excellent diplomat and negotiator. He had an elegant, upscale image that contrasted with the sometimes crass and less polished personalities of more typical early ACEP members. Mills knew wines and fine dining. His friends all called him "an Anglophile." He loved British culture and would travel with his wife each year to London for several weeks to take in the theatre and other cultural events.[45] In the early years of ACEP, Mills did not think highly of the hotels selected for ACEP meetings. Wiegenstein remembers,

> When I was president, we went to a lot of unusual places, inexpensive places, and when he became president he announced, "This is the end of the Holiday Inn era!" So our first board meeting was at the Ritz-Carlton in Boston. I went into the bathroom in my room. I saw this little bulb just hanging bare…so I kidded him. I said, "I thought this was a ritzy place, Jim. There is a bare bulb hanging in my bathroom!" He said, "Did you look at the fixture? It's gold."[3]

Mills aristocratic leanings were counter to his sentiments for the poor and common people he advocated for in medicine. He was revered by his co-workers, particularly nurses, orderlies, and paramedics. He was regarded as a father figure by students and younger colleagues. Now this compassionate aristocrat, along with his new friends, was focused on making emergency medicine a specialty. Wiegenstein notes,

> He was a master at getting consensus and getting people together. He was level headed and he was quick to point out—he would congratulate you for a job well done, and then he would tell you what was wrong with it![3]

The wisdom of the early leaders to choose as their first two presidents men who had airs of propriety and great diplomatic skills served the developing specialty well (see insert, Figure 12). Overly aggressive, hotheaded leaders would not have been received well by the AMA and elsewhere in the house of organized medicine. Wiegenstein and Mills were perfect agents for a persistent, professional approach to legitimacy for the field of emergency medicine.

It is difficult to say when ACEP leaders moved from the goal of merely forming a specialty organization to a push for a full-fledged medical specialty in the American Board of Medical Specialties. For a few early members, it was when R. R. Hannas gave his first talk about requirements for a medical specialty at Reinald Leidelmeyer's national organizing meeting in November 1968. For some, it was after the first organizational meeting at the Downtowner in New Orleans in 1970. That meeting was Karl Mangold's first, and he remembers coming away feeling like he was,

> Shot out of a cannon, because I found some other guys who thought like I did. It was so validating…I said to my wife, "I'm going to make this a specialty. We are going to have a specialty society, we're going to have boards, we're going to have residencies, we're going to be another specialty." I said, "It will take about 5 years of running around the country. Five years—alright, the kids are 7 and 5." So you figure it will be 5 years—it took us 10.[44]

By 1971, ACEP was officially pursuing a track toward specialty recognition through its efforts to have emergency medicine named as a section in the AMA. The ACEP board, on the recommendation of Ron Krome and his subcommittee on graduate education, endorsed the concept that certification in emergency medicine would be by exam only. This approval was tempered by comments that the field was still a long way away from certifying emergency physicians with a sanctioned board exam. The next phase for ACEP, its founders, and newer leaders like Podgorny, Krome, and Mangold, was to play the national politics of organized medicine in the quest for specialty status. In doing so, they would eventually link up with the academicians, who had lagged behind ACEP, but were just beginning to play a role in emergency medicine. By 1972, a handful of emergency medicine residencies had tenuously developed, and the first resident had completed training.

5 Training Emergency Physicians

The notion that it would be desirable to train physicians to practice in emergency departments (EDs) dates to at least the 1950s when Robert H. Kennedy, M.D., the surgeon who advocated for better trauma care through the American College of Surgeons, mentioned this in his addresses and writings. But Kennedy and other early leaders in emergency medical services did not feel the need for training as acutely as those pioneers who first left their practices to work full time in EDs. The first emergency physicians realized that they lacked the training to be able to handle the great variety of critical and noncritical emergency cases and had to learn on the job. R. R. Hannas may have been the exception. He had some surgical training and a vast amount of experience as a general practitioner (GP) with little backup. This allowed an easier transition to his ED work. But, although he felt comfortable in the ED, Hannas was a champion of the idea that education had to be the main thrust of early organized emergency medicine. This meant training the current practitioners and promoting the development of residency training programs so that future emergency physicians would be far better prepared for their practices than the pioneers who left other fields to pursue emergency medicine.

Every early emergency physician had knowledge gaps. For someone like George Podgorny, who had extensive training as a general and thoracic surgeon, it might have been pediatric medical conditions. For someone like John Wiegenstein, who was general practice–trained, it was trauma care and orthopedics. As William Haeck noted before, he sought to improve his skills in radiology.[1] The usual method for correcting deficiencies in practice knowledge involved self-identifying problem areas and then seeking tidbits of knowledge in that area from offerings at medical meetings, at conferences, or in textbooks or the medical literature. A big problem was that most specialists who wrote about emergency conditions did not practice in EDs and frequently did not provide a practical approach to the emergency care of medical or surgical conditions. As Karl Mangold remembers, "I couldn't find any textbook. The only textbook I could find then was a British textbook on accident and casualties."[2] The inadequate infrastructure for furthering their education frustrated the early emergency physicians.

Before residencies were started, even before the formation of the American College of Emergency Physicians (ACEP), ideas for providing a more concentrated period of training for practicing emergency physicians were surfacing. The first appears to have been Eben Alexander's grant proposal to the U.S. Public Health Service in 1965 to 1966 for a 1-year, postgraduate training program to prepare physicians to become ED directors. Alexander, a faculty neurosurgeon at Bowman Gray School of Medicine in Winston-Salem, North Carolina, had seen the desperate need for trained physicians to at least direct EDs and was familiar with George Podgorny's interest in emergency care. The grant was not funded, and some of the protagonists who might have helped Alexander move his plans forward, including Podgorny, moved across town to begin their emergency practices at Forsyth Hospital. Like almost all emergency practitioners of their times, their training would come on the job.

The first consistently operating program for postgraduate emergency medicine training came, somewhat surprisingly, out of Massachusetts General Hospital (MGH). MGH was a highly regarded training institution with strong programs in internal medicine and general surgery. The MGH ED was typical for an urban academic teaching hospital in the late 1960s—compartmentalized into medical and surgical sections and run by eight to 15 unsupervised interns and residents. The ED patient volume had grown precipitously. John Knowles, M.D., trained at MGH and remembers being assigned there as an intern in 1951, then observing the ED in 1965 in an administrative role. He notes that the ED census was 18,000 patients per year in 1951 and had grown to 65,000 per year in 1965. In 1966, he wrote of the Mass General ED,

> *People continue to come in growing numbers with growing hopes and expectations...More and more come because of social and psychic disease, but they are matched by those with disease and injury—heart attacks, ruptured blood vessels, accidents, suicides, accidental taking of poison, strokes, cancer, and so on. Whatever the need, the people give the best care to the injured and to the sick, whether the problems are social, psychic, or somatic in origin. It is an incredibly successful function of the modern hospital.*[3]

It is unlikely that the unsupervised interns and residents at Mass General always gave "the best care," but it appears that the hospital provided the resources in terms of nursing, x-ray, and money to make the department work.

Two physicians at MGH, Steven Goldfinger, a gastroenterologist, and a young internist, James Dineen, were approached in 1966 or 1967 by three GPs from Lynn, Massachusetts, who had retired from their practices and were forming an Alexandria Plan–type emergency medicine group to staff a local hospital ED. They called themselves "old retreads" and recognized the need for additional training before they tried to practice full time in the emergency setting.[4,5] Goldfinger and Dineen developed a 2-week course designed to train practicing physicians in aspects of emergency and critical care. After the initial trio went through, the course continued to attract experienced physicians who were practicing in EDs. Dineen noted in 1971 that the average age of physicians who had taken his course was 50 years. Participants were required to obtain credentials for MGH and to take an initial exam to help identify areas of weakness. Those who took the course threw themselves into the experience. They were scheduled to work 30 hours per week in the MGH ED, finishing their shifts at 9 PM, but Dineen noted that "frequently they are there until midnight or 1 AM. They really get turned on."[4,5]

Karl Mangold, who had been practicing emergency medicine in California for about 3 years, took the MGH emergency medicine course in 1969. He remembers, on meeting Dineen and Goldfinger, "I think I finally met somebody in academic medicine that sees what I see." If Mangold had entered a residency, as he had initially intended, he would have been a fourth-year resident in 1969. His work in the MGH emergency medicine fellowship brought him in contact with residents and fellows in internal medicine and surgery. Mangold discussed the new field of emergency medicine with these residents, telling them, "This is going to sweep the country, can't miss, we have to have residents, people like you." Mangold remembers, "The fellowship was long days, it was very well organized."[2]

> *...[T]hey gave us lectures and we went in the lab and we did arterial blood punctures, we put chest tubes in. It was like an academic experience that really filled in holes for me. We'd get to put endotracheal tubes in...put nasal trachs in...did cricothyrotomies on cadavers and it was just very good for me but the big thing that I came out it of was, I worked shoulder to shoulder in the emergency department with the senior residents and I was holding my own with these guys. I figured if I could hold my own at Mass General Hospital never having gone through a residency but being very interested in learning, I said this is alright.... So I went there, had a great time and that kind of let me know that I was doing okay on my intellectual progression to be the best possible emergency physician I could be.... Goldfinger and Dineen were academically far ahead of a lot of people.*[2]

When Mangold returned to California, he recognized how other physicians who were staffing his EDs might benefit from the type of training provided by the MGH emergency medicine fellowship. He encouraged his emergency physicians to apply for the MGH fellowship,

> I got very involved in trying to upgrade the skills of the docs because we'd get surgeons, they didn't know anything about asthma, acute myocardial infarction, on and on. Then you'd get internists, "Okay what do you mean, we've got to put in a chest tube?" …I came back and sent a lot of people there. Some got in, some didn't.[2]

From the late 1960s to the early 1980s, the MGH emergency medicine fellowship trained hundreds of early emergency physicians in the basics of critical care. For the many physicians in that time who came to emergency medicine with only internship training, the most frightening part of practice was dealing with critically ill patients with cardiac or respiratory illness, or severe injury. Although it was a brief training period, the fellowship was intensive and well taught. It also gave practitioners the right to say that they had a training experience in emergency medicine at the MGH. This imbued them with credibility when they sought jobs or interacted with residency-trained physicians in other specialties. By 1970, other institutions were attempting to recreate MGH-type courses for "second-career" emergency physicians. The Pennsylvania Medical Society held a special conference to plan and develop courses in emergency medicine.[6] Ironically, emergency medicine did not progress at MGH, despite the widely acclaimed work done by Dineen and Goldfinger. It was not until nearly 25 years after the MGH emergency medicine fellowship that emergency medicine residents and emergency medicine–trained faculty would care for patients in the MGH ED, and as of 2004, the ED was still directed by a surgeon.

Cincinnati: Birthplace of Emergency Medicine Residency Training

By late 1969, at least 1,000 American physicians considered themselves full-time emergency physicians and probably two or three times that many practiced part time in EDs. ACEP was a new but rapidly expanding organization. The American Medical Association (AMA) had an active Commission on Emergency Medical Services. The federal government knew about the growing professional practice of emergency medicine. Emergency care was in the national consciousness, sometimes as a promising new venue for medical advances, sometimes as an eyesore or embarrassment. Many people had ideas about how to improve emergency practice. Even a Vermont medical student, Phil Buttaravoli, as previously described, could see where the field was going and that a great need existed to formally train physicians in emergency care. The problem was widely acknowledged—inadequate physician training in emergency care. The solution was obvious: develop residency training programs in emergency medicine. But the creation of the first residency programs was surprisingly unplanned and serendipitous. Although the early Alexandria practice pioneers and ACEP leaders were on the record as favoring emergency medicine residencies, they lacked the academic wherewithal and connections to make this happen. People like Wiegenstein, Rupke, Hannas, Mills, and Haeck became masters at organizational medicine, but they did not walk comfortably in the halls of academe. The early surgeon converts to emergency medicine like Wagner, Krome, and Podgorny were in academic settings, but in 1969 were not quite ready to advance residency training programs. The sequence of events that led to the first emergency medicine resident was a strange confluence of individual aspirations and institutional pragmatism.

In the late 1960s, the University of Cincinnati had a well-respected medical school and an attached traditional large teaching hospital, the Cincinnati General Hospital, which was run by the city of Cincinnati. The "General" sat up on the plateau above downtown Cincinnati. Between the downtown and the General Hospital was a neighborhood called "Over the Rhine." This was a tough section of town, with a large, indigent, primarily black population who used General Hospital for most of their medical needs. Cincinnati experienced the typical post-Medicare boom in patient volumes. The ED census of Cincinnati General Hospital climbed rapidly until in 1968 to 1969 it was around 100,000 patients per year. The staffing of the ED was solely by interns and residents. In the late 1960s, race riots hit Cincinnati, like many other large cities, and some black citizens complained about the long waiting times and poor quality of care they received at the General Hospital ED. At least once, demonstrators with picket signs lined up outside the hospital to protest.[7] The administrators and powerful department chairs decided that something needed to be done. Internal medicine was appointed the task of making the ED better. The person who was tagged to carry out this huge undertaking was Herbert Flessa, M.D., a bright, young academic internist and hematologist. Like many other junior faculty members around the country, Flessa found that he had been put in charge of a burgeoning, unstructured clinical mess. Flessa describes how he came to be in charge of the ED,

> The wish was that somebody could try to make sense out of a very complicated, stumbling along operation, both in clinic and the Emergency Unit [EU].[7] Being the new kid on the block and having an hour or two to spare, you're given extra jobs, and one of the extra jobs I was given was to run the clinic services and emergency services…with no help and no money! What we did in the late sixties was try to figure out a way to improve emergency services, not only in General Hospital but thinking over the long term…Department directors and many residents and interns stomped their feet about working in the EU, saying it was a waste of time…More and more people were going to emergency units not only at our hospital but in hospitals around the country because Blue Cross and Blue Shield would pay for emergency unit visits but wouldn't pay for doctor visits in some contracts. So they came to the emergency unit and got their care that way. And I think we recognized the need to train people to try to cover emergency units. It wasn't very complicated I thought we just needed it.[7]

Flessa went to Dr. Joe Lindner, Jr., the powerful chief of staff at the Cincinnati General Hospital in 1967, and the two discussed the idea of training emergency physicians. The first step was to obtain support from the other departments. Flessa met with the chairpersons of internal medicine, surgery, and other departments. He found them "warmly enthusiastic…because it would relieve some of the pressure from their residents who didn't want to work in the ED."[8] The impetus for the program on the medical center side was to put more physician bodies in the ED, but there was also the interface with an angry community. Richard Levy, who would later lead the Cincinnati program for more than 20 years, remembers asking Flessa and Lindner why the program arose so quickly, and concluded,

> The only reason for a training program here was to put out a fire that was burning, and burning very, very hot in Cincinnati, Ohio…It was to do something political. To try to in some fashion to placate a local population. It was an idea, then the idea started to take on some meat around that bone, which was a reactive bone.[9]

The sequence of events that occurred next is not clear, but it seems likely that Flessa contacted the AMA to determine how a residency becomes certified. He either attended or reviewed the proceedings of the AMA Commission on Emergency Medical Services National Conference, "The Community and Emergency Medical Services," in San Francisco in January 1968. If he attended, he would have been in the same room with John Wiegenstein and John Rupke, who were there as interested, practicing emergency physicians, but would not found ACEP for another 8 months. At that time, the AMA Council on Education was the primary certifying body for residencies. The Accreditation Council for Graduate Medical Education (ACGME) had not yet formed, and the process for starting a residency in an existing specialty was not onerous. The problem for Flessa and his colleagues was that emergency medicine had no certifying board, and was not a recognized specialty. It had no section council and no political capital in the AMA. Flessa explored various ways to have an emergency medicine residency approved. He remembers,

> Ultimately, after hundreds of phone calls and letters the agreement was reached that, yes, this would be an official emergency medicine training program under the

aegis of family practice…and if your young people come into the program they will get a certificate saying that they are emergency medicine trained.[7]

Flessa, Lindner, and H. Paul Lewis, a neurosurgeon who had just finished his residency and was for some reason interested in the ED and a residency, put together a 2-year curriculum for an emergency medicine residency. It mattered little to them that it was approved by the AMA under general (family) practice. These individuals were focused on developing an emergency medicine training program primarily to address a local need. They were not concerned with a creating a specialty or promoting the idea of a specialty board and did not have the connections to do so. The Cincinnati physicians had almost no contact with ACEP as they were developing and starting the residency. John Wiegenstein, who was ACEP president at the time, remembered, "No, we didn't have any communication with him at all. He came out of the blue."[10] The plan was for the residency to begin after a rotating internship. In the first year of residency, the emergency medicine trainee was required to do 2 months in the emergency unit, 2 months each on in the internal medicine and pediatric wards, and 1 month in coronary care, anesthesiology, and respiratory care. The second year had no assigned months in the emergency unit, but added rotations in orthopedics, surgery, neurosurgery, and at "other medical facilit(ies)." One month of elective was allowed. The original plan also called for a fellowship year after the 2-year residency with rotations in surgery, coronary care, respiratory care, anesthesiology, neurosurgery, and neurology with 1 month of elective time. It appears that Flessa and colleagues believed that some physicians who had done other residencies or who had been out in practice might do 1 year of the emergency medicine residency followed by a fellowship year.[11] The rationale for training emergency physicians and the curriculum was written up by Flessa, Lindner, and Lewis in a "white paper" on the "The Emergency Physician." Through the AMA, Flessa learned that ACEP had formed, and he was invited by the AMA to attend the first national strategic planning meeting for ACEP at the Palmer House in Chicago in February 1969. This meeting was the result of John Wiegenstein and John Rupke's desperate trip to Chicago to seek help from the AMA in organizing ACEP. Flessa presented his white paper to the group and instantly became regarded as a national expert on training emergency physicians. He did not reveal that his residency was actually classified by the AMA as a family practice residency and that he was covertly calling it an emergency medicine residency. Because there was no certifying or specialty body in emergency medicine at the time, it made little difference. The important thing was that physicians could become residency trained in emergency care. Now all Flessa had to do was find his first recruit.

Bruce Janiak was then a fourth-year medical student at the University of Cincinnati. As mentioned in Chapter 4, he had moonlighted in an ED as a student and found the work exciting. While doing a fourth-year rotation at Jewish Hospital in Cincinnati, Janiak asked an attending physician if training was available in emergency medicine. The attending said he had heard that Herb Flessa and others were exploring that idea at the University of Cincinnati. Janiak knew Flessa, more from flag football games than academics, and sought him out:

I had a couple of meetings with him…the upshot of it was that…he found a guinea pig to launch an idea he had. I didn't even know about the Alexandria plans. All I knew was that this sounded like an interesting thing to do. I had no thought about finances or structure or where you would do it or how you would do it, it just seemed like, "Gee, what a fun thing to do." I knew that there was work to do, you could see it at Cincinnati General. There were doctors in the emergency department doing things so it was obvious to me that somebody might want to do that, but they would need to know how to do it. I just asked if there was training and…ACEP—I never heard of it, never heard of R. R. Hannas or any of those people. It wasn't until actually I think I got closer and closer to actually beginning the three years of training that I began to understand there was an organization…The agreement was that I would stay at the General, listing them first on a match for a rotating internship. If I did that then they would work with me during that internship year to develop a 2-year curriculum in emergency medicine training. That is exactly what happened. I did agree to list them and I was accepted as a rotating intern, clearly I chose my rotations to augment emergency medicine and during the year we had meetings and worked with other hospitals, the Good Sam[aritan] being one, for various rotations.[12]

Janiak did his rotating internship at Cincinnati General Hospital from July 1969 to July 1970 (see insert, Figure 13). The residency had to be officially approved, and Janiak remembers,

The approval process was in general practice by somebody from the Residency Review Committee in general practice for the AMA: one-person interview, 20 minutes— approved residency![12]

When Janiak started residency, he sported a new nametag that declared him an emergency medicine resident. Only Janiak really knew what that meant, and he was largely making it up as he went along. It was up to him to educate others on his pioneering role. As he rotated on other services, he would explain what his training entailed and what he hoped to gain from each rotation. Sometimes he would be clever and inform his supervisors on surgical services that an emergency medicine resident did not go to the operating room for long, complicated cases, but was best utilized working up surgical problems in the ED,

… [F]or instance in orthopedics, I don't believe I ever went to the operating room during my 2 months of orthopedic rotation, but I did take care of, when I was on duty, every fracture in the emergency department. I put more people in traction from hip fractures…I put 10,000 pins through knees and set them up in traction and of course the orthopedic residents thought this was the greatest thing ever, and actually it turned out that I was offered an orthopedic residency in the middle of that rotation, which made me feel pretty good. I turned it down because I was really into emergency medicine but I got to do everything. I've always been a wheeler-dealer so that's what I would do. I don't want to go to the operating room, but I'll make life easy for you down here in the emergency department. I did the same thing on emergency surgery. Let me evaluate the patient and think if they might have a surgical abdomen and then you come down. I'll do all that for you, and by the way I'll have a cold beer available for you. Which I did.[12]

When Janiak was assigned to rotate in the ED, he was "the King in the emergency department during those 2 years."[12] He was given an office, and nurses looked to him to help solve administrative problems. It was also his social base, stocked with beer, and Janiak notes, "You will never write down what I did in that office!"[12] The Cincinnati General emergency department was typical for its time in that attending or faculty physicians did not supervise residents, and the establishment of an emergency medicine residency did little to change that. Janiak recalls,

Herb, as I remember, rarely came to the emergency department, as a matter of fact I can tell you…the one interaction I had with a faculty member in 2 years in the emergency department. That was when…the student health physician…walked by, put her hands on this patient's abdomen and said to me, "Ah ha, the classic doughy abdomen of abdominal tuberculosis" and walked away. That was my one interaction in 2 years. I still to this day say, "What the hell is a classic doughy abdomen of abdominal tuberculosis?"[12]

It turned out that the physician was wrong. Janiak was left to train himself in the ED during his emergency medicine residency. He remembers gaining valuable critical care training at nearby Good Samaritan Hospital, where he and an internal medicine resident ran the intensive care unit during that rotation.

Reliance on other disciplines to educate emergency medicine residents was the unavoidable paradigm in all the early residencies. The few practicing emergency physicians in the early 1970s were mostly in nonacademic practices. Almost no one in the academic world had the experience to teach emergency medicine residents how an emergency physician functioned in an ED. Those who started emergency medicine programs were routinely not emergency physicians and were usually consumed with administrative duties and had little time to teach. The men who might have been able to provide the most practical knowledge and teaching to early emergency medicine residents—Mills, Hannas, Wiegenstein, and others—were not yet focused on the academic side of the field.

In the first year of the Cincinnati residency, Flessa went back to being a hematologist, and handed over the reins to James Agna, M.D., another respected internist who had no sense of what emergency medicine training should be and no national connections with the field. Agna was the head of the Department of Community Medicine, under which the emergency medicine residency was now assigned. In 1972, Agna noted that he was receiving "rather grumpy letters" from the AMA Council on Medical Education, reminding him that the "emergency medicine" residency was really a pilot project and that it remained classified as a general practice residency.[13] Despite this nebulous status, residency classes were recruited to follow Janiak. The members of the second class were Phillip Buttaravoli, William Teufel, Timothy Allen, and Keith Blankenbuehler. As Buttaravoli describes it, Flessa "...birthed this baby and then suddenly it was a foster child. Jim Agna arrives and is handed this big screaming baby, which is what we were."[14] Shortly after Agna assumed his position, he named Thomas Blum, a physician who had only completed an internship, as the emergency medicine residency director.

Phillip Buttaravoli was the prescient medical student at University of Vermont who wrote a senior treatise on what emergency medicine must become. He did his internship in 1970 to 1971 at Santa Clara Valley Medical Center and found the ED, run by a full-time physician director and ACEP member named Liz Fields, to be well run. During his internship, Buttaravoli traveled to the second ACEP scientific assembly in Las Vegas. He remembers meeting the early ACEP leaders and was especially impressed by Bill Haeck and his views on what the specialty might become. Buttaravoli had been accepted into the Cincinnati emergency residency over the telephone without doing an on-site interview. He expected great things as he traveled to Cincinnati for the first time to begin his residency. At this point, Buttaravoli was much more knowledgeable about emergency medicine than Bruce Janiak had been as an intern, and he had well-formed ideas of what quality emergency care should be. He would not find it in Cincinnati:

> After the internship, coming to Cincinnati was a bit of a disappointment. Here I pretty much was anticipating having everything that I dreamed about as a medical student, as to what emergency medicine should be, and where we are going, and...really, what I envisioned, was something that probably didn't happen at Cincinnati for 20 years. I thought it was going to be all in place when I got there. Of course, there was nothing in place. It was a terribly run emergency department. The worst you could ever imagine. There was no leadership...Jim Agna, he was Community Medicine, and he had this dream of setting up outreach clinics and Tom Blum was going to be one of his helpers to help with these outreach clinics. Tom Blum only had an internship. He was no better trained than any of the residents that were there, and his orientation was towards [sic] community medicine service to clinics in managing indigent care and that kind of thing. Jim Agna was just a magnificent man, a magnificent person and yet the first time we met with him, the first day all of us got together with Jim Agna, I can remember very distinctly trying to convince him that there was a reason to have a specialty of emergency medicine. He couldn't see what the need was to have a specialty of emergency medicine. This was our new director. This was the new chairman of our department, the head of our program and he basically didn't think that we needed a specialty of emergency medicine![14]

Bruce Janiak had relatively modest expectations for his residency training, and in his happy-go-lucky manner made the best of the situation. For Phil Buttaravoli, who was more exacting, more intense and had big dreams for the specialty, the conditions at Cincinnati were difficult to bear. The actual, assigned time in the ED was limited to just a couple of months for the entire residency. Perhaps Flessa and the other originators of the program understood what a poor learning environment the

Cincinnati ED was. They seemed to put their faith in the off-service rotations to provide emergency medicine residents with the essentials of emergency care in each area. Buttaravoli, like Janiak, found that the only teaching that occurred during his residency was on his off-service rotations:

> I thought it was a good thing that we weren't in the emergency department because there was no teaching in the emergency department. It was learn through your mistakes, which is how it was in medical school and everywhere else. I mean it is one way to learn, but it is not really fair to the patients that you are taking care of. So, I was happy to be on the various rotations.[14]

The five residents in emergency medicine at Cincinnati in 1972 were often spread out on different rotations and did not see each other much. This prevented Janiak from serving as a role model for the other residents. It was difficult to carve out space for the residency program, especially when the physician leaders of the program were not true advocates for the cause of emergency medicine. Even simple things to improve the quality of the residency fell to the residents to do themselves. For example, Buttaravoli believed the emergency medicine residents needed a space where they could work, read, or discuss things in private. No such space existed—apparently, Janiak's "office" had gone by the wayside. When Buttaravoli took this matter to Tom Blum and James Agna, they were not helpful, so Buttaravoli went to work with his classmate Tim Allen. They decided to convert one of the gynecology rooms in the ED to a resident's room. In the middle of the night, they carried the gynecology exam table out of the ED and down into the "catacombs" that lay beneath Cincinnati General Hospital. When the tunnel terminated in a dark room with a dirt floor, they deposited the exam table, thinking that no one would be able to find it to bring it back to the ED. Next they went upstairs in the hospital and "borrowed" two nicely upholstered leather chairs and a table and brought them to their new emergency medicine resident office in the ED. Buttaravoli knew that their residency director, Tom Blum would not have the power to undo their night's work.

> We knew that Tom couldn't make any change occur, nothing ever changed when Tom was there. So, what we figured was that if we changed it, it would stay that way. And…it was a resident's room for at least as long as we were there.[14]

Buttaravoli also found the Cincinnati ED to be "terribly understaffed," with nurses who were "unhelpful." He claims that the head nurse was schizophrenic and the department ran that way. It was split into different areas—medicine, surgery, and psychiatry—and patients were triaged to an area where a resident physician would provide care:

> They had this enormous need in that department for someone to take charge and make good things happen and bring it about. Although the university at the time was good enough to embrace the concept, they were not prepared to put the money, effort, and personnel behind it to make it happen. We were sort of just struggling on our own with very little in the way of leadership and personnel.[14]

Just as a military experience can bond people together, the early emergency medicine residency at Cincinnati hatched strong friendships. Early residents like Buttaravoli invoke war terminology to describe their resident tour of duty, saying it was "quite a battlefield in that emergency department." But somehow they learned and came to know each other well. Buttaravoli's overall disappointment with the residency was ameliorated by this:

> I still thought I got excellent education and there was an enormous camaraderie. We were different than everybody else. We were the soldiers of fortune that were trying to battle our way within this big medical center. Nobody understood who we were, what we were doing. So we had an enormous bond.[14]

The Cincinnati residency made it through its first 3 years, alive but not thriving. In 1973 an idealistic young man, fresh out of the Harvard Public Health School interviewed at the Cincinnati emergency medicine program. Tom Blum, the residency director, was immediately impressed with Richard Levy, admiring his background and knowledge of emergency medical services and his academic interests. He offered him a residency position with a handshake. Levy had also looked at David Wagner's Medical College of Pennsylvania (MCP) program, but it was very new and untested. When Levy visited Cincinnati he remembers seeing an emergency medicine resident perform an intubation. The resident "seemed to be very much in control" and Levy "was very impressed." For Levy, who had come out of rural Kentucky and attended medical school at Louisville, the masters program in public health at Harvard was eye opening. After seeing how the federal government was highly interested in emergency medical services (EMS) in the early 1970s, Levy became

> …interested in emergency medicine as a system kind of issue and then it occurred to me that this is a place that Richard Levy could make a high-impact contribution to changing the world.[9]

Levy, as a member of the fifth class of emergency medicine residents at Cincinnati, found a slightly improved educational experience. Most mornings at 8 AM, Jim Agna or another faculty member would gather the emergency medicine residents who were available in the orthopedic "cast" room of the ED to give a brief conference. Another 1-hour conference was held each week. In his senior year of residency, Levy developed an orientation program for the new residents and provided lectures nearly every day for a month to prepare the residents for what they would encounter in the ED. But the Cincinnati emergency medicine residents continued to spend precious little time in the ED—only 3 months of their 36 months of a rotating internship and 2-year residency. Early residents felt in some ways as though their entire residency was a rotating internship. When they were assigned to the ED, they found the same disorganized conditions as their predecessors. A few physicians were hired in 1973 to 1974 as faculty to see patients in the Cincinnati General ED. One, Judy Daniels, was trained as an anesthesiologist, and the other, Louis Pagani, was an Argentinian who had trained as a neurologist and was a brilliant diagnostician. However, the ED was still resident run and a dysfunctional, dangerous place. Richard Levy remembers:

> I can tell you that it was wild and woolly, it was the Old West compared to anything that anybody could imagine today, it was unsupervised, it was not good, it offended me. I didn't like it because I was always worried about hurting people and I knew that other people were making mistakes that could be harmful, and I knew that was happening, but there wasn't any supervision and I also knew that it was for another generation that was out there to bring some order to all of this and be able to make it work with some instruction.[9]

Mel Otten, who had been a Vietnam medic and then became a medical student at the University of Cincinnati, probably had a greater role in teaching the early emergency medicine residents at Cincinnati than did the faculty. The Cincinnati General Hospital hired medical students to do much of the menial work in the ED—suturing and wound care, electrocardiograms, drawing blood, and transporting patients. Otten, as a medic, had good skills in wound care. He remembers,

> …I went to medical school from 8:00 in the morning 'til 4:00 in the afternoon and then from 4:00 in the afternoon 'til midnight I worked as a suture doctor making $1.05 an hour so it was pretty good pay. Then from midnight 'til 8:00, I slept in the emergency room in the on-call room. So I never had to leave the emergency room. This was in 1973 so the emergency medicine residency was only 3 years old and the first residents basically were still there so I got to meet a lot of the original residents in emergency medicine and the attendings in those days, none of them were trained obviously in emergency medicine and most of them didn't know anything about emergency medicine and a lot of them actually were more harmful than good to the practice of emergency medicine. One thing, I got to know the residents. By the time I was a second- or third-year medical student I was actually teaching the residents how to

suture and how to—I was doing posterior tibial nerve blocks, things like that—because you just got so good at it 8 hours a day, 5 days a week—you got kind of good at all kinds of minor wound care.[15]

Otten decided that he, too, wanted to train in emergency medicine. Despite being their teacher as well as a student, he remembers looking up to people like Janiak and Buttaravoli, "As Gods. Some of those guys were just like my idols...They were training in emergency medicine. They knew so much." When Otten told the Cincinnati faculty that he wanted to do an emergency medicine residency, but was only applying to the Cincinnati program, the faculty asked him what he would do if he were not selected. He recalls, "I said, I'll just apply again next year. And I guess they felt, oh my God, we don't want to interview this guy every year we'd better let him in and get it over with."[15] Of course, the faculty viewed Otten as an experienced, excellent residency candidate. He had the typical negative response from other medical school faculty, particularly in internal medicine, when he told them he was training in emergency medicine:

Emergency medicine was thought of for people who were stupid, people who didn't speak English, people who were bad, who got in trouble, maybe were drug addicts or drunks or things like that, that's the people who went into emergency medicine. Real doctors were either internists or surgeons.[15]

But many of the physicians who chose emergency medicine started in the "real doctor" residencies. Otten remembers that almost all of his coresidents at Cincinnati transferred from medicine, surgery, or other residencies or came back from community practice in another field before choosing emergency medicine.

The early emergency medicine residents were part of something new and exciting, but they were also viewed as outsiders and were constantly questioned about their decisions to pursue emergency medicine training, by their colleagues, family, and friends. Richard Levy experienced this frequently:

There was always the undercurrent of, what's a smart guy like you doing in this? Why are you doing this? What's wrong with you? In a similar fashion, my father asked the question, "How does this fit into the house of medicine?" My mother, I thought asked a more insightful question, "Why would you want to do this?" Which was actually a much tougher question to answer. What I'm saying is people outside also couldn't understand why a bright, energetic, smiling human being would go into something called Emergency Room because it also had a terrible reputation and that's where losers are. It was almost like a general concept of losers. Losers hang out there...[A]nd that was part of what shaped me. If you think of my personality as a Chair, part of what shaped me—maybe put a little bit of a chip on my shoulder.[9]

Kenneth Iserson, another Cincinnati-trained emergency physician, also remembers a difficult time with his family and the concept of emergency medicine.

The biggest problem the first few years, actually the first decade, of being an emergency physician for me, was trying to explain to my mother what I did. "Aren't you ever going to have a real office?"[16]

Those who pursued emergency medicine residency training in the early 1970s faced an insecure future. They were training in an unrecognized medical specialty, without a specialty board, and no guarantee that the field would persist. As Iserson notes, they were,

Gamblers, very much risk takers—we were risking our whole career on something that could pay off big, but everybody was telling us that it was never going to happen. Every single day of my residency at least one time someone would say, "Why don't you go into a real specialty?" They offered—I got offered to go into every specialty I rotated in. The only one I actually laughed at was when the neurosurgeons asked me—Oh my God![16]

Richard Levy and his wife loved to travel, and after finishing his residency, they embarked on a 6-month trip to Southeast Asia and thought they might settle in the

Northeast when they returned to the United States. While they were away, the Cincinnati emergency medicine program began to implode. Tom Blum, the residency director who had never completed a residency himself, became frustrated both by his own deficient training for his role and by the lack of support of the hospital and medical school for the emergency medicine residency. He announced that he was leaving in early 1977 to do an internal medicine residency at the Mayo Clinic. No one was eager to assume his role in directing the residency. James Agna, who was the chair of the Department of Community Medicine and had overall responsibility for emergency medicine, did not show much interest in maintaining emergency medicine under his realm. The emergency medicine residents and faculty wanted their own department in the medical school, with a national search for a qualified chair. The dean of the Cincinnati medical school, Dr. Robert S. Daniels, did not like this approach and announced that he would make emergency medicine a division of surgery and let the department chief of surgery run the emergency medicine program. The emergency medicine residents saw this as a death sentence.

Kenneth Iserson, who was just finishing his first year of residency, was politically savvy about what might influence the dean. He knew that the lucrative EMS (ambulance) contracts held by Cincinnati General Hospital could be transferred to another institution. He met with the director of the ED at Good Samaritan Hospital, which was already a teaching site for off-service rotations for the residency, to discuss transferring the program and the EMS contracts to that institution. He and some of his resident colleagues then met with Dean Daniels and pleaded with him to create a department of emergency medicine and recruit a qualified chair. Daniels was steadfast, and Iserson remembers:

> I stood up right across from him and I said, "Look, we've got a deal already in the works, you either do what we ask or we are moving the whole department, the whole residency program, and our EMS contracts to the other hospital." Then he stood up and he was red in the face, screaming, and saying, "This is my medical school, don't you threaten me!" And he walked out. The next day he appointed a committee to search for the chair and appointed me—I was shocked—appointed me the resident member on the committee.[16]

Meanwhile, Richard Levy was on the island of Fiji with his wife, not much concerned with how things were back in Cincinnati. Somehow, Judy Daniels, one of the junior faculty who worked in the Cincinnati ED contacted Levy, telling him "The program is falling apart and this program may go out of existence." The dean had asked the faculty to suggest someone who might be able to temporarily run the program, and Levy had the support of the faculty. Judy Daniels begged Levy to hurry home, and he and his wife skipped the last leg of their long vacation to return to Cincinnati. Levy remembers:

> …[G]oing in and seeing Dean Daniels who met with me and said, "Are you willing to hold this together? I don't know if it will take 2 months or 6 months until we can hire somebody. Are you willing to hold it together?" I said, "Yes, but I need a couple of things to be done," and…I think they gave me an office and a couple more things. That was the deal. It was very much a holding action on the part of Dean Daniels, the College of Medicine, and the hospital. That was my job. To hold things together.[17]

Levy did much more than hold the program together. He stayed and created a strong academic framework and developed a plan that made the department financially very successful. After its tenuous first few years and near extinction, the Cincinnati emergency medicine program emerged under Levy's leadership to become one of the most influential and highly regarded programs in the country.

MEDICAL COLLEGE OF PENNSYLVANIA: A DIFFERENT APPROACH TO EMERGENCY MEDICINE TRAINING

In the late 1960s, David Wagner was plugging along as director of the ED at the Medical College of Pennsylvania while still working as a surgeon (see insert, Figure 14). Wagner began to see how emergency medicine was expanding in community hospitals, and he started to think about training physicians in "acute care." As his ideas developed, he would need, like Herbert Flessa in Cincinnati, to find a volunteer to be the first trainee. Wagner has a way of describing the early people who chose emergency medicine:

> *I often call them "the wagon train riders." They were the people who would have jumped on a covered wagon and gone West 100 years earlier, and they had decided that this was something that piqued their interest and curiosity and so they just appeared.[18]*

For Wagner, the first wagon train rider, in keeping with MCP's history as Women's Medical College, would be a woman named Pamela Bensen. Bensen was a member of the last all-female, 66-member class at MCP.

Pam Bensen was raised in Princeton, New Jersey, about a block from the campus. As a young girl, she saw Albert Einstein walking the streets of the neighborhood "with an ice cream cone and that hair flying."[19] Bensen wanted to be a doctor from her very early years:

> *I was probably about 4 years old, and it is a very vivid memory—somebody asked me what I wanted to do when I grew up and I just looked at them and said I was going to be a doctor, and they patted me on the head and said, "Girls aren't doctors, girls are nurses." I just looked at them and said, "You want to bet?"[19]*

Bensen spent her girlhood making up concoctions for her cousins and friends to ingest as they played doctor. She bandaged them like casualties and made them lay on the lawn for a photograph. Bensen remembers studying hard in the second and third grades because she knew she would need good grades to become a doctor. She did well in college and got married just a few days before she started medical school. One of the reasons she chose MCP was that in the interview process the school did not ask about her plans for marriage and a family. Bensen was interested in the field of genetics and initially planned to become a medical geneticist. However as a freshman medical student she had a good friend who was a second-year medical student. One night when her friend was working in the ED, Bensen brought her dinner. Once Bensen saw the ED, "It was like, pow, I like this! From then on in it was like nothing else existed for me…Nothing else mattered."[19] Bensen did medical school over a 5-year period. She had a child in her second year of medical school and took a semester off when her husband was sent to Vietnam. Early in her fourth year, she was pregnant and planned to practice in emergency medicine after some period of residency training. One of the reasons that emergency medicine appealed to Bensen and her supportive husband was the opportunity for scheduled hours, which would make it easier to manage their family life. Although Bruce Janiak had started his emergency medicine residency at this point, Bensen was not aware that the Cincinnati program existed. She thought that she would do a rotating internship, followed by a year in medicine and a year in surgery as preparation to practice emergency medicine—"and when I think I know enough we'll go out and I'll work."[19]

Bensen knew David Wagner from working with him during her surgery rotations during medical school, and he had done minor surgery on Bensen's daughter. She did not know that he was playing with the idea of emergency medicine or acute care training. Wagner knew a little bit about ACEP, and may have been aware of the Cincinnati program, but at this point, he had not attended any ACEP meetings. Wagner had discussed his ideas for emergency medicine training with Ethel Weinberg, M.D., an associate dean at MCP. One day in November 1970, Wagner and Weinberg were having lunch and exploring these concepts further. Pam Bensen, quite pregnant, was looking for an empty seat in the crowded MCP cafeteria. She found one next to Wagner and Weinberg:

> *I sit down and they are being polite and they turned to me and they say, gee Pam, what is it that you'd like to do? I said well, the thing I want to do doesn't exist. I want to be an emergency physician. Now, if it was a movie all the music would have stopped and everybody in the room would have turned to look at me while I said this because*

David and Ethel were discussing starting a residency but didn't know whether there would be any students that would do it. What were the chances, I mean, this was like fate. So, basically that was the beginning of the three of us working to, by the time I finished school 6 months later, to have a program put together.[19]

The protagonists at MCP, like their counterparts in Cincinnati, discovered that the approval process for a new internship was through the AMA. Wagner and Weinberg had an advantage because Glen Leymaster, who was in an administrative position at MCP, was involved in the Council on Medical Education at the AMA. Leymaster would become a central figure in the AMA as emergency medicine pursued specialty status. After meeting to discuss a curriculum, Wagner and Weinberg agreed that Pam Bensen should go to the AMA to make the pitch for the new acute care internship. Bensen was no stranger to the AMA. She had previously traveled to Chicago to protest when the AMA decided to drop the childbirth section from its program on disaster management. This was during the cold war, when disaster planning was primarily for a nuclear attack. As Bensen notes, "we were going to be underground for 6 months," and she felt strongly that childbirth should not be omitted.

Bensen returned to Chicago to present the acute care internship proposal. She remembers a stark contrast between herself, a young woman in the third trimester of pregnancy, and the panel before which she presented: "The average age in the room was 70, the average gender was 100% male." The AMA did not give immediate approval, but promised to discuss and consider the proposal. Bensen returned to Philadelphia and her daughter was born 6 weeks early, around Thanksgiving of 1970. The baby had Potter syndrome, and died shortly after birth. Like R. R. Hannas and his wife, who experienced the tragedy of losing a child when he was a medical student, Pam Bensen and her husband got "some experience with death and dying"[19] (see insert, Figure 14).

The AMA finally approved the MCP acute care internship in the late spring of 1971. Bensen had an alternate plan to do a rotating internship in Germantown, Pennsylvania. When the letter came from C. H. William Ruhe, M.D., from the AMA, Bensen remembers part of the explanation for approval was "so women could have scheduled hours." This irritated Bensen, but she kept quiet, happy to be able to train in the manner she wanted. In the late 1980s, when she was a leader in ACEP, Bensen was assigned to attend a meeting of the National Board of Medical Examiners. The meeting was in part a retirement party for Dr. Ruhe. Bensen remembers:

I get in the reception line and I shake his hand, take his hand in both of mine, and look him right in the eye and say, "Dr. Ruhe I just want to thank you for approving the MCP Acute Care Internship so that we women could have scheduled hours, it's been a wonderful career for me."[19]

Wagner and MCP did not initially receive approval from the AMA for additional training beyond the acute care internship. However, Bensen and other early trainees decided that they needed more training, and signed on for additional years. David Wagner attended the ACEP winter meeting in Sarasota in 1971 where he met the early ACEP leaders, and spent time discussing residency training issues with Ron Krome, who was thinking about developing a program in Detroit. Wagner and Krome had a common background as surgeons who had ventured into emergency medicine. Wagner's program did not receive funding from MCP or government sources for additional residency years. All the residents were funded from practice revenues. After completing internship, the emergency medicine residents were licensed and certified, and because he received no other funding for these residents, Wagner billed in their names for services provided when they rotated at EDs at MCP and outside hospitals. This created a problem later on when the program was formally reviewed.[18]

Pam Bensen jumped into her acute care internship in July 1971. Wagner had recruited three other acute care interns, all men, to join Bensen. Only two of the original four, Bensen and John Wasserberger, ended up practicing emergency medicine. The MCP ED was newly built, but poorly designed for emergency care. It had the traditional organizational split into medical, surgical, and gynecology areas. Bensen remembers an experience on the first day of her internship:

> …[T]he nurses called me…there was a young man seizing, he was probably some-where in his 20s and it was 8:05 day one. I'm now Dr. Bensen, and I'm thinking, no way. I froze. The nurse took one look at me, her name was Nell, and she said, "Dr. Bensen do you want 5 or 10 mg of IV [intravenous] Valium for this patient?" I said, "You had better bring 10, we might need it." That was my introduction to the fact that the nurses were going to save my ass. They were also going to save my patient, but I had to listen to them. I have never forgotten that….[19]

Although David Wagner had a bigger presence in the MCP ED than the early faculty in Cincinnati, the ED was resident run, with almost no faculty supervision. Wagner or another faculty physician would make rounds at 8 AM, review the cases from the night before, go over charts, and review x-rays. When she was not in the ED, Bensen found, like her early Cincinnati counterparts, that she had to explain to residents and physicians in other fields what she was doing. Her function on off-service rotations was largely determined by her own assessment of what she needed to learn:

> People would look at me and say, "Bensen what the hell is an emergency physician?" I'd say, "Well, I just want you to teach me how to take care of your patients between 2 AM and 8 AM so you can sleep."[19]

Bensen remembers functioning in a manner very similar to that of the early Cincinnati residents. When she was on surgical services like orthopedics, she spent most of her time in the ED working up patients rather than in the operating room or wards. She knew that her training experience was fresh and novel, but also had the sense that it could be much better than it was. Bensen would have the chance to promote improved emergency medicine residency training on a national level at an early stage of her career (see insert, Figure 15).

Early in her internship, David Wagner made Bensen aware of the upcoming ACEP meeting in Miami, Florida. He encouraged her to go. Bensen remembers it being a tough decision, but she went:

> … [W]e have one child, my husband is working three jobs, we have no money, we sometimes wonder how we are going to eat, and I go home and say I need to go to Florida. Okay, we'll put it together, so I end up going back to Dave and saying I'm going to the meeting, I've signed up for it and he says well, I'm going to give you the name of somebody that I want you to meet there…since you are going to do this, you need to know these people. So, I go down to the Fontainebleu Hotel in Miami Beach Florida, and I'm one of the most naive and from-the-sticks type girls. You know I've gone with the same guy since I was 15, I'm married to him now, we've got a kid, I'm totally naïve, so I'm in the lobby of this hotel and every time I'd meet somebody from this meeting I'd say do you know—and I'd pull this name out of my pocket and ask, do you know this guy and about the third person I asked they said, oh yeah, come on, I'll introduce you to him and this person…introduced me to Ron Krome. Now, I cannot tell you a better way to get started in ACEP than to be introduced to Ron Krome as the first intern in emergency medicine. That man didn't let go of me for the rest of the meeting. I never bought a meal, I was introduced to everyone, John Wiegenstein, Jim Mills, you name it, I mean top to bottom, anybody who was there, I got to meet. I was dragged to the board meeting, I was asked to speak at the board meeting and to comment on education for emergency physicians and what was going on in my program, etc. I was encouraged to raise my hand and speak at the board meeting.[19]

Bensen was appointed to the ACEP Graduate Medical Education Committee. The 1971 Miami ACEP meeting was momentous in that it was the first time that physicians who were in postgraduate training in emergency medicine had a chance to meet. Bruce Janiak, Phillip Buttaravoli, and Tim Allen were a few months into their training in Cincinnati emergency medicine residency program and had been allowed to attend the ACEP meeting. They found Bensen, and on a beach in Miami they sat and began "…talking about what we are going to do with the future and what part we were going to play in all this." Bensen also had the chance to meet other women who practiced emergency medicine at the Miami meeting. She remembers seeing Vera Morkovin from Illinois and Elizabeth Fields, from California. The atmosphere was very accepting toward women in emergency medicine, but Bensen remembers it was also "a typical male convention." While respected, the women "were pursued for not necessarily altruistic reasons."[19] When Bensen returned to Philadelphia she was exuberant:

> I'll tell you, I came back, I became an ACEP junky. I mean, I was free-basing ACEP…I…was just so full of, of my God, there are people like me, this is gonna work, I have chosen the right thing! I just was flying. I was just flying. I didn't have many doubts to start with, but any I had were totally gone when you meet people like Jim Mills and John Rogers and Ron Krome and John Rupke…George Podgorny. I mean all of these people. Bill Haeck, Karl Mangold, that whole list, I met them all. In fact…it was like I got handcuffed to somebody and they just passed my handcuff around. I was their future and they knew it, and they were wonderful. I'll never forget because at one of the dinners, when they paid for my dinner I said, "You know guys I've got to pay you back for this," and…Jim Mills just looked at me and said, "Pam you can never pay us back, just pass it on."[19]

Pam Bensen got pregnant during internship and had a child during her residency year. After her internship and 1 year of residency in emergency medicine, she decided to practice emergency medicine to restore a bit of order to her life and to finally earn a decent income. She, her husband, and two small children settled in rural Maine, where Bensen intended to practice for a couple of years before returning to academics to become a residency program director. She had many offers to do this as she left MCP. But Bensen was the type of person to become immersed in her immediate world. She spent the next 25 years developing the field of emergency medicine and EMS in Maine and became an active leader in ACEP. The MCP residency, with its emergency medicine internship followed by 2 years of residency, became the first to train residents in a 3-year format. The program, despite being poorly resourced, grew steadily under David Wagner's guidance and began to recruit residents from around the country. By the middle of the 1970s, it was viewed as one of the best places to train in emergency medicine.

LOS ANGELES COUNTY/UNIVERSITY OF SOUTHERN CALIFORNIA: THE WESTERN FRONT OF EMERGENCY MEDICINE TRAINING

Given its distance from Virginia and Michigan, California had become relatively advanced in terms of early emergency practice by the early 1970s. The first American textbook of emergency medicine by Thomas Flint came out of Northern California in the 1950s. Karl Mangold had started to work in and provide physician staffing for EDs in Northern California in 1966 and others like Richard Stennes, M.D., soon followed his lead in Southern California. As noted before, the Santa Clara Valley Medical Center, run by Elizabeth Fields, M.D., was state of the art when Phillip Buttaravoli did his internship there in 1970. Many California hospitals saw their EDs as key portals to their hospitals and potential money-making enterprises. However in the large county hospitals such as Los Angeles County/University of Southern California Medical Center (LAC/USC), the mission was to provide care to all. The LAC/USC Medical Center is the type of building that invites nicknames. Some called it "the Great Stone Mother," others referred to it as "Big County."[20] The hospital is a magnificent, old, vanilla-hued structure, perched like a palace or fortress on a knoll in Los Angeles. Construction was finished in 1932, and in the foyer, above the large entrance doors is engraved:

> Erected by the citizens of the County of Los Angeles to provide hospital care for the acutely ill and suffering to whom the doctors of the attending staff give their services without charge in order that no citizen of the County shall be deprived of their health or life for lack of such care and services.

Richard Bukata, one of the early LAC/USC emergency medicine residents, remembers interviewing at LAC/USC and beholding the building for the first time:

> I just remember this enormous frigging hospital...it's built on a hill so it looks like it's even bigger than it is. It seemed enormous. It looks like the walls are about 4-feet thick on the thing. I just remember looking up the steps of the place and saying, "Holy smokes!" ...I'd never seen anything like that. I remember going to the emergency department and people were, they were just screaming and yelling and it was like God, what am I getting myself into?[20]

The noble calling of the physicians and staff of Big County was stressed to the limits by the same factors that increased hospital visits across the country in the post–World War II period. ED visits increased so sharply, with primarily indigent patients, that by the late 1960s there was a genuine crisis in emergency care. LAC/USC Medical Center was handling an astounding 1,000 patients a day through its ED. The ED was a massive intake area for true emergencies and countless nonemergent patients who presented there because they did not have a physician or did not know how else to access health care. It was staffed by interns and residents, supplemented by a pool of 250 moonlighting physicians.[21]

Gail V. Anderson, Sr., M.D., was in Southern California even before the boom of the 1960s. An obstetrician gynecologist by training, he became the first full-time faculty member in obstetrics and gynecology at LAC/USC in 1958 and was named a professor and director. Anderson was very interested in gynecologic emergencies, and the ED of LAC/USC Medical Center was especially rich in gynecologic pathology. About 20% of the patients who were admitted to the hospital from the LAC/USC ED had gynecologic or obstetric problems. Anderson had become an expert in surgical procedures for dealing with pelvic infections and abscesses. He was also very aware of how gynecologic emergencies could be mismanaged in the ED by untrained physicians— "patients with ectopics were going to medicine to be worked up for anemia of unknown etiology, toxemia patients were going to neurology, it was a mess."[21] He assigned his gynecology residents to shifts in the ED to try to provide better care for these patients. Anderson understood that emergency care in the1960s was almost uniformly of poor quality. As a medical student in the 1950s, he had worked as the "doctor" at a "storefront" ED clinic in Alhambra. As an intern in Washington, D.C., he remembers a major highway accident, with victims presenting to the ED and private surgeons being unavailable to care for critically injured patients.[21,22]

In 1968, the county opened a new Women's Hospital a block away from the main LAC/USC hospital, and Anderson directed a new emergency area in the Women's Hospital that saw 100 patients a day. The LAC/USC Medical Center ED in 1970 was run by an internist named Ann Elconin. Elconin had identified the immense need for more medical coverage in the ED and sought a way to do this. She looked for federal help. Roger Egeberg, M.D., had been the dean at the USC Medical School and was at that time undersecretary for health in the Nixon administration. Elconin worked with Egeberg to develop a grant to help fund the training of physicians and physician's assistants in emergency care. She applied for and received grant support from the Department of Health, Education, and Welfare to begin training three emergency medicine residents per year in 1971. The residency would consist of 2 years of training after a rotating internship. Elconin announced that she was leaving just before the residency was to start. This created a leadership crisis in the ED, and the administration scrambled to find a replacement. Robert Tranquada the medical director of LAC/USC Medical Center knew Gail Anderson, Sr., well and respected the high quality work that Anderson had done with gynecologic patients in the ED. Anderson remembers that around May 1971, Tranquada came to him and said, "We've got a problem, would you help us fix it?"[21] Anderson was preparing to go to Peru to help the Peruvian Navy start a residency in obstetrics and gynecology. He found the idea of directing the ED intriguing, particularly because his home department had not treated him well. By 1970, the USC medical school was trying to become more nationally prominent in cutting-edge obstetrics and gynecology areas like infertility and high-risk obstetrics. Anderson's skills in gynecologic surgery became less valued. Although he had been the first full-time professor in obstetrics and gynecology at LAC/USC, others were elevated to more powerful positions at the new Women's Hospital. It was a good time for a change in his practice, but only if certain conditions could be met:

> So I said if you guys are serious, and I didn't have a notion that these guys would do what I asked them to do…if you really want this thing to go, establish a department and if you will make me chairman and professor and give me 10 faculty… I would seriously consider it, but I didn't really think that this could ever come off. But, I spent the month in Peru…The day I got back…Bob approached me and said, "They gave you virtually everything you asked for." And I said, "No kidding!" At that moment, I didn't know what I was going to do with it, but I had made this commitment so that was the beginning of my second career.[21]

In this inauspicious manner, Gail Anderson, M.D., became the first chairman of the first department of emergency medicine in a U.S. medical school in October of 1971 (see insert, Figure 16). He assumed control of three emergency medicine residents who had started their residency in July. He had received permission to hire 10 faculty members. He believes that other departments agreed to give up faculty spots to his new department because they thought that the department of emergency medicine "wouldn't make it anyway, so there was no big gamble." Anderson had negotiated well and he gained a key concession in control over who determined when and where patients were admitted.

> One of my stipulations of taking the job was that besides the space, faculty, the one thing I stood firm on was that I had to have absolute admitting rights to any service…so I said whatever we admit is going to be admitted, you guys can fight it out the next day whether it's an appropriate admission or not. That was very important in those early days….[21]

Anderson still had a huge task ahead of him in bringing some organization and quality to the resident-run ED. The day before he was to start as chairman and director of the ED he gained a first-hand view of his new department as a patient:

> I slit my finger in my backyard and…I came in here as a patient…I tried to tell them starting at the guard down here that I was in charge of the department, and they said, "Oh sure, yeah, I'm President Nixon, too." It was a comedy of things like that, and I played the game for about 1½ to 2 hours and the final blow was when I was in there washing my finger in Betadine in the minor trauma area…and a fairly solid individual, by that I mean academically solid, was talking to me and was taking care of my finger and some second-year resident walked in from orthopedics and started talking about how he would screw somebody in a dorm, and whatever, and I said, "Wait a minute this doctor is taking care of my finger and I don't want you interfering with my treatment." He said, "Who the fuck are you?" I said, "Well go out there, pick up the phone and call your chairman…and ask him who Gail Anderson is." So he went outside and called and came back in, "Oh I'm so sorry." Anyway, that's quite an experience to go through all of that.[21]

Anderson at this point had no knowledge of ACEP or of the existence of the Cincinnati residency program, but he quickly became familiar with the key figures in the field. Like Pam Bensen, he attended his first ACEP meeting in the fall of 1971 in Miami. Bensen went as a starry-eyed intern, but Anderson went as the freshly crowned chair of emergency medicine at USC, and director of the busiest ED in the country. He found that people like Wiegenstein and Mills were looking to him for advice and leadership on how emergency medicine could advance in the academic world. Anderson certainly cut the figure of a leader: handsome and tall with a strong, sure voice and a pleasant, light Southern accent from his boyhood in Pensacola, Florida. But he was not yet prepared to lead on a national level—his local responsibilities would take all of his time for the next few years. Anderson's role was as a full-time administrator, managing the crises that were part of day-to-day life in the busy LAC health system. His job was to keep the ED afloat and the residency alive. He never assumed a major role working shifts in the ED and did not claim to be an expert in the broad field of emergency medicine. He was well versed in gynecologic emergencies and septic shock and taught residents in these areas.

Anderson endeavored to help the City of Los Angeles develop its EMS. The inadequacies and disorganization of EMS in Los Angeles were made apparent in 1968 when Robert Kennedy was shot at the Ambassador Hotel while campaigning as the Democratic presidential candidate. The City of Los Angeles ambulance personnel operated out of a receiving hospital that did not have good emergency or trauma capability. Kennedy was transported by an ambulance crew who passed by a qualified hospital on the way to the receiving hospital. Anderson remembers that at the receiving hospital, "There was nobody there to take care of them and then they had to go back."[21] Kennedy died of his wounds, and a grand jury investigated the emergency services response. As a result of this, the City of Los Angeles stationed EMS providers at firehouses around the city and approved paramedic training programs. When Anderson took over in 1971, he agreed to train Los Angeles paramedics at LAC/USC Medical Center and put his department squarely in the middle of EMS in Los Angeles. Anderson later developed a Medical Alert Center to coordinate helicopter services, a hyperbaric chamber, and other rescue programs out of the LAC/USC ED. Anderson's approach was to take on new activities and responsibilities—to be in the mix of anything that had to do with emergency services in Los Angeles—and then to try to hire people who could do the detail work. He even agreed that the department of emergency medicine would run the jail ward, a 50-bed unit in the LAC/USC Medical Center. His faculty conducted studies on toxicology and other diseases in this unit.

One of Anderson's first moves was to hire Robert Dailey as the residency director. Dailey was a tall, lanky, intense, but perpetually smiling young physician who was working as the junior associate chief of the ED at Highland Hospital in Alameda, California. Dailey grew up in New Jersey as a "white, Anglo Saxon, Protestant, upper-middle-class suburbanite" who attended Amherst College and Cornell Medical School. Despite this traditional, privileged course, Dailey emerged as something of a nonconformist. He did his postgraduate training in internal medicine at four different institutions, including a 2-year stint in the Air Force in Idaho. He took a year off to travel around the world. Eventually he started practice as an internist with the Kaiser system because he wanted to be near San Francisco. It took only 4 months for Dailey to realize that he was not happy, which prompted a "great self-revaluation that I was temperamentally unfit for internal medicine and I had to undergo a very painful if brief soul-searching to decide what I was going to do for a career." Dailey had always enjoyed his time in acute care and EDs during his internal medicine training. He inquired about jobs in the area, and as he prepared to leave on a 6-week ski vacation, "jobless and without a care in the world," Dailey got a call from the director at Highland Hospital ED. He interviewed, accepted the job, took the ski vacation, and returned in 1970 to start his job.[23]

Although it was in many ways a typical county ED, Highland Hospital had a good reputation in emergency care. Dailey, who had always enjoyed teaching, was delighted to be responsible for many interns and residents. He remembers:

> At that time it was a hospital that was, in many ways, way ahead of its time. For instance, the emergency department was the tail that wagged the dog. It was very busy, two thirds of the admissions were from the emergency department; all of the house staff spent a great deal of time in the emergency department because service needs were great. It was a full hospital department low and behold. It had two full-time staff at a time when the hospital had five full-time staff...So it was a wonderful introduction to emergency medicine and interestingly Highland Hospital through the years produced many, many emergency physicians before emergency medicine ever existed...It was very easy for them to like emergency medicine. Many of them with a year of internship started a career in emergency medicine. Not many of those at that time achieved "prominence" or involved themselves in the national scene in emergency medicine, but by golly, they sure provided a lot of practitioners in California especially.[23]

Some of the physicians who worked in the breeding ground of Highland Hospital ED in the 1960s and early 1970s did go on to achieve national prominence. Peter Rosen, who finished his surgical residency at Highland in 1965, was about to embark on his academic career in emergency medicine in the early 1970s. Dailey would go on to become a key figure in the early development of residency training programs in emergency medicine, and later a close friend of Rosen. Michael Callaham, M.D., another East Coast boy who came to San Francisco for the weather and the late 1960s' culture of the Bay Area, attended medical school at the University of California, San Francisco from 1966 to 1970. Callaham did his internship at Highland and worked with Dailey in the ED. He remembers, "after finishing a flexible internship it was considered logical that I would be eminently qualified to be director of an emergency department." Callaham was hired by Karl Mangold, the original Bay area emergency medicine entrepreneur, to be the ED director at Fairmont Hospital in San Leandro. He later followed Dailey to LAC/USC where he did his residency in emergency medicine. Callaham would go on to become the highly regarded editor of *Annals of Emergency Medicine*. At a time when all major teaching hospital EDs were resident-run, the Highland Hospital ED seemed to function better than most. It was busy, yet did not overwhelm the residents. Supervision was lacking, yet the ED was organized enough to make working there fun rather than frustrating. The Highland ED experience planted a seed in many young physicians' minds that emergency practice might be a career option worth pursuing.

It did not take long for Bob Dailey to realize that his decision to leave internal medicine for emergency medicine was a good one. When he started work as an internist, his parents bought him a desk nameplate for his practice and expected that he would one day hang out his shingle. Dailey notes, "I wasn't going to hang out a shingle, I was going to hang out in the emergency department."[23] Dailey quickly became a leader in the Highland ED. His boss, the director of the ED was not involved in the clinical workings of the ED. Dailey remembers that his boss, "Mostly sat in his office, rolled his own, and...dabbled at administration because he was near retirement age and that was a good venue for it." Dailey managed the interns and residents and it occurred to him, just as it had to Herbert Flessa and David Wagner that it might be a good thing to train physicians to practice only in the ED. Dailey found out about ACEP and attended the Winter Symposium in Las Vegas in 1972.[23] He met R. R. Hannas, who then was the chair of the Commission on Education for ACEP. Because Dailey was very involved in intern and resident education at the Highland Hospital ED, Hannas asked him to become a member of the Graduate Medical Education Subcommittee. Dailey also met Gail Anderson, who was desperately seeking faculty members for his new academic department at LAC/USC. Anderson offered the position of residency director to Dailey, who jumped at the chance.

Dailey came to LAC/USC in 1972 as residency director and found a different environment than at Highland. The ED was truly out of control, bursting with patients, and it was not clear who was in charge. Emergency medicine residents fought with medical and surgical residents to manage critical cases. The LAC/USC hospital had a legendary practice of giving "red blanket" treatment to critically ill patients. The practice began pre–World War II as a way of identifying patients on the hospital ward who promptly needed tests or attention—a red blanket was placed on the foot of the bed of these patients. The term "red blanket" came to be used whenever a very sick patient needed something done immediately—so that even today emergency medicine residents upon encountering a critically ill patient, will call out: "We need to R.B. this guy!"[24] The "C-booth" area of the LAC-USC ED has been used for resuscitating patients since 1946. William Mallon, M.D., a current faculty member says, "Over the last 50 years, more people have probably died, and been saved, in this little space than anywhere else in the country."[24]

But in the 1970s, the emergency medicine residents at LAC/USC ED, who were the new kids on the block, had to assert themselves to be involved in the care of sicker patients. The pioneer residents in the LAC/USC—Richard Goldberg, Marilyn Boitano, and Joseph McDougall—had even greater challenges than Bruce Janiak at Cincinnati and Pam Bensen and her classmates at MCP. One problem was the sheer magnitude of patients to be seen and the relatively small impact that the one or two emergency medicine residents on duty had in a milieu that included scores of residents who were assigned to the ED or came to the ED to consult on or admit patients.[22] The early LAC/USC emergency medicine residents could become lost in the shuffle, and because Anderson, as the leader of the department, did not work clinical shifts, he was not often there to advocate for or support the residents. Another problem was the "red blanket" treatment for critical cases at LAC/USC. Patients who were critically ill or injured and designated "red blanket" cases were descended upon by medical or surgical teams from the hospital wards and rapidly moved to intensive care units. The role for early emergency medicine residents was minimal in such cases.

As the new residency program director, Bob Dailey attempted to put some order into emergency medicine resident education. He developed a curriculum that had more ED time for the residents than residents at Cincinnati and MCP were experiencing. He developed a didactic program. The training program was still subject to almost monthly modification by the residents. Michael Orlinsky, M.D., did his residency from 1974 to 1976. Like many of the other early residents, he had been out in the world, working for 2 years as part of the Public Health Service on an Indian reservation before coming back to do emergency medicine residency. Orlinsky remembers that half of his residency months were spent in the ED and that emergency medicine residents were not allowed to rotate on surgical services because the chairman of surgery did not believe in the concept of emergency medicine training. Orlinsky quit his obstetrics and gynecology rotation after 1 day because he believed he would not learn anything new. Teaching by faculty in the ED was spotty at best. Orlinsky remembers one faculty member was a pediatrician, but was better known as an acupuncturist.[25] Michael Callaham remembers an emergency medicine faculty member

…who always wore sneakers and jeans…an eccentric kind of guy who would just kind of wander through the emergency department. But again, in those days, to have an attending nonpresence wasn't even slightly remarkable. In a lot of programs you didn't expect to see the attending, so we didn't, it was a self-teaching program.[26]

Richard Bukata, who came to the residency just after Callaham, also found the quality of the faculty to be quite poor, except for Bob Dailey:

They were a hodgepodge of doctors who had come from this or that kind of thing. Their skill sets were generally very weak, but the star of the program was Bob Dailey. He had the charisma and the interest and the passion and the leadership so that he was the program in terms of why people would go there, in addition to the fact that they had this extraordinary pathology. But, in terms of the training program, there were so many weird doctors who were faculty…a lot of them honestly were misfits that seemed to kind of gravitate there and found a job. They were nice enough people but it certainly in terms of their ability to teach you very much they were very weak.[20]

The LAC/USC ED was a place where the unexpected happened on a daily basis. In a walk through the ED, Anderson points to a stretcher where he remembers a patient who took a direct route to his ED care. A depressed man was hospitalized in the twelfth-floor psychiatric ward, part of the hospital that towers over the ground-floor ED. Anderson remembers he was in the ED teaching a group of students how to suture. The patient jumped out of a window from this height and plunged through a skylight of the ED to land roughly on a stretcher where Anderson had just finished teaching. The man was successfully resuscitated as a trauma patient.[21] The experiential nature of training in the LAC/USC emergency department created residents who by the end of their training were confident and felt like they had seen it all, even if they had not learned it all. William Mallon, M.D., who trained in emergency medicine at LAC/USC in the 1980s remembers coming to California as an East Coast medical student and, "…being interviewed by a resident who wore a butcher's apron with blood stains all over it, and a muscle shirt underneath." I thought, "This is the toughest motherfucker I have ever seen!" During his residency, Mallon remembers a faculty member giving a lecture on airway management "with an inch of ash hanging off his cigarette."[24]

Although some early residents were not clinically strong, and some did not even stay in the field of emergency medicine, the LAC/USC emergency medicine residency of the early 1970s produced many physicians who would later become leaders in emergency medicine, including Gerald Whelan, Richard Bukata, Ronald Stewart, and Ronald Crowell. Bukata would become the father of emergency medicine continuing education. Stewart would go on to develop a strong emergency medicine program at the University of Pittsburgh and cofound the National Association of Emergency Medical Service Physicians (see insert, Figure 17). Crowell would become the EMS director of the state of California. As other residencies began to develop in Southern California, some medical students opted for a less busy ED for training. Jerome Hoffman, M.D., who became a leading academic figure at the University of California at Los Angeles (UCLA) Medical Center, started his residency at LAC/USC but was dissatisfied and left to finish his residency at UCLA when that program started. For Bob Dailey, 2 years as a residency director at LAC/USC was enough. As might be expected for someone who was new to a residency director position in that frenetic environment, Dailey never figured out how to deliver a solid educational program to his residents and was bothered by the lack of support for the residency. In a manner similar to Phillip Buttaravoli, who came to Cincinnati with such high expectations, Dailey was an idealist who could not tolerate the conditions at LAC/USC. In 1974, he moved to Valley Medical Center in Fresno, California, as the director of the ED, with a promise that he could start a residency program in emergency medicine. Rich Bukata remembers the group of residents at LAC/USC "was pissed because he was the residency."[20] When he left LAC/USC, Dailey jumped out of the fire and into a frying pan.

Dailey arrived in Fresno to discover that the Valley Medical Center ED was staffed by resident physicians who had a certain stake in their ED work:

> Well, before I showed up for work I was moving into my apartment the day before and a pleasant young man volunteered to help me unload my car which I thought was really nice and I was asking about who he was and he said he was the chief surgical resident at VMC. I said how interesting, because I'm coming as chief of emergency medicine. Whereupon his face took on a different aspect and a friendly helping hand was replaced with a glower of admonition, and he told me not terribly politely that I would be wise to take what bags I had taken out of my car and place them back in the car because the idea of an emergency residency which has been circulated at the hospital was an anathema and that they would ride—the house staff as one—would ride me out of town on a rail if I so much as suggested an emergency residency. I said, how so? The how so was that the residents at the time were probably making $15,000 a year, only they were all moonlighting in the emergency department and picking up an extra $7000. So, if we start an emergency residency, developed with the funds that were being used for moonlighting, we would in one stroke not discontinue their obligation to working in the emergency department. Number two, would remove 33% of their current salary…and number three, they would have another department in the hospital which had potential for conflicting with their own interests. Well, all of these were true. So, within the first week of my tenure at Valley Medical Center I was to have a meeting with the medical director and the executive committee of the house staff. When I showed up in the cafeteria, low and behold, virtually every house staffer was there. The only thing that was missing was the large pot in which to throw the missionary. But, in effect what happened was they said what do you intend to do Dr. Dailey? I told them exactly what I intended to do, and to a man and woman they said, "Oh no I wasn't!" I said, "Oh yes I was!" Well, it was one against something like 150, and the rest is history because we, fortunately, the administration and the medical director already made the decision that it was going to happen…It was simply divined and…it was tough for about 2 years.[23]

Dailey, with the help of Michael Callaham, who followed him from LAC/USC, developed a solid emergency medicine program in Fresno with a residency that produced more emergency physician leaders, like Robert Knopp, who became the long-standing chair at Valley Medical Center. Then, like the closure of a loop of California medical history, Dailey and Callaham returned to Highland Hospital in the late 1970s to establish an emergency medicine residency at the place that had provided the early spark for many who went into emergency medicine on the West Coast.

The career change of Gail Anderson from gynecologist to emergency medicine administrator was the sentinel event in a groundswell of academic activity in emergency medicine in the Western United States. Many refer to Anderson as "a figurehead," but in the good sense of the word. Anderson knew that he would not, after having a successful career as a gynecologist, be able to retool as an emergency physician, but he did come to believe passionately in training people to deliver high quality prehospital and ED care. Like John Wiegenstein, he was a tall, white-haired, "elegant statesman" who could successfully negotiate with deans, hospital directors, city administrators, and local politicians to advance the cause of emergency medicine. His approach for his own department was to hire good people and let them do their work. After a few years, this formula was successful, and the LAC/USC program thrived in a very challenging environment. Anderson would then go on to play a significant role in helping to form the American Board of Emergency Medicine.

CULTIVATING EMERGENCY MEDICINE RESIDENCIES IN THE HEARTLAND OF AMERICA

After the first emergency medicine residencies became established in the Midwest (Cincinnati), the East (MCP), and West (LAC/USC), the next new wave of residencies, from 1972 to 1975, came out of the Midwest. In Louisville, Donald Thomas, the rollicking red-haired, gun-toting anesthesiologist, who ran the Louisville EMS system and was known as "the Chief" by the legions of Louisville EMS providers he had trained in the 1960s, began to push for the academic development of emergency medicine in his hospital in 1970. In a manner almost identical to what happened with Gail Anderson at LAC/USC, Thomas was asked by his medical center to shift his administrative role from his primary field to emergency medicine. Thomas was asked to become the director of the ED at Louisville General Hospital in September of 1970, and he petitioned for full departmental status in the Louisville medical school. This was granted in 1971. Thomas's emergency medicine residency started in July 1972. An article in the *Journal of the American College of Emergency Physicians* noted that Thomas used the "Proposed Essentials of a Residency Training Program in Emergency Medicine" to develop the program. This demonstrates that although the "Proposed Essentials...," which were developed by ACEP in 1970, had been rejected by the AMA in 1971, they were still used by early programs as a guideline for structuring an emergency medicine residency. The Louisville program was a 2-year program after an internship. Louisville also offered an emergency medicine internship with 4 months of ward medicine, 2 months in the ED, and 6 months of elective time, but the internship was still considered a separate training experience.[11]

R. R. Hannas led the charge in the realm of education for ACEP from its inception, but it was a big step for him to formally return to the world of academic medicine and direct a residency program. Hannas, regarded as a prime mover by many of the national medical organizations, was wary of pedagogues and high-minded academicians. His role in the American Academy of General Practice (AAGP), ACEP, and the AMA brought him to the attention of the American Hospital Association (AHA). He was asked to be a member of a Blue Ribbon Committee that was responsible for studying U.S. health care and making recommendations. Hannas's work for this committee was in ambulatory and emergency care. The committee produced a report in a smartly bound little yellow book called the "America Plan" that was sent to Congress, but there was no significant action on the elements of the plan. Through his work with the AHA, Hannas met administrators at Evanston Hospital in Illinois, who recruited Hannas to come in and clean up their emergency services. Hannas agreed to come if he was allowed to start an emergency medicine residency. He moved from Kansas City to Evanston in 1971, and quickly applied for a residency program. He started three physicians in July of 1972 as interns as part of a 3-year training program in emergency medicine. Only one of the three ended up practicing emergency medicine. One example of how loose the residency structure was in the early days of emergency medicine was Hannas's agreement to allow a physician who had completed a residency in internal medicine to do only 4 months of training in order to graduate from the Evanston emergency medicine residency. Because there was no regulatory body for emergency medicine residencies, physicians who had done internships or portions of other residency programs, or who had been out in practice, were permitted to make individual deals with emergency medicine programs on the duration of their emergency medicine training. R. R. Hannas stayed at Evanston just long enough to see his first graduate, but he found that support for emergency medicine was waning in the hospital. He remembers when he started at Evanston Hospital,

> …three guys…were my supporters there, one was head of surgery, one was head of medicine, another was the assistant administrator. All physicians, all solidly behind me. So…about the fourth year…two of them retired and the other one quit medicine for a while. What did they do? They made the ED run by a committee that had a pediatrician that hated my guts, an obstetrician [who] didn't know anything about it, a surgeon [who] was absolutely against us and that was the committee. That was bullshit, so I told them sorry about this fellows and I made arrangements to leave and I took a job then down in Austin, Texas.[27]

Hannas's brief sojourn into academic medicine ended in 1975 when he became the director of the ED at Brackenridge Hospital in Austin, Texas, a place he refers to as "a zoo." Hannas struggled in Texas with bureaucratic problems and a high indigent patient load. His plans for an emergency medicine residency at this new site fell through, and he lasted only a little more than a year. Hannas's next stop was also a new and different setting. St. Joseph Hospital in Kansas City was in an impoverished part of the city and served a poor, primarily black community. Hannas knew of St. Joseph Hospital from his previous time in Kansas City and remembers when the director of the Emergency Department Committee at St. Joseph Hospital, Clarence C. Reynolds, "a big old black guy, C. C. Reynolds" called him in Texas: "R squared?," this big deep voice, 'This is C squared—get your ass up here!' I did, and I knew I had it."[27] Hannas found professional and personal happiness back in Kansas City. He worked with mostly black physicians caring for the poor of Kansas City. He and his second wife, Kay, traveled extensively and were often the animated life of the party at ACEP functions. Conditions improved when a new St. Joseph Hospital was built in a better location, with a new, modern ED. Hannas worked at St. Joseph Hospital for 21 years and retired in 1987 at the age of 69 (see insert, Figure 10).

At the same time that R. R. Hannas was starting his residency program at Evanston Hospital, Peter Rosen was a stone's throw south at the University of Chicago. Rosen, who had his career as a Western surgeon abruptly halted by two heart attacks, returned to Chicago, where he had done his internship, to become the director of the ED. Rosen, at the age of 36, was made an associate professor of surgery with tenure and suspects "there were no other applicants" for the job.[28] Ironically, this would be the only job in his career in which Rosen would achieve tenure. Before returning to Chicago, Rosen and his family took a vigorous summer vacation, driving around the western part of the United States.

> I guess it was sort of a stress test, if that didn't kill me it would be all right to go back to work…While I was on that journey I found an article…about the Cincinnati residency and I had thought that was a brilliant idea, obviously, to train people to be there that want to be there. I'd met a couple of guys in Wyoming who had done emergency medicine in other locations and had heard that that was beginning to occur and it seemed to me a very logical solution to the major problem which was there was no labor pool. There were a lot of other problems but that to me was the number one problem because when I went back to look at the job at the University of Chicago where I had interned, they were still working out of the same small Emergency Department that had been there when I was an intern that saw fewer than 10,000 patients, and now they were seeing 56,000 patients. Instead of staffing with one intern, they were staffing with two interns and two first-year residents. That was it. There were no faculty, the [director] never set foot in the emergency department. I guess his job was to make out a schedule and that was about it. And of course it was an unbelievable

mess and I decided on that trip that I was going to start a residency as soon as possible because there was no way to get manpower there.[29]

Rosen was not greeted with open arms. He remembers,

The first month that I was at the University of Chicago there was a faculty meeting. It was the only faculty meeting in the 6 years that I was there that had 100% attendance. The subject was the emergency department. I presented my plans for the emergency department and before I ever said a word, the chair of surgery, the department I had been appointed in, stood up and said anybody who would do full-time emergency medicine was demeaning to this faculty.[29]

Even in his own department, Rosen was in a bad situation, but his position was tenured, and he never backed down from a battle. Most surgical residents were displeased with spending any time in the ED and were livid when they were pulled off surgical or research rotations to help with the increasing emergency patient volumes. Rosen first attempted to hire surgical faculty members to provide supplemental staffing to the ED.

The president of the university gave me special funds to hire surgical faculty to cover the surgical side of the emergency department. I could pay them $25 an hour and I had a full professor who would call 5 minutes before a shift and say, "I forgot about a dinner party tonight, I can't come." When they did come they were so scared of seeing patients that they would hide in the doctors' work room while the first-year medical residents saw all the patients.[29]

When it became apparent that piecemeal staffing would not solve the great need for physicians to work in the ED, Rosen went back to his initial plan to start an emergency medicine residency. He again met with the department chairs and administrators at the University of Chicago.

I gave them several alternatives and why I didn't think they would work. It's clear that we can't keep doing what we have been doing. There is not enough manpower, the residents in other specialties are neither interested in the emergency department, nor do they want to spend time there, and their respective services keep pulling them. I said we could hire an outside group, which is what they thought they were getting, that I would come in and run it like a student health service. I said we could do that and probably do it pretty quickly but you won't live with that and the reason you won't live with that is because you will not give that group what they have in an private hospital, namely admitting privileges and the kind of clinical support that you haven't given anybody in this emergency department. I said the only real alternative for this university is to create an academic program in emergency medicine just like every other specialty and we will train people to be there, we will teach them to be there, and we will teach them how to be emergency physicians, and they will teach others. So they accepted that.[29]

Around this time, a tragic case of a missed diagnosis in the University of Chicago ED helped Rosen to advance his cause:

It was my first year at University of Chicago and it was the incident over which the emergency medicine residency program was approved at the University of Chicago. It was in 1971. I went…for a ski trip over Christmas and while I was away there was a graduate student who came in with belly pain. The first-year resident in medicine consulted the first-year resident in surgery and they didn't realize that he had a perforated ulcer and they sent him home and he died. The first-year radiology resident hadn't read his film correctly, which was a difficult film because his free air was in the lesser sac rather than under the diaphragm. Well, the response to that was to fire all three of the residents. I went to each department and I said this is absolutely hypocritical. You don't provide any teaching to these people. You don't provide any supervision, you're not available to them when they get a difficult case, and this was not an easy case, and then you want to punish them for making a mistake that they couldn't help making. They weren't trying to harm this patient, they weren't being lazy, they were seeing 56,000 patients between the two of them and where were you? You were in bed and you will not fire someone from my department who was working unsupervised. So they didn't fire any of them. That was when I began to realize that (although it took me a few years longer) that you needed to have 24-hour attending supervision and that the house of medicine was filled with hypocrisy.[29,30]

The negative publicity from this case along with Rosen's strong stance forced the university to act.[28,30] Rosen was allowed to hire five faculty members and to develop a 2-year, postinternship emergency medicine residency with 16 residency slots. This was a major accomplishment considering that the university had a hiring freeze on for faculty at that time. Rosen visited the University of Cincinnati residency program, which was in its second year, and as noted before, was not a stellar training program at that point. He met Tom Blum, and realized that Blum did not know any more about training emergency medicine residents than he did. One of the things that Rosen least liked about the Cincinnati residency was the lack of time spent in the ED

At the time I saw it, the bulk of the residency was rotating on other people's service and it looked like 3 years of rotating internship. I just felt that you don't learn how to do surgery by rotating on the medical service, and you don't learn emergency medicine by rotating on an inpatient service, you learn it by taking care of patients in an emergency department, which was the model I learned surgery from. You learn surgery by doing surgery under the teaching, in my case, of senior residents because we didn't have any faculty.[29]

Rosen's approval process was similar to what other early emergency medicine residencies had experienced. He wrote to the AMA to ask how a residency becomes listed in the "Green Book," the catalogue of all U.S. residency programs. He never got a reply. Rosen started with one resident in 1972 and then a full residency class of eight residents in 1973. He had great difficulty hiring qualified faculty, and despite his intention to train residents well, he admits that in the first few years the education was meager. University of Chicago residents, in a manner very similar to Cincinnati, LAC/USC, and MCP, learned by "taking care of some mighty sick patients—56,000 of them—under the guise of a faculty that was not there 24 hours a day and wasn't very well trained themselves"[29](see insert, Figure 18).

Rosen hired the best people he could from other fields to serve as ED faculty. One of his early hires, Beverly (Bonnie) Fauman, a psychiatrist, credits Rosen as her "first real mentor." Rosen supported Fauman's interests in emergency psychiatry, and she went on to help found the discipline of emergency psychiatry. In 1999, Fauman received the American Association for Emergency Psychiatry's highest award and devoted a significant portion of her remarks to Rosen's role in her development:

Peter was instrumental in further development of my career because of his unique leadership. He has been very nurturing to several generations of physicians, encouraging us to develop, write, teach, and so on, stating that the more we achieved, the better he looked. Further, he believed that the only way to establish emergency medicine as a credible specialty was to do studies and publish…He felt that his responsibility at the University of Chicago was to "teach the teachers," not to train the troops. His goal was to select the best physicians, who would lead emergency medicine into the next decades, not to train doctors simply to run emergency rooms in the suburbs.[31]

It might have been surprising to those who were mentored by Rosen in the early 1970s that he had been a community-based surgeon only 2 years before. Rosen notes, "…it took me probably about 3 years to stop thinking of myself as a surgeon, but it took me exactly a month to realize that somebody trained in a conventional specialty cannot practice emergency medicine just because they trained in another specialty."[32] Rosen's identity change was hastened by his combative nature. Because surgeons opposed and offended him as he started to build his emergency medicine program, they became worthwhile adversaries, and the fact that he had been one of them just a few months before did not seem to matter. He was fueled to a slow boil by the insults and slights at the University of Chicago and nationally, and this made him one of the most outspoken and effective leaders in emergency medicine over the next two decades. Harvey Meislin, one of Rosen's first residents notes, "Peter…was an evangelist for the specialty."[33]

Meislin was a bright and talented surgery intern on the fifth Harvard Surgical Service. The surgery program at Harvard was a 7-year commitment, including 2 years of laboratory time. Meislin's training was done at a variety of Boston hospitals, and in 1973 he met Jeb Boswell, M.D., who had started an emergency medicine residency at the busy Boston City Hospital. Boswell's first resident was Elliot Salenger, M.D. Meislin rotated at Boston City Hospital and was drawn to the work of the overrun ED. After talking with Boswell and Salenger, Meislin thought that training in emergency medicine might be useful, even though he was looking at the field more from a trauma surgery perspective. Meislin got information from Boswell on emergency medicine residencies and interviewed with Bob Dailey at LAC/USC and Peter Rosen at the University of Chicago. Meislin remembers his interviews with Dailey and Rosen:

> I really was impressed with both of them. I really liked what they had to say. They had a vision that was refined, it was focused, it was very similar between the two of them. You could see it—you could almost see the road of where it would be.[33]

At the time, Meislin's future was uncertain because he was drafted to serve in Vietnam, starting in July 1973. He had opted out of the Berry Plan because it would have meant adding years to his surgical training. As Meislin went through his draft physical and was preparing to go to Vietnam, the war was winding down, and in April, it was announced that the draft was not mandatory. He rented a U-Haul truck and drove from Boston to Chicago to start a new life as an emergency medicine resident. A difficult first year would await him as an emergency medicine resident at the University of Chicago (see insert, Figure 18).

> I can tell you very honestly that I was very disappointed in the quality of teaching of education. I'm not sure what I expected, but I kind of expected what I experienced in medical school and at Harvard, and I thought University of Chicago would be like that. It was rough. There were several times I accused Peter of selling goods that weren't real. He and I went at each other several times, in fact I remember calling him up at night and telling him how angry I was about having to be in Chicago and next morning Peter ended up in the coronary care unit. I felt so guilty. I sat vigil. I was at his bedside.[33]

Meislin's experience mirrored the struggles of other early emergency medicine residents at Cincinnati and LAC/USC. One difference in Chicago was the uncommon degree of animosity from other services toward the emergency medicine residents. Meislin describes how bad it could become:

> I mean you'd literally almost come to blows to get some patients admitted. We would do things…we were pretty aggressive because Peter has a surgical background. We would do thoracotomies all the time. You didn't die right away, you got a thoracotomy. Well, occasionally we'd bring one back. If we had some penetrating wound to the chest and he was losing his vital signs, you did a thoracotomy and bring him back and the surgeon said, "I guess we are going to admit him?" The chest is open, you are full of blood. Literally many times, I mean I'm not sure I'd ever do this today, but I'd grab the guy by the throat—I'm physical—I grab the surgical resident and say, "He's coming in or you and I are going outside!" I mean that is how it was and I can tell you there was an event where one of the surgical attendings hit one of our residents, knocked him out. It was rough. It was rough from the neighborhood, it was rough from the abuses you took both externally and internally, …you know, where a year ago I was in a great program, and now I kind of went from the top of the heap to the bottom of the heap. It was rough, those were very rough days.[33]

Many of the problems in the ED stemmed from the unresolved nature of the medical environment at the University of Chicago in the 1970s. This renowned university sits in a beautiful old southside neighborhood in Chicago, with lovely boulevards and Frank Lloyd Wright–designed homes. But surrounding the university neighborhood was a tough, poor, crime-infested section of the city, with roaming gangs like the Blackstone Rangers. Peter Rosen and his family initially lived in this area—in Hyde Park—but his wife and children were victims of threats and a mugging, and Rosen moved his family to a different part of town. The University of Chicago Hospital and Medical School saw itself as a tertiary care, research-based, institution. But, many of its patients were the poor, distressed citizens of its neighborhood, and an uneasy alliance existed between what the University of Chicago Hospital wanted to be and the reality that it functioned like an inner city, indigent care hospital. These tensions often played out in the ED, where the burden of indigent care and diseases of abuse, neglect, and violence were most apparent. Although the University of Chicago Hospital was glad to have someone running and adding some organization to the ED, there was an almost-constant subversive friction that threatened to erode Peter Rosen's initiatives. Meislin notes, "We were a reflection of what the university didn't want. They didn't like emergency medicine, they didn't like the emergency department, and we were filling up the hospital."[33]

As the first University of Chicago emergency medicine residents faced the challenges at their institution, they developed a "band of brothers" mentality. Most lived on the north side of Chicago, and they would car pool to work. Meislin recalls,

> I think our class was a very good class. There were people who were interested in quality care and the academic side of it. And as time went on we started publishing and we started doing research and even though we had no funding for it, and we didn't have time for it, we were working a million hours a week, but we started doing academic things. We would have good teaching conferences, we'd bring people in, so slowly the new unit changed what was going on…we chipped away. We allowed doors to be opened that would otherwise be unopened.[33]

Working with some residency classmates, Meislin remembers developing a proposal to upgrade the EMS system in Chicago to modular ambulances with paramedics. At the time, the Chicago Fire Department ran all ambulance services, which consisted of Cadillac hearses that were configured to transport patients but could provide little in the way of emergency medical care. Meislin and his group made a presentation to the Chicago Fire Departments' famous Commissioner Quinn. After hearing their proposal, Quinn said, "I think the good citizens of Chicago deserve a ride in a Cadillac at least once before they die," and vetoed the proposal. Upgraded ambulances for Chicago would have to wait a few more years.[33]

In addition to developing educational programs, Peter Rosen and other academic leaders had to address the sorry state of their academic EDs. The crowded, resident-run EDs of urban teaching hospitals were rife with patient safety problems and were often impersonal and insensitive to patients. At the University of Chicago, rape victims might be announced in the ED as "we have an alleged rape here!" Rosen issued a memorandum in March 1972—"New Procedure for Care of Rape Victims." Rosen wrote that "effective immediately…all rape victims will be referred to as 'Code R' patients; the words 'alleged rape' will not be used."[34] This more humane treatment of sexual assault victims was just one example of the hundreds of changes that were required to improve care in teaching hospital EDs.

STRENGTH IN NUMBERS, BUT NOT IN THE WORLD OF MEDICINE

The number of emergency medicine residencies tripled between 1972 and 1973, from five to 16 residencies. By 1975 it was up to 32 (Table 5.1). Ron Krome, who like Rosen and David Wagner was a young surgeon in charge of a busy ED, started a program at Detroit Receiving Hospital with Brooks Bock, M.D., as its first program director. Krome was assuming a more important role in ACEP as the chair of the Graduate

TABLE 5.1   Emergency Medicine Residency Programs as of January 1975

Akron City Hospital
Akron General Hospital
Albert Einstein College of Medicine (New York, N.Y.)
Baptist Medical Center of Oklahoma
Bowman-Gray School of Medicine
Charity Hospital (New Orleans, La.)
Denver General Hospital
Evanston Hospital (Evanston, Ill.)
Georgetown University Hospital
Grady Memorial Hospital (Atlanta, Ga.)
Hennepin County General Hospital (Minneapolis, Minn.)
Hershey Medical Center (Hershey, Penn.)
Johns Hopkins Hospital
Kansas City General Hospital
Los Angeles County/USC Medical Center
Louisville General Hospital
Medical College of Pennsylvania (Philadelphia, Penn.)
Medical University of South Carolina
Methodist Hospital (Indianapolis, Ind.)
Northwestern University (Chicago, Ill.)
Providence Hospital (Portland, Ore.)
Royal Victoria Hospital (Montreal, Canada)
St. Anthony's Hospital (Denver, Colo.)
St. Francis Hospital (Peoria, Ill.)
St. Lawrence Hospital (East Lansing, Mich.)
St. Louis City Hospital
St. Vincent's Hospital (Toledo, Ohio)
University of Chicago Hospitals
University of Cincinnati Medical Center
University of Kentucky
University of New Mexico School of Medicine
Valley Medical Center (Fresno, Calif.)

From Emergency Medicine Residency Newsletter, published in *J.A.C.E.P.*, Jan/Feb 1975, page 73.

Education Subcommittee and would become a driving force in the organization of academic emergency medicine. He served as the key link in the 1970s between the academic and nonacademic worlds of emergency medicine. Kendall McNabney, the Vietnam War surgeon who was interested in the development of emergency medicine, also started a residency in emergency medicine in 1973 at the Kansas City General Hospital.

The directors of the early residency programs became acquainted from ACEP meetings. The knowledge that they were not alone was comforting amidst the immense challenges of running the early emergency medicine residencies. As Bob Dailey describes,

> You can ask the next question, which is: "When did the fun start?" Of course the fun started almost immediately because there were a lot of people involved in emergency medicine who were nationally involved and who were starting residencies under the worst of circumstances…I mean starting a residency program was akin to lifting yourself up by your boot straps. I mean the idea of faculty was ludicrous. Yet you had to have faculty. The idea of receiving institutional monetary and academic support was ludicrous. So the idea of the emergency department as anything other than that dreadful place down on the first floor that you always had letters of complaint from, and other problems with, suits, etc., etc., and bitching from the house staff about being there—it was nothing but a problem. It was a wart on the ass of prosperity, no question about it.[23]

Dailey called the early program directors together to discuss the condition of their "warts" and other issues in late 1972. Seven residency directors, including Tom Blum, David Wagner, and Peter Rosen, came to Los Angeles and had wide-ranging discussions about how to successfully run a residency. They formed a loose organization, and Dailey was named the liaison to this group by ACEP.

The great majority of the early emergency medicine residencies were developed at institutions that were not considered the elite training sites for American medicine. Cincinnati led the way in the Midwest, and the emergence of other Midwest programs fueled the rapid expansion in emergency medicine residencies between 1970 and 1975. Of the 32 U.S. programs in existence in 1975, 15 were in midwestern states and only five were in the Eastern United States (Table 5.1). The first city to have two emergency medicine residencies was Akron, Ohio. The Akron General Hospital program was started in 1973 by Gus Roussi, an early ACEP leader, and friendly competition undoubtedly caused Akron City Hospital to start its own emergency medicine residency in 1974. John Wiegenstein followed R. R. Hannas's lead as an early ACEP leader with a residency program by starting an emergency medicine residency at his workplace, St. Lawrence Hospital, in 1974. With the exception of Rosen's program at the University of Chicago and a struggling program at Johns Hopkins University, most of the renowned medical schools did not have emergency medicine residencies and had no plans to move in this direction. These institutions had a large corps of residents who covered their EDs and the marginal, unsupervised care that occurred in resident-run EDs was often not much different from the unsupervised care that occurred on the hospital wards. So emergency medicine programs sprang up at St. Francis Hospital in Peoria, Illinois, Hershey Medical Center in central Pennsylvania, Methodist Hospital in Indianapolis, and St. Louis City Hospital, but not at bastions of medical education like Duke University, the University of Pennsylvania, the University of Michigan, Washington University in St. Louis, or the University of Washington in Seattle. Jeb Boswell, M.D., an ACEP member started an emergency medicine residency at Boston City Hospital in 1973, but it lasted only 1 year. Harvard and Massachusetts General Hospital, despite the well-known minifellowship for practicing emergency physicians run by Goldfinger and Dineen, had no institutional interest in starting an emergency medicine residency (see insert, Figure 19).

At nearly all of the big medical school teaching hospitals, EDs evolved that were segregated into medical, surgical, pediatric, and obstetrics/gynecology areas. Residents from each discipline ran the areas, and a faculty member from the corresponding department might provide some administrative support. How the ED functioned was more dependent on the professionalism and dedication of the nursing and ancillary staff than on the residents. If anyone was "in charge" of the whole ED, it was usually a junior surgery faculty member. It is not surprising that this system did not serve as a stimulus for emergency medicine residency training. The ivory towers were somewhat insulated from the two critical factors that drove emergency medicine development elsewhere—service needs and patient complaints and demands. The solution to increasing ED patient volumes in academic centers was to assign more residents to the ED or to hire moonlighting residents, fellows, or itinerant physicians to meet staffing needs. Large urban teaching hospitals continued to struggle with immense patient volumes. Cook County Hospital in Chicago was seeing as many patients as LAC/USC—up to 1,000 new patients per day. A 1971 *Time* magazine article described how Cook County handled patients who presented for emergency care:

> Instead of a traditional all-purpose emergency room, it has an admitting department run by a doctor who serves as a triage, or sorting officer. He sees each patient within 2 minutes of admittance, makes a quick decision as to where the patient should go for treatment. The system means that people will not be served in the order or their arrival, but it should go a long way toward providing prompt and proper attention for serious cases—which is what an emergency room is supposed to offer.[35]

It is very likely that the Cook County admitting doctor was a first- or second-year resident. This type of plan to unload the ED was common in the early 1970s—if a teaching hospital did not develop an emergency medicine residency or have enough qualified physicians to manage the ever-increasing volume of emergency patients, attempts would be made to shunt the patients elsewhere. In most cases, this was like trying to push floodwaters back into a swollen river. The other outpatient areas where patients might be shunted also had limited capacity, and in many cases, this was why patients showed up in the ED—because they were turned away from crowded clinics.

Even if emergency care was not the best, the administration at the large teaching hospitals did not have to worry. Most ED patients at the major urban teaching centers were indigent, uninsured, and lacked a voice or the power to change poor quality care.[36] An implicit understanding existed that the teaching hospital would provide essentially free care for many of their patients, and in turn those patients would accept inefficiencies and indignities without complaining. The situation was different in smaller hospitals that had fewer residents or in those few places like Cincinnati, MCP, and LAC/USC where the solution became to train emergency physicians as a way of dealing with the ED problem. As R. R. Hannas remembers, "We met a public need, a hospital need, and a medical staff need."[27] Each hospital that started an emergency medicine residency was reacting to the service demand by putting fresh, working bodies in their EDs to see a caseload of emergency patients that seemed to be perpetually expanding.

The evolution of emergency medicine training in response to service needs was different from what had occurred in other medical fields. In fields like ophthalmology, otolaryngology, internal medicine, surgery, and pediatrics, the boom in science and research of the early and mid-1900s created silos of knowledge, and it made sense that experts would emerge who would manage these silos and train others to do the same. The leading academic medical centers and medical schools were the natural places for residency training to develop in other medical specialties because that was where the teachers, researchers, and technological advances were based. A cadre of academicians and teachers existed to train those who first sought formal training in these fields. Experienced faculty internists trained resident internists and faculty surgeons trained resident surgeons. It was different in emergency medicine, where the cart seemed to be in front of the horse. Emergency medicine residents were enrolled in training programs where only one or two faculty might have actually practiced in an ED for any amount of time. In emergency medicine, the early leaders were mostly nonacademicians. It was also harder to define the content of the field. The early advances were in systems delivery rather than in medical science, and this was of more interest to hospitals and government than it was to medical schools. Although the early emergency medicine leaders came up with a specific definition of the specialty, and some began residency programs, the rest of medicine was not buying into the idea.

The development of emergency medicine residencies was similar to what occurred in family practice, an immediate predecessor to emergency medicine in the quest for medical specialty status. After family practice was approved as a specialty by the American Board of Medical Specialties (ABMS) in 1969, residencies began to proliferate at medium-sized and smaller hospitals around the country. Like emergency medicine, family practice was largely shut out of mainstream academic medicine in its early years. The traditional disciplines such as internal medicine, surgery, and pediatrics had established their footholds in the major academic centers and were not welcoming to new residencies that might challenge their departments for space, patients, and limited medical school or hospital resources. For the field of family practice, which had a mandate to train physicians for community care, there was less impetus to push for development in the traditional academic centers. Most family practice leaders were content with having a large number of residencies at smaller medical centers and hospitals. Graduates of these programs were more likely to stay and practice in the communities they served as residents. While this approach was instrumental in bringing more family doctors into practice in the United States, family practice remained on the fringe of academic medicine. In the hospital-based field of emergency medicine, the path of least resistance was also in the smaller, less-acclaimed hospitals and academic centers, but the early leaders realized that for the field to become credible, it would eventually have to break the embargo in the major teaching centers.

Physicians who completed family medicine residencies in the early 1970s had a couple of advantages over residency trained emergency physicians—their residencies were approved by the AMA, and they could take a board exam and become certified in their specialty. Because emergency medicine was not an officially approved specialty, its residencies were not listed in the "Green Book," the annual catalogue put out by the AMA of all U.S. residencies.[37] Most of the early emergency medicine residents were mavericks who for the most part did not care about the formal approval of organized medicine. They had made a risky choice to embark on a new path, with no guarantees, and seemed to relish, in a near-sighted way, the uncertainty that was part of forming a new field. Beverly Fauman, who as a psychiatrist and emergency medicine faculty member at University of Chicago interviewed candidates for the emergency medicine residency, noted,

> I often regarded this first residency class as pioneers or "cowboys." They were taking a chance that they were training in something which would become a specialty, but the groundwork was only then being laid. They had been in the service as general medical officers or had run emergency rooms, or simply wanted to be generalists but were too action-oriented to consider family medicine. Many of them had very action-oriented hobbies, were pilots, skiers, or skydivers, and looked for excitement in their medical careers.[31]

Those residents who were more plugged in to what was happening in the field saw that a certifying board might come, but they were not too worried about the details. Pam Bensen, when asked if it bothered her that no emergency medicine board existed when she was training, replied, "Not in the least. All I wanted to do was practice and I knew it was coming. It was just time. There was no doubt in my mind that it would happen...."[19] Some of the early emergency medicine residents viewed boards and certification as the accoutrements of a stodgy medical establishment. The early graduates could obtain fine jobs immediately out of residency, often as directors of EDs, or were hired into faculty level jobs in academic centers. Many thought, why do we need a board? Ironically, it was the older emergency practitioners, who also did not need a board for their own sakes, who saw the bigger picture and realized that residency training without an eventual certifying board would be a dead-end career path for future emergency physicians. As the early residency programs matured and the organizational quest for specialty status moved forward, the emergency medicine residents of the middle to late 1970s came to expect that ABMS Board certification in emergency medicine would be available, and as will be seen later, they protested when it appeared that it would not.

The Organization of Emergency Medicine Academics and Residency Training

THE AMERICAN MEDICAL ASSOCIATION AND EDUCATION IN EMERGENCY MEDICINE

At the same time that the AMA Board of Trustees was approving a provisional Section Council for emergency medicine (1973), the AMA Council on Education twice stubbornly refused to approve ACEP's Proposed Essentials for Residency Training in Emergency Medicine. In 1971, the Council on Education referred the "Essentials" to the section on family practice for review and consideration. This was particularly distressing to emergency medicine leaders. In an address at the ACEP-sponsored Symposium on Community Medical Services and the Design of EDs in February of 1972, James Mills, Jr., was aware that the heads of the AMA Commission on Emergency Medical Services and the Committee on Community Emergency Services were in the audience. He remarked that the image of the AMA "has been that of the Boston Brahmin who gazes disdainfully over his pince-nez at the turbulence of life in the real world," and offered the AMA "an opportunity to partially dispel that image" through approval of the "Proposed Essentials for Residency Training in Emergency Medicine." Mills accused the AMA Council on Education of being woefully out of touch with what was happening in the field of emergency medicine. He claimed that at ACEP's interview with the council, members "asked such basic questions as: 'Doesn't the emergency department just do triage? Aren't you just talking about emergency department directors? You don't mean you work 11 PM to 7 AM? You don't mean a full-time job, do you?'"[38] The AMA was simultaneously giving a warm handshake to emergency physicians as a credible political group in medicine and a cold shoulder to the idea of training emergency physicians. It was in this uncertain climate that emergency medicine was invited to participate in a major AMA conference to attempt to resolve some of the issues surrounding emergency medicine education.

The AMA Council on Medical Education and its Committee on the Emergency Room Physician developed and hosted a 3-day "Workshop Conference on Education of the Physician in Emergency Medicine" at the Marriott Motor Hotel in Chicago in July 1973. The scope of the workshop conference was very broad, as was the list of participants. Seventy-eight people attended. ACEP was well represented, with men like Wiegenstein, Rupke, Mills, Haeck, and Mangold playing an important role. ACEP also cleverly maneuvered for more representation by having R. R. Hannas listed as a representative of the American Academy of Pediatrics, and not under ACEP. The early academic surgeon/emergency physicians were there—Wagner, Podgorny, Krome, and Rosen—as well as 10 surgeons from the University Association for Emergency Medical Services. Bob Dailey represented residency directors in emergency medicine. Oscar Hampton from the American College of Surgeons (ACS) was present, as were representatives from most other medical specialty societies, the ABMS, the American Hospital Association, and the American Association of Medical Colleges. The newly formed Society of Critical Care Medicine had four representatives, led by the prominent resuscitation researcher, Peter Safar. Government officials from the Bureau of Health Manpower Education attended. For the first time, most of the stakeholders in U.S. emergency care were gathered at one meeting, and the stakes were especially high for ACEP and the early residency leaders in emergency medicine. George Podgorny remembers,

> ...it was the first meeting about emergency medicine, not called together by emergency medicine. First time, rest of the house of medicine took a note that something is happening, and...that was the meeting when it became abundantly clear, or crystal clear as Nixon used to say, to everybody that for emergency medicine to progress from the viewpoint of emergency physicians we need a great deal of formal education and training, because until then even many emergency physicians were talking about maybe 6 weeks. You know, we will go and have a preceptorship for 6 weeks. We are going to take a surgeon and we will teach him EKG [electrocardiogram]. We will take an internist and we will teach him how to suture. So that's it, what else do you need to know? ...And that meeting was very rancorous, if I may use that word. Clearly, showed the other specialties that there is such a budding thing as emergency medicine, and that they are most likely not going to go away. They became interested in emergency medicine, people we educated, though they had a different idea how we should be educated. But both sides fought and were not friendly so to say, both really came to the same conclusion—education. How and what is the curriculum was an absolute, you know, a one hundred eighty degree difference.[39]

The goals of the workshop conference were broad and lofty—"to identify and define services provided in emergency medical care and in critical care medicine, to identify...the roles of the medical specialties..., to identify the educational needs of the physician who provides...emergency medical care... [at] ...the undergraduate, graduate, and continuing medical education levels, identify the type of educational standards or essentials which would best meet the educational needs...."[40] One of the "two sides" referred to by Podgorny was the nonemergency practitioners, many of whom believed that emergency medicine was not a legitimate medical specialty, that separate residency training in emergency medicine was not necessary, or if it did become common, that the training should be directed by the other medical specialties. The other camp consisted of the early emergency physicians and some of the academic leaders in emergency medicine. But, some academic leaders, usually young surgeons who were put in charge of teaching hospital EDs were ambivalent in their support of training in the field.

The conference began with a keynote address by R. R. Hannas, who tried to explain emergency care to the nonemergency physicians in the audience by showing a figure that charted the spectrum of care in medicine and the relationship of physician skills, types of health states, and the type of physician that was needed to care for patients in each category. He then presented, in a manner that would not be viewed as typical for him, an erudite, formal, scholarly discussion of the various models of patient/physician interaction, the rationale for emergency care and emergency medicine training in America, the current state of the field, and how all Americans could benefit from emergency medical technicians (EMTs), medical students, residents, and practicing physicians who were properly trained in emergency care.[40] The conference participants were assigned to one of four workshops that covered medical student education, resident education (chaired by Ron Krome), the critical care physician, and the "second career" emergency physician (chaired by William Haeck).

Two key acknowledgments came out of the meeting. The first was an agreed on definition of an emergency physician as "as a specialist in the immediate recognition, evaluation, and response to acute illness and injury, and in the administration, teaching and research in all aspects of immediate care and disposition of any patient." This definition had been previously used by ACEP. The second acknowledgment came out of Krome's workshop, which "agreed unanimously that there should be residency training for emergency medicine." Although several residency programs in emergency medicine were operational by this time, the legitimacy of residency training in emergency medicine was still a point of contention. The agreement to support residency training at this conference gave the green light to the creation of emergency medicine residencies on a large scale. Krome did note in his report that "a very small minority" of participants (most likely led by Oscar Hampton of the ACS) did not support the definition of emergency medicine as a distinct entity or specialty. Another contentious area was who should train emergency medicine residents. Krome notes that a compromise was reached between those who believed that emergency medicine residents could be adequately trained by other specialists and those who believed it was essential to have emergency medicine residents trained by emergency physicians, primarily in the ED. The compromise acknowledged the key role of "certain specialists" in teaching emergency medicine residents, but that "the integration and application of the material learned would have to occur in the emergency department." An indication of how strong the opposition was to the concept of emergency physician faculty training emergency medicine residents is Krome's statement, "A significant minority, however, felt that the education of the emergency resident would have to be placed in the hands of the emergency physician and that if there was to be specialty status, it would be necessary to train a cadre of educators who were emergency physicians."[40] The emergency physicians in Krome's workshop group were clearly outnumbered; they represented only about one third of the participants. Another key result of Krome's workshop was the inclusion in the final report of ACEP's "Guidelines for Residency Training in Emergency Medicine." These were the revised version of the "Proposed Essentials of a Residency Training Program for Emergency Physicians" that ACEP had submitted, and the AMA had rejected, in 1971. The AMA Workshop Conference legitimized these guidelines, and allowed ACEP to claim a small triumph. This was important not only as a moral victory, but as part of the path to specialty recognition, because AMA approval of "essentials of residency training" was required for a specialty to be officially recognized.

The workshop on the education of the second-career emergency physician, chaired by William Haeck, made several important recommendations on determining emergency physician numbers and need and providing adequate educational courses and continuing medical education for practicing emergency physicians. The report stated, "a goal of all 'second-career emergency physicians' should be official certification of their capabilities. Organized medicine should make provision for their certification." This was the first time that a national level report broached the subject of a specialty board for emergency medicine. The final report contained an extensive "skill group list" itemizing the practices and procedures that all emergency physicians should master.

The critical care component of the AMA workshop was a bit of a tangent at a meeting that dealt with emergency medical education. Peter Safar was the driving force behind attempts to link emergency medicine and critical care as national attention became focused on emergency care. Safar, who was a leading researcher in resuscitation in Baltimore and then at the University of Pittsburgh, strongly advocated for fellowship training and a medical specialty in critical care. He viewed the role of critical care physicians as extending from the prehospital environment to the intensive care unit and frequently noted that only 5% of ED cases were actual critical care cases. ACEP already had liaisons with Safar and the Society for Critical Care Medicine before the AMA workshop. The recommendations of the workshop were to recognize that critical care is "a multidisciplinary endeavor," and therefore, a critical care fellowship should be encouraged for any physician who plans to focus in this area, and emergency medicine training followed by a critical care fellowship "was considered highly desirable."[40] This final, common-sense recommendation proved the most difficult to implement, and to this day, emergency medicine–trained physicians are excluded from doing critical care fellowships that lead to certification by the ABMS.

The product of the AMA's "Workshop Conference on Education of the Physician in Emergency Medicine" was an 85-page "Blue Book" report that was a national consensus of the current state of emergency medicine education and plans and hopes for the future. The Blue Book was widely disseminated and was available for purchase through ACEP for $3. The Blue Book was referred to extensively and served as a voucher of credibility as emergency medicine tried to make progress in education and specialty recognition. The 1973 AMA workshop conference is still regarded by the early leaders in emergency medicine as one of the most crucial events in the first decade of the field. The recognition by the rest of the house of medicine that emergency medicine was not going away, and in fact would be expanding its influence in education, hospitals, and organized medicine, paved the way for a flurry of activity in the next few years. The Blue Book meeting, with its areas of contention and lively debate, also was a harbinger of the significant opposition that other areas of medicine would mount as emergency medicine tried to move forward.

DEVELOPING A RESIDENCY REVIEW PROCESS

In late 1972, still smarting from the failure of the AMA Council on Education to approve the Proposed Essentials for Residency Training, ACEP approved a review process to certify residencies. This was another required component in the move to reach specialty status. All approved specialties have a Residency Review Commission (RRC) to provide this function, but emergency medicine was not yet in this position. Proceeding with the structure of specialty development without the approval of the AMA or other bodies would become the modus operandi of ACEP and the early emergency medicine leaders. The attitude was, "If they won't approve us, we'll do it on our own." James Mills, as ACEP president in 1973, reviewed for the ACEP Council the 12 required steps for emergency medicine to "receive proper AMA recognition" (Table 5.2). In the middle of

---

TABLE 5.2 The 12 Steps for American Medical Association Recognition Presented by James Mills, Jr., M.D., October 23, 1973

1. Listing as a national scientific medical society.
2. Establishment of scientific section in the AMA.
3. Definition of a specialty content.
4. Establishment of essentials for residency.
5. Establishment of residencies.
6. Establishment of a residency review mechanism.
7. Approval of the AMA Council of Medical Education.
8. Development of a specialty examination.
9. Approval of the Liaison Committee on Medical Education (Council on Medical Education of the AMA, Association of American Medical Colleges, and American Hospital Association).
10. Approval of the American Board of Medical Specialties.
11. Establishment of a certifying specialty board.
12. Approval of the AMA House of delegates.

AMA, American Medical Association.
From ACEP Board of Directors meeting minutes.

the list were three aspects of residency training: establishment of essentials for a residency, establishment of residencies, and establishment of a residency review mechanism. The first of these three steps was on hold, the second was happening, even though the emergency medicine residencies had quasi-approval from the AMA, and the third was initiated by ACEP, because there was no other body capable of certifying residencies. The Residency Review Committee, as it was originally called, was part of the ACEP Graduate Education Committee and was charged with reviewing and approving or denying emergency medicine residencies at a cost to the programs of $200 per day per reviewer.[41] This committee started in a hole—at least 15 residencies were functioning before the RRC was ready to start, and the number of new programs was growing exponentially. Only two programs were reviewed by the original RRC. In 1974, ACEP announced a new residency endorsement procedure. Robert Dailey was the leader of these initiatives. He describes how he developed the criteria that emergency medicine residencies must meet to be endorsed the review committee:

> …we were really an ad hoc operation and there wasn't even a clear vision of what emergency medicine was as a specialty let alone…what a residency program should be…We rapidly saw…if you were going to judge something, you had to have confines by which to judge it. I can distinctly remember the day in Fresno, I sat in my apartment on a sunny day and I was pondering the upcoming committee meeting and…I realized that we were in a bit of bind because we were going to make judgments about residencies when we had no criteria. So, I sat down in about 15 minutes, I outlined on a piece of paper about 10 to 12 principles that had to be obtained in order to have a proper educational process for residents. I rank ordered them.[23]

Dailey's criteria included the requirement of 2 years of training, with a split between ED and off-service rotations, and the requirement that residents should have a graduated increased in their level of responsibility in the ED. Dailey clearly remembers that the

> two most important things that were at the top of the list—there should be adequate pathology for an experiential learning base that within the 3 years you had to have the adequate number of sick people and diverse patient pathology to develop the skills necessary to practice in any emergency department venue… [T]he other…was that there had to be on-site supervision by faculty. Because it was not only in my experience, but also other peoples' experience that there was always a lie there. That training was not training…it was primarily experience with little supervision. Not that it ended up with catastrophe, but it wasn't truthful, and I realized particularly in emergency medicine patient care, decisions have to be made on site and that therefore decision making had to be on site…So, these were really the two principles that were, if you will, the inviolate principles…and then I did…some genius secretarial work, and derived the forms that the residency programs would have to fill out.[23]

Most of Dailey's principles, scratched out in 1973 in the Fresno sun, are used today in reviewing and approving emergency medicine residencies.

ACEP also came to realize that it could not independently review residency programs. The University Association of Emergency Medical Services (UA/EMS) had formed in 1971 and was beginning to develop a credible voice in national emergency medicine circles by 1973. Although few of the surgeons who were leaders in the UA/EMS were associated with emergency medicine residency programs, they did have influence in medical schools and teaching hospitals. Dailey crafted a new residency review organization in 1975 that he named the Liaison Residency Endorsement Committee (LREC). The LREC had equal representation from ACEP and UA/EMS, and when the American Board of Emergency Medicine was incorporated in 1976, three members of ABEM were added. The LREC was very active, visiting and approving more than 30 emergency medicine residency programs in its first 2 years.

Although the LREC created a formal process for residency review, the actual site reviews were not always rigorous. Peter Rosen and Bob Dailey were the "least compromising" members of the LREC and were most likely to hold programs to the standards outlined in the residency endorsement documents.[23] One of the most difficult requirements for early programs to meet was 24-hour faculty supervision. George Podgorny notes, "[I] cannot tell you that all the programs were wonderful programs, they were not."[39] A natural tension existed between the desires of the early leaders (many of whom were reviewers for the LREC) to see many new emergency medicine residencies approved and the desire, best expressed by idealists like Dailey and Rosen, to require high standards for the new programs. The fact that the reviewers and program directors were part of a small cohort of physicians in academic emergency medicine meant that an unbiased review was difficult to achieve. Judy Tintinalli remembers, "You would go and see your friends, you would have dinner at their homes."[42] Programs could receive full endorsement, provisional endorsement, or no endorsement. Provisional endorsement was for programs that had been in existence less than 2 years or for programs that had "serious but correctable weaknesses," and would be rereviewed in a year.[43] In the first 3 years of LREC reviews, all programs were given full or provisional endorsement.

THE UNIVERSITY ASSOCIATION FOR EMERGENCY MEDICAL SERVICES

Surgeons had their hands in emergency medicine in the United States before there was such an entity as an emergency physician, and the field of surgery continued to play a parallel role to the pioneer emergency physicians in the late 1960s through the late 1970s. The origin of the University Association for Emergency Medical Services is traced to October 1968 when a group of six young surgeons who were each in the position of ED director at their teaching hospitals met for lunch at the ACS meeting in San Francisco. The six were Alan Dimick from the University of Alabama, Charles Frey from the University of Michigan, George Johnson from the University of North Carolina, James McKenzie from McMaster University in Ontario, Raymond Mathews from the University of Toronto, and Robert Rutherford from the Johns Hopkins University. As these six explored their common challenges and problems in ED management, they sought to expand their ranks and organize, and a charter meeting for UA/EMS was organized for March 6, 1970, at Dimick's institution—the University of Alabama in Birmingham. A surprisingly large number of academic surgeon ED directors attended the meeting. One hundred-thirty eight participants came, representing 96 of 119 U.S. and Canadian medical schools. Workshops were held on "movement of the acutely ill or injured patient to the emergency department," "the emergency department," and "planning of emergency medical services."[44] An organizational caucus was held in June 1970, and Charles Frey was elected the first UA/EMS president.

The charter meeting of UA/EMS was held in Denver in November 1970. A constitution and by-laws were approved, and 125 charter members were inducted into the organization. Sessions were given on "the nonemergent patient in the emergency room." Alexander Walt, who was Ron Krome's boss and chair of surgery at Wayne State Medical School and Detroit General Hospital, delivered a talk in the form of a fairy tale called "The Administration of the Emergency Room." The minutes of the meeting note that "ten new workshop groups were then formed to discuss methods whereby the fairy tale could become reality." It is interesting to note that although Ron Krome had been given the responsibility of running the ED at Detroit General Hospital, Walt was the representative at the early UA/EMS meetings. However, within a year, Krome was an active member of UA/EMS. He was the first UA/EMS member who also held a key position in ACEP. Krome remembers the collection of early UA/EMS members:

> I would say that the group was split along several different lines. Some of the surgeons perceived that they were stuck running the emergency room but they thought it was an academic wasteland and they wanted to get out of it as soon as they could. They were doing it because their boss asked them to, but they could see no research opportunities and they wanted to get out of it as soon as they could. Others were stuck with but may not have had a promising academic career anyhow, and they were just trying to make the best they could out of it. Then there were others…who saw that given enough hard work and diligence you could do things, academically, not just service-wise.[45]

The first UA/EMS president, Charles Frey, was an example of a surgeon ED director who had a sincere interest in improving ED care and developing an academic approach to the field. Frey was at the University of Michigan and had been assigned as ED director at an early stage of his career. Frey was curious to understand how nonacademic EDs functioned, and he knew Karl Mangold—he was a surgical resident at Cornell when Mangold was a medical student. Mangold remembers inviting Frey to come and see his community ED in California:

> I had him come out and work, I had him credentialed at our hospital, he was very interested in emergency medicine, and I got him to work with me in the ED on some incredibly busy Saturday and Sunday afternoons. He was as an academician, saw the need for front-line–quality doctor of first contact, and actually over the years became a very big ally in a group where he had to keep his mouth shut, but the College of Surgeons were just vociferous in their opposition to us and they're very politically powerful...Charlie Frey came and I so respected Charlie because he said let me come out and see, work with you, let me get credentialed at your hospital. He had a California license and I thought, you know, Charlie you're all right. As an academician you're going to step out of your—he was a big pancreatic researcher—but he wanted to get his hands dirty with me. He lived in my house and...we worked together and then after that we took our children and went backpacking in Yosemite National Park.[2]

Frey eventually moved to the University of California at Davis, left emergency medicine, and became a prominent academic surgeon and researcher.

UA/EMS was, like ACEP in its first few years, a small organization with a budget of several thousand dollars, but with big ideas and potential for interaction with an endless number of organizations and individuals who were interested in emergency medical services. The early UA/EMS leaders looked to make liaisons and influence policy in the federal government, AMA, critical care, emergency nursing, and ACS. They were broad in their ideas and unfocused in their agenda. The membership quickly rose to around 300 members, which included almost all of the academic surgeons in the United States and a few from Canada who had ED duties. The overall pedigree of these surgeons was superior to that of the early emergency physicians. However unlike ACEP, which had a pool of thousands of practicing emergency physicians from which to recruit new members, UA/EMS had a much smaller pool. After the initial jump to 365 members, membership did not increase much over the next few years. UA/EMS noted early in its existence that the organization was not restricted to surgeons and that any physician who held an academic appointment and worked in an ED might qualify for membership.[46]

UA/EMS, because of its academic base and the reputations of some of the early surgeon members, may have had higher credibility with government and other medical organizations than ACEP. Even if it had a vague mission and objectives in its early years, UA/EMS was frequently asked to be at the table when major emergency care policies were discussed. An early assistant for UA/EMS remembers "there was this vast number of organizations" interested in emergency medicine and EMS and "everybody was liaisoning and setting up these links with each other."[47] UA/EMS was in some ways overinvolved given its small base and the relatively junior status of its members. By attempting to deal with all the other groups and organizations in emergency medicine and EMS, it did not have time to develop its own mission or agenda.

UA/EMS was in a strange position when it came to supporting residency training for emergency physicians. Because none of the early leaders except Ron Krome, David Wagner, and Peter Rosen (who was minimally involved in UA/EMS in its first few years) had emergency medicine residencies at their institutions, they were tepid in their support for residency training. In 1971, Ron Krome appealed to UA/EMS to help ACEP in supporting the creation of emergency medicine residencies. Meeting minutes note that one UA/EMS member "expressed concern that the ED was now being asked to train a number of professional and paraprofessional personnel and questioned whether there was simply room enough for everybody to be there for such training." Another comment was that "training in family practice should also be included, since all patients coming to emergency departments were not true emergencies."[46]

Full endorsement of emergency residency training created a paradox for UA/EMS. If the organization came out strongly in support of training a new type of physician for emergency care, it would mean that surgeons would eventually have to relinquish their control of academic EDs. If UA/EMS withheld support, it would be seen as resisting the movement to provide better emergency care in the United States. The result was that UA/EMS, in the first few years of its existence, stayed at the periphery of the residency training issue, neither fully supporting nor opposing the boom in emergency medicine residencies. UA/EMS was also ambivalent on specialty status and a certifying board for emergency medicine. Minutes of the December 1972 UA/EMS Executive Council meeting note that "[t]here were varied opinions" on the issue of board status for emergency medicine and that a poll would be taken of the membership in 1973.[48] Peter Rosen remembers from his early contact that UA/EMS was not supportive of residency training in emergency medicine:

> They were totally scornful of it and they were pretty hostile to it. I mean they were surgeons and emergency medicine was a surgical specialty and it was going to be surgeons who controlled it and not guys who didn't have training in anything. They were opposed to residency training. They were not very helpful...and they refused to address any of the real issues of the field which was how do we train people, how do we get recognition for that training, how do we insist that quality of care improve and it has to be independent of other specialties.[29]

As membership reached a plateau, and the organization struggled financially, UA/EMS began to look for a way to support its administrative and executive functions. The busy academic surgeons did not have time to produce meeting minutes, answer calls and send letters to other organizations, or to coordinate new member applications. The leaders first looked to the federal government for grant support, but none was forthcoming. UA/EMS knew of ACEP and had invited ACEP leaders to speak at its early meetings. John Wiegenstein remembered attending the first annual UA/EMS meeting, hosted by Charles Frey at the University of Michigan in Ann Arbor in May 1971. Karl Mangold also attended, representing ACEP's Committee on Education, and Wiegenstein remembered that Mangold "in his usual flourish" stood up and boldly addressed the group of academic surgeons:[10]

> I am 33 years old and have done emergency medicine for 6 years...I would like to make a very blunt plea. It is time for you gentlemen to get on your feet and take care of 60 million people who are coming to emergency departments...Were are now getting communications from medical students, from interns and residents, who want to join us full time. There are no standards. There is no training. I had to travel 3,000 miles to take Jim Dineen's course...If you gentlemen, who are the directors of the university departments don't do it, who will?[13]

Wiegenstein also remembered that in the first years of ACEP, he was looking for someone to become the membership representative for ACEP in Alabama. Alan Dimick, the founding member of UA/EMS who worked at the University of Alabama–Birmingham, had "secretly" joined ACEP. When Wiegenstein asked him to become the Alabama membership representative, Dimick said, "I don't really think I can do that, John."[10]

Overlooking ideologic differences, UA/EMS turned to ACEP, which by 1972 had an executive office in Lansing and was doing better financially. With some trepidation, UA/EMS signed a contract with ACEP for management services to start in January 1973. Like a stepson from a new marriage, UA/EMS operations moved into ACEP headquarters. Art Auer, the ACEP executive director appointed another ACEP staffer, Fred Towns, to be the executive manager of UA/EMS. Mary Ann Schropp, who started work at ACEP in 1976 on her nineteenth birthday, functioned as an administrative assistant for ACEP and ended up doing much of the work for UA/EMS:

> I remember in particular their membership records—it could take a year to get approved as a member in UAEM, they were horrible at it. So, they badly needed

administrative support and I think Art…could see the writing on the wall, ACEP was going to be a big organization but ACEP was made up of clinical practitioners of emergency medicine and at that time UAEM was considered sort of the people in the know.[47]

Thus began a strange, symbiotic relationship between ACEP and UA/EMS that would last about 8 years. UA/EMS, as a small organization with limited resources, benefited from ACEP's organizational largesse and ACEP benefited by gaining some access to the academic world. One of ACEP's motivations in this relationship with UA/EMS was to monitor and influence an organization that could serve as a competitor, and possibly an opponent, in aspects of emergency medicine development.

UA/EMS continued to be a small, poorly funded organization that was nonetheless at the table in most discussions on the big picture of emergency medicine in the United States. Membership hovered around 300 and concern was expressed in 1973 that membership was declining. Slowly, the emergency physician members of UA/EMS began to exert their influence. In a December 1973 meeting, Ron Krome urged UA/EMS to strongly push for departmental status in universities and medical schools. Robert Rutherford, one of the UA/EMS founders who was a surgeon at Johns Hopkins University, cautioned,

If you state outright that this must have university departmental status, you will develop great resistance. Get residencies established and certified; get things going; all things will come in time.[49]

This type of reasoned advice from an experienced academic surgeon contrasted with some of the rhetoric that came from UA/EMS against the movement of emergency medicine toward specialty status. As was noted earlier, UA/EMS members who attended the 1973 AMA "Blue Book" Conference on Education of the Physician in Emergency Medicine in Chicago did not warmly endorse the idea of residency training. UA/EMS had paid homage to Robert H. Kennedy, M.D., who pioneered surgeons' involvement in emergency medical services, by naming a lecture after him at their Annual Meeting. In 1974, Oscar Hampton from the ACS was asked to give the Robert H. Kennedy Lecture at the meeting in Dallas, Texas. Hampton gave a long and acerbic review of emergency medicine. His lecture was titled, "Emergency Department Physicians: Their Capabilities, Contributions, Education and Future Status." Hampton acknowledged that emergency practice was established in the United States, but described "the incompetency of some ED physicians." He noted,

A surgeon in a western state recently reported that one ED physician merely stuck an open 16-gauge needle into the pleural cavity, ostensibly to correct a clinically diagnosed pneumothorax. If the diagnosis was not correct before, it certainly was afterwards![50]

Hampton apparently did not understand that appropriate initial emergency treatment for a tension pneumothorax was exactly what he described. Hampton also acknowledged that ACEP was a powerful organization, with excellent leaders like James Mills and John Wiegenstein. He said, "If I wanted to form a new medical organization and needed a large membership and almost instantaneous recognition for it, I would attempt to hire John and Jim to do the job." But he criticized ACEP's use of the name "College" and its lax standards for membership, noting that early members had to have "interest" in emergency medicine and not necessarily full-time practice in an ED. He also complained about ACEP's cosponsorship of the 1973 AMA "Blue Book" conference on education of the physician in emergency medicine and believed that ACEP had stacked the deck in influencing the recommendations of the conference. Indeed, this had been the case—ACEP had inserted ACEP members as representatives into other organizations that were invited to the Conference, thereby increasing their influence. Hampton was particularly opposed to the requirement that teaching faculty in an approved emergency medicine residency should be specialists in emergency medicine, noting that surgeons and other specialists would not have a role in educating emergency physicians. He called for another conference to consider the "unresolved problems"[50] (see insert, Figure 20).

Oscar Hampton used the Kennedy Lecture at the UA/EMS meeting as a bully pulpit to question the legitimacy of emergency medicine as a specialty, and to politically appeal for a greater role for surgeons in the training of emergency medicine residents. Many in the audience agreed with his viewpoints, and a few did not. UA/EMS was an organization that shared an executive headquarters with ACEP and was allowed to announce its meetings in the *Journal of the American College of Emergency Physicians*, but was still trying to figure out if it supported the same concept of emergency medicine as ACEP. But even as Hampton spoke in 1974, UA/EMS was beginning to change. Many of its members realized that residency training in emergency medicine was rapidly developing and that the academic surgeons could best improve emergency care by supporting the training of residents, medical students, and practicing physicians. In 1975, George Johnson, Jr., M.D., a vascular surgeon from the University of North Carolina gave the UA/EMS President's Address at the fifth annual meeting in Vancouver, Canada, and his tone was much more conciliatory than Hampton's. He spoke of the how important it was that those with "academic credentials" teach medical students, residents, and practicing physicians, but that skill training alone would not be enough and trainees would need the "basic science–oriented system of physician education." He supported emergency medicine residency programs that could teach basic science concepts and a scholarly approach to the field. Johnson stopped short of endorsing one of ACEP's objectives, saying: "I am not sure, however, that I agree with the ACEP that all medical schools need training programs for the emergency physician."[51] David Wagner attended the Vancouver meeting, listened to Johnson's address, and encountered some of the founders of UA/EMS in the hallway:

> I remember getting dragged into a room because I had been sort of on the outside of this group…They said, you know somebody with a training program ought to get involved more in the leadership.[18]

Wagner was quickly elected to the executive council of UA/EMS, and by 1976, he was president of UA/EMS. One of the first things he did as president was change the name to the University Association of Emergency Medicine (UAEM). He remembers how he was able to get the name change approved:

> …it went through because, as you well know in those business meetings, nobody shows up. Afterwards I remember taking a bit of flack and hearing people say wait a minute, what did we do, what happened here? I think…looking back, that was a critical watershed because we were previously…focusing on emergency medical services and that was sort of a nebulous term…now all of a sudden there was a name in front of you: emergency medicine.[18]

The name change was also a sign of transition of the organization's focus and the makeup of its membership. Since its inception, UA/EMS had been very involved in the delivery of EMS and ED management. After the name change, the focus began to slowly shift to the profession of emergency medicine and the role that academic emergency physicians could take in advancing research and education in the field. Many of the surgeons who founded UA/EMS or were early members had a choice to make: They could declare their allegiance to the field of emergency medicine and join the rush of activity or they could go back to being surgeons and leave the work of academic emergency medicine to the newer members. Wagner saw UAEM members "using it as a spring board," either landing in the emergency medicine pool or landing "back in the operating room."[18] The transition was not rancorous—it was more like an evolutionary process. Mary Ann Schropp, the administrative assistant for ACEP who was assigned to UAEM, remembers the exodus of the surgeons, "…they just stepped aside, I don't remember resentment, I don't remember people leaving in disgust, they slowly filtered away."[47] Ron Krome was UAEM president in 1978, and Kendall McNabney was the president in 1980. Then in a landmark year, one of McNabney's emergency medicine residency graduates, Joseph Waeckerle, M.D., succeeded his former boss in 1981 to become the first emergency medicine residency–trained physician to lead UAEM. McNabney remembers George Johnson, Jr., saying to him about Waeckerle: "Joe is a trained emergency physician—we've got to turn this organization over to people like that."[52] It took only a decade for the academic association to change its demographics from a surgeon-dominated organization to one led by emergency physicians.

THE EMERGENCY MEDICINE RESIDENTS ASSOCIATION

Given the active, energetic nature of early emergency medicine residents, it was natural that an organization for residents would develop. The Emergency Medicine Residents Association (EMRA) was formed in late 1974 to "provide representation to ACEP and UA/EMS, and to express the members' viewpoints on various Resident social, economic and ethical matters relative to their chosen specialty."[43] The words "chosen specialty" convey a strong sense that the early residents, even though they did not have a certifying board, considered themselves specialists in emergency medicine. Robert Wolfensperger, M.D., a resident from St. Louis was the first president of EMRA and early board of directors members included James Roberts, M.D., who was a resident in David Wagner's program at MCP, and Michael Tomlanovich, M.D., who was one of Peter Rosen's first residents at the University of Chicago. Joseph Waeckerle, one of Kendall McNabney's first trainees in Kansas City, was already a resident leader in UA/EMS and served as a liaison between EMRA and UA/EMS. Rosen and Wagner encouraged residents to get involved in the national organizations of emergency medicine. The Cincinnati residents, despite coming from the first emergency medicine residency were minimally involved in EMRA and ACEP at this time due to the faltering leadership in their program (see insert, Figure 19).

EMRA was supported administratively by ACEP. This made sense, because ACEP wanted all EMRA members upon graduation to become ACEP members and was eager to have emergency medicine residency–trained individuals become active in the organization. Just a few days after the formation of EMRA, Ron Krome, as chair of the ACEP section on education, moved at an ACEP board of directors meeting that an EMRA member be included on the ACEP board of directors. R. R. Hannas noted that this would require a change to ACEP's constitution, and Krome withdrew the motion after some discussion.[53] The ACEP board did agree to appoint an EMRA member to the ACEP graduate education committee and to pay that person's way to ACEP meetings. George Podgorny was the designated ACEP board of directors member who served as a liaison to EMRA. This close relationship allowed ACEP to monitor EMRA activities and sentiments regarding ACEP policies. ACEP's approach with EMRA was similar to its relationship with UA/EMS—by keeping the other organization close and financially dependent on ACEP, a certain amount of authority and control was ceded to ACEP. As an early ACEP staff person notes, ACEP, and Art Auer, its executive director, functioned like a "kingdom builder," with many organizations besides ACEP running out of the Lansing, Michigan, headquarters.[47] However, ACEP's budget was also tight in the mid-1970s, and in 1975, it was noted that EMRA was collecting membership dues "in an attempt to replace ACEP funds currently being spent in support of EMRA."[54]

THE SOCIETY FOR TEACHERS OF EMERGENCY MEDICINE

Another organization was added to the mix of academic emergency medicine in 1975. The Society for Teachers of Emergency Medicine (STEM) was created by ACEP as a "paper organization" to gain access to the Council of Academic Societies (CAS) in the American Association of Medical Colleges (AAMC). The CAS is only open to those academic medical societies that are considered nonprofit, medical education foundations and are designated by the Internal Revenue Service as 501(c)(3) in their tax status. ACEP and UA/EMS were designated as nonprofit educational organizations, with a 501(c)(6) tax status. The AAMC was a 501(c)(3) organization. The big difference in this seemingly small status change is that 501(c)(6) organizations are able to lobby for their causes in the federal government, but 501(c)(3) medical education foundations are not. Also 501(c)(3) organizations are required to have a membership that is open to the public; this was a requirement that was not always fully implemented by medical organizations. UA/EMS initially pursued 501(c)(3) status, but in 1974 settled for the other designation. It was important for ACEP to have the ability to lobby, but in preserving this, the organization was effectively barred from the AAMC. Although a voice in the AAMC was not an absolute requirement in the quest for specialty recognition, emergency medicine needed to be at the table in the CAS if it hoped to develop as a credible academic discipline.[49,55,56]

The other major reason for the formation of STEM was ACEP's lack of confidence and trust in UA/EMS to represent the interests of emergency medicine in the academic sphere. In 1975, UAEM still had a few vocal surgeons who resisted the idea of an independent specialty for emergency medicine. Mary Ann Schropp, who was an ACEP staff person at the time, remembers being told by a senior ACEP staff member that

> ...they developed STEM to keep UAEM out of the AAMC. They were afraid that if you got the UAEM people in with the other traditional specialists at the AAMC, that emergency medicine would not do well.[47]

ACEP turned to the cadre of known teachers of emergency medicine who were not heavily involved in UAEM to develop STEM. The emergency medicine residency program directors had been meeting regularly since Bob Dailey's initial meeting in Southern California in 1972, but had never formed an official organization. This group was approached by ACEP leaders in 1975 and asked to form an organization. In May 1975, the group first met during the UA/EMS meeting in Vancouver, British Columbia. David Wagner was asked to be the chairman of the organizational meeting of STEM. This was a busy few days for Wagner—as mentioned previously, he had been taken aside and strongly urged by UA/EMS leaders in Vancouver to become a leader in UA/EMS. Now he was being asked by ACEP to form a new academic society, albeit a "paper" organization. As Wagner opened the meeting, he explained to the 35 emergency medicine educators in the room that STEM was being formed primarily because of the tax code implications and noted "it is felt that, to further emergency medicine, representation is needed with the AAMC." Those at the meeting included Bruce Janiak, Ron Krome, George Podgorny, Gail Anderson, and W. Kendall McNabney. Nonsurgeons who were involved in emergency medicine, like John H. Stone, M.D., a cardiologist (and well known writer and poet) who started an emergency medicine residency out of Grady Hospital in Atlanta, felt more at home in STEM than UAEM. By-laws were approved at the organizational meeting, and Bob Dailey was elected as the first president of STEM, and his friend Peter Rosen was voted in as president-elect. STEM was incorporated and an application was submitted to the AAMC Council of Academic Societies, and two representatives (Gail Anderson and Ron Krome) were elected to represent STEM on the CAS. Dues for STEM members were set at $25 per year.[55]

STEM started out with two simple purposes—to represent the specialty at the AAMC and to hold an annual meeting to help educate emergency physicians on how to train residents. Dailey, as the first president of STEM was not exuberant over its formation. He remembers feeling, "It was a politically necessary organization for tax purposes and such and I had really no interest. I remember saying, 'Oh my God, not another organization!'"[23] Despite the transactional approach to its formation, STEM was not destined to remain a paper organization. Its members were some of the most dynamic early emergency physicians. In STEM they found the proper forum to discuss what was near and dear to their hearts—how to develop and run an emergency medicine residency. The bonds that formed among STEM members were made stronger by the fact that they faced similar adversities and enemies, and at the annual meeting could commiserate and plan for how to combat these hostile elements back home. Kenneth Iserson, the Cincinnati residency graduate who developed an emergency medicine residency at the University of Arizona, and later served as President of STEM, remembers:

> *We didn't have a lot of illusions that we were that distant from ACEP. I think the attitude of the membership of STEM was probably the most important. It was very collegial. Extremely collegial, there is nothing like that in emergency medicine any more. Everybody knew everybody else, it was really fun to be there. The people who are now considered real leaders around the country in academia were little kids. In STEM you got a chance to help them develop things…we sat around these tables…and we discussed real issues on how to solve the real issues and it was just give and take and that was really valuable…but that was really where faculty development was happening, within STEM.[16]*

The type of collegiality early STEM members felt at their meetings contrasted with their involvement in UAEM. Iserson remembers a not-so-welcoming attitude when he attended a UAEM meeting:

> *…we all would go to the UAEM meeting, most of us would, also. I came in and we were at the registration desk and this big guy was waving his arms and saying something like "How could the hotel let those damned emergency docs in here at the same prices we are?" It was Ken Mattox. He was president of UAEM at that time. Boy, I remember that.[16]*

Mattox was a famous trauma surgeon and EMS leader out of Texas.

STEM gradually assumed a consistent and visible presence in the world of academic emergency medicine. Yearly educational sessions were presented at the UAEM and ACEP meetings, and STEM published a newsletter with helpful news and information for program directors and other faculty. STEM was a forum for faculty to share ideas, stories, and frustrations, but it went beyond this by helping to develop faculty in emergency medicine. Unlike ACEP or UAEM, which were broad in scope and less focused on individual member career development, STEM's limited scope made it a respite for faculty to engage in academic discourse and hone their educational knowledge. STEM produced the "STEMLETTER," a quarterly 10- to 20-page newsletter stuffed with information, discussion, letters, opinion pieces, announcements of research studies, and opportunities for faculty. In keeping with one of the original purposes for forming STEM, the group represented emergency medicine at the AAMC annual meeting, where the role of emergency medicine in medical student education was discussed. As UAEM became less "surgical," many STEM members also became UAEM members. By the end of the 1980s, it was clear that the two organizations had the same mission and goals and were offering much the same thing to members. The organizations merged to become the Society for Academic Emergency Medicine in 1989.

A FOOTHOLD IN THE ACADEMIC WORLD

By the mid-1970s, emergency medicine had secured a foothold in U.S. medicine. A critical mass of training programs was established, and medical students were demonstrating interest in the new field. UAEM, STEM, and EMRA provided some strength in numbers and solace for emergency medicine faculty and residents. The AAMC, AMA, and the federal government were paying attention to emergency medicine as an academic entity in medicine. Somehow, with a dearth of trained faculty, crowded and underresourced EDs, and significant obstruction from other fields, emergency medicine residents were being trained in America. Whether the training was of high quality is debatable, but the intense, concentrated time spent in busy EDs certainly made the first emergency medicine residency graduates better prepared than their predecessors. As Harvey Meislin notes of his training at the University of Chicago:

> *We learned a lot. We did it ourselves. A lot of it was our Journal Clubs, we taught each other, and we learned things, we did learn. I think, as I look back at it, as rough as it was, it was really a good education. I felt very, very clinically confident.[33]*

Most of the early emergency medicine residency graduates went out to practice in community hospital EDs, where they were in high demand. The early residency-trained emergency physicians could command high salaries, and it was a common practice for graduates from a residency to form small groups and secure a contract with one or more hospitals. Meislin remembers,

> *The private practice opportunities in those days were phenomenal. There was a ton of money in emergency medicine. If you had somebody trained, you could make millions of dollars....[33]*

Those residency graduates who chose to stay in academics made significantly less money. Meislin's starting salary as a faculty member at University of Chicago in 1975 was $30,000 per year. Like a number of other early residency-trained emergency physicians, Meislin went from being a resident one day, to being a residency director the next. For Richard Levy at Cincinnati, it was from resident to director of emergency medicine. Just as they learned emergency practice by doing it, people like Meislin would learn academics by being thrust into roles for which they had almost no preparation. This underscores the importance of the organizations—STEM, UAEM, and ACEP—as nurturing grounds for young faculty in emergency medicine. In many cases, these organizations were the only place to turn for advice, counsel, and training on how to be an emergency medicine academician.

The elephant in the closet for emergency medicine in the early 1970s was the fact that for all the development and initiative in education of emergency physicians, the field was still just a field—not a full-fledged medical specialty. Although some emergency medicine residents, with their caution-be-damned attitudes, did not dwell on the lack of specialty status, many were concerned about their futures. They could have satisfying practices and make money in emergency medicine, but on a visceral level, they were concerned about perpetual second-class status. Training alone could not erase the 1950s stigma of the "ER doc" as an undedicated, unprofessional, for-hire physician, who functioned outside the mainstream of American medicine. Fortunately for those early emergency medicine residency graduates, the pioneers of emergency practice, who never had the chance for formal emergency medicine training, were leading a parallel movement to the advances in emergency medicine training. Wiegenstein, Hannas, Mills, Podgorny, Krome, and others were buzzing around the landscape of organized medicine, working to make emergency medicine the next medical specialty.

6 | Becoming a Specialty

By 1973, the campaign to form a specialty of emergency medicine was at a no-turning-back stage. After initially questioning the value of seeking specialty status, the Alexandria pioneers, especially James Mills, Jr., were now solidly behind the process. In fact, it was Mills who reiterated the steps that would be required to gain specialty recognition when he was president of the American College of Emergency Physicians (ACEP) in 1972 (Table 5.2). George Podgorny wrote in 1980 that the early leaders had "the idea that emergency physicians occupied a unique spot in the spectrum of medical care in the United States and deserved to be recognized as such."[1] The drive for specialty status became a "unifying theme" for almost everything ACEP did in the early 1970s.[1] The University Association of Emergency Medical Services (UAEMS), despite being the academic organization was more ambivalent about specialty status when it first formed, but as more emergency physicians joined and became leaders, UAEMS became the University Association of Emergency Medicine (UAEM) and supported the specialty drive for emergency medicine. Joseph Waeckerle, M.D., who as an emergency medicine resident attended his first UAEMS meeting in 1974 said, "I went because I didn't want a bunch of surgeons determining our future."[2] Even the public was unofficially acclaiming emergency medicine— a 1965 *Reader's Digest* article was titled, "Emergency Service: Medicine's Newest Specialty."[3] As emergency medicine surged forward in the early 1970s, both facilitating and suppressive forces determined the movement toward specialty status.

Emergency medicine emerged in the era of the flower children. It is not surprising that Robert Dailey, the free-spirited emergency medicine residency director at Los Angeles County University of Southern California (USC) Medical Center who had spent his early career in San Francisco, used a flower analogy to describe emergency medicine. Dailey was asked to do a presentation at one of the first UAEMS meetings. At this point UAEMS consisted largely of surgeons who were trying to gain more information on training programs and the move toward a specialty, and what role they would play in this process. Dailey had the Art Department at University of Southern California make a picture of a flower with many petals, emerging from the dirt. He showed this picture as a slide during his presentation, using the metaphor that emergency medicine was a young flower, growing out of the detritus of organized medicine (Figure 6.1). Emergency medicine was sprouting in an area that had been neglected, or viewed as refuse. The petals of the flower were the other medical specialties united by emergency medicine, which was the central portion of the flower. Dailey's flower lecture was adapted and later published in an emergency medicine textbook as *A Metaphor*. Dailey wrote,

> *A new flower is growing in medicine's garden of specialties. Botanists argue whether it is a true flower or simply a weed. And even those claiming it a flower question its legitimacy, wondering whether it's simply a hybrid, formed by cross-pollination of the other flowers in the garden. However, many classify it a genuinely new strain, its seed blown into the garden by the winds of necessity...Astute observers have noted the flower takes root only in the most arid soils where other plants cannot and have not grown. Some fear it will crowd out and supplant the other flowers; but rather than displace, it appears to complement them, to fill gaps in the garden previously not even recognized...So that now it remains to be seen only whether it will remain neglected as a runty sport, or whether instead, it will be cultivated, to blossom and become an accepted part of medicine's garden.*[4]

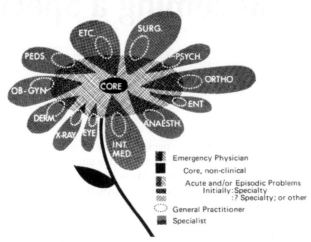

Figure 6.1 *Robert Dailey's flower symbol for emergency medicine. (From Daily RH: The emergency physician and his residency training. In: Jelenko CI, Frey C, eds. Emergency medical services: an overview, Bowie, MD, 1976, Robert J. Brady Company, a Prentice-Hall Company.)*

As Dailey remembers, "everyone was trying to define the field" and his flower presentation "touched a nerve" with the surgeons at UAEMS and others.[5] Dailey's presentation and flower analogy were referred to and critiqued in the Presidential Address at the 1975 UAEMS Annual Meeting.[6] Dailey used his flower theme in other presentations, and many in emergency medicine adopted the flower symbol— a sign of the times—to promote the field.

Emergency care was in the national consciousness by the mid-1970s. Media reports on emergency care highlighted both the deficiencies and the problems. Articles in *Time* magazine in 1971 and *U.S. News and World Report* in 1972 described increasing emergency department (ED) patient volumes, and the lack of trained providers, but also noted the new emergency medicine training programs and what was being done to improve emergency care.[7,8] In 1970, a journalist and writer named Ann Cutler wrote a book that was a scathing indictment of poor emergency care in the United States. Her investigation of the quality of medical care available for victims of heart attacks and injuries was called *Four Minutes to Life*.[9] Cutler noted that half of U.S. ambulances were run by undertakers and that EDs were staffed by "inexperienced interns" or "careless rotation of physicians." The book included chapters entitled "The Scandal of Our Emergency Rooms" and "Lives Imperiled by Ambulance Services." Cutler relates the story of a Chicago man gasping for breath and dying in the ED waiting room while an overwhelmed intern was suturing a wound. In Boston a 7-year-old fell from a roof and was impaled by a picket fence. He died in the ED from hemorrhage "on his mother's lap crying softly while he waited in hope of seeing a doctor." A case from Cleveland is described where a 14-year-old boy brought to the ED by his mother for altered mental status and attended to by "the nurse in charge, harried and harassed...she dismissed him." The boy was taken home and died in his sleep. Cutler relates a particularly disturbing case from Memphis of a 16-year-old boy who was in a motor vehicle crash, along with his mother, and became disoriented as he went in to shock from internal bleeding while waiting on a stretcher in the ED. The intern on duty mistakenly interpreted the boy's agitation as intoxication and ordered him to be restrained. He was "wrestled down by nurses and ambulance attendants who flipped him onto his stomach...Charles's injured mother could hear him scream, 'Please don't! Stop! You're killing me!'" The intern then ordered that the boy be transferred to a municipal hospital that "handles drunks." Charles died in the ambulance during the transfer, bleeding to death from a severely lacerated liver.[9] Although it exposed the poor quality of emergency care with vivid examples, Cutler's book did not have much impact on a national level. Cutler largely neglected the nascent emergency medicine movement that was gaining steam in the United States by 1970. She did quote Reinald Leidelmeyer and James Mills in her book, but to a lay journalist the successful emergency practices of these physicians were just a couple of bright twinkles in a black night of dreadful emergency care in America.

A book for young readers called *Emergency Room* by Anita MacRae Feagles was also published in 1970, providing an account of a community hospital ED through the eyes of a teenaged girl volunteer. The book provides an interesting look at the ebb and flow of activity in a smaller ED—in one section of the book the doctor on duty is napping on a stretcher because "For 2 hours…not a single patient has come in." But the typical mix of heart attacks, motor vehicle crash victims, alcohol-intoxicated patients, and domestic violence seen in today's EDs is described.[10]

Newspapers in many cities around the country ran articles critical of emergency room care in the 1960s and 1970s. A few, such as those in Cincinnati, had positive news to report as the emergency medicine residency developed. All this attention, even if largely negative, was helpful to the pioneers of emergency medicine. As the problems were enumerated, one obvious solution was to train physicians, nurses, ambulance workers, and other allied health professionals in emergency care. Men like Wiegenstein, Hannas, and Mills felt like they had the solution to the problem—emergency medicine residencies, strong continuing medical education in emergency medicine, and specialty recognition to give the field a stable platform on which to develop.

Of course, people would need to find the field an attractive career alternative. In the early 1970s, most physicians who chose to do emergency medicine residencies were viewed as out of touch with mainstream medicine. Work in emergency medical services (EMS) was also poorly understood at the time. However, a 1970s television show produced by Jack Webb changed America's understanding and opinions of emergency medicine. *Emergency!* premiered in 1971 as a 2-hour movie and became a weekly show on NBC in 1972. It was one of the most popular and successful shows on television for six seasons, and stopped when Webb turned to other endeavors, not because of failing television ratings. It was then syndicated and broadcast widely for years—the show still runs on cable television. *Emergency!* was roughly split in terms of characters and content into scenes of paramedics responding to emergencies, and emergency room, and hospital scenes. The paramedics ran out of Squad 51 and took patients to the Rampart Hospital emergency room (ER). Characters were well developed and not aggrandized, but the overall feel was one of Californian excitement. Countless young people could identify with Johnny Gage, the paramedic; Dixie McCall, the ER head nurse; and Dr. Kelly Brackett, the head emergency physician at Rampart Hospital.[11] The show was quite authentic in its portrayal of EMS and ED work. More than a dramatic series, it dealt with the problems and controversies in emergency care and educated viewers on emergency lifesaving techniques and EMS systems. Webb did a good job of hiring advisers and even some EMS actors for the show. One of the main consultants was Ronald Stewart, M.D., and it is thought that at least one of the doctors on the show was patterned after Stewart.

Ronald Stewart, M.D.: From Nova Scotia to Los Angeles

Ronald Stewart's life is almost fit for a television show. Born in the sparsely populated, picturesque northern island of Cape Breton in Nova Scotia in 1942, Stewart's Scottish father was a miner. He remembers his father wanting him, as a good Scottish lad, to learn how to play the bagpipes,

> *My father…arranged for my private lessons at $2 a lesson with a guy whose main credential was that he survived the war as a piper, which was very unusual because they would march these guys out playing the pipes right out in front of the armies advancing the infantry. But he did, and he had every reason to need to drown his sorrows and memory, I'm sure. We used to have to get him out of the pub, which was the first thing on Saturday morning, and by the time we would get to him he'd be quite drunk and we'd go back to his house, he'd take the pipe down from the wall and play a tune or two and then give them to me to play a tune or two, following in his foot steps in more ways than one. By the time I would get them they would be totally*

saturated with alcohol fumes and so I was inhaling these and the pulmonary circula-
tion was just besieged with alcohol molecules which quickly added to the central
circulation and I became a drunk as a lord and would pass out every lesson. This was
considered to be the sort of price one paid for learning the great Highland Bagpipe.[12]

Stewart went to Dalhousie Medical School in Halifax and then went into family practice in Neils Harbour, the most remote part of the province. He suffered a serious brain injury in a motor vehicle crash in "a blinding blizzard in April," and was left with "a serious impediment in my speech. I was aphasic." He found it difficult to continue his practice and decided that he would pursue training in emergency medicine, an area he had learned a bit about in medical school. He interviewed in Cincinnati in January, but found it as cold as Nova Scotia, "but without the snow," and then headed for Los Angeles to interview at the Los Angeles County (LAC)/USC program. Stewart remembers meeting Gail Anderson, "with his flying white coat starched, bright white, and Southern charm, and I just thought the world of him." In July of 1972, he loaded up his Volvo and drove diagonally across North America to Los Angeles to join the second emergency medicine residency class at LAC/USC. Stewart "was afraid of the freeway," and when he got to Los Angeles he "mistook the Sears store in East LA for the hospital."[12]

Stewart lived in the interns' quarters in the hospital and worked with speech pathologists on his language impediment and slowly improved. Like the other early residents at LAC/USC, he found the teaching to be abysmal, except for Bob Dailey, whom he greatly admired and respected. Stewart rapidly developed an affinity for EMS, and "had a real interest in translating medical stuff to lay people." As a resident he went to the Fire Academy and took the course to understand the basics of fire training. When he finished his residency in 1974, Stewart stepped immediately in to a new job as medical director of the Los Angeles County Paramedic Training Program. He also worked shifts in the emergency departments at LAC/USC, and two other hospitals, but EMS became his life. Stewart immersed himself in teaching paramedics and created a system that became almost instantly famous. He lived out of a boat docked at Long Beach Marina, with a Jacuzzi on board. It served as a "party boat" for paramedics and physicians, although Stewart was "in the streets all the time" rather than on his boat.

The LAC paramedics were approached to serve as advisors for the *Emergency!* television show, and Stewart was also asked to participate. He helped with script generation and script review, and sometimes went to the set of the show to help explain medical issues, or advise the actors. Many of the early scripts were stories from Stewart's experiences, which he "sanitized," made confidential, and gave to the writers.

Emergency! was viewed with some skepticism by some early ACEP leaders. William Haeck, who was on the ACEP board of directors at that time remembers:

The original reaction from a bunch of people in ACEP was, "Gee this is terrible,
there is so much that is shown here that's wrong." I said, "Look guys, this is going to
be the biggest piece of PR [public relations] that we can ever get, you just need to
thank God that it is there." That was the case.[13]

Emergency! did more for recruiting young men and women in to emergency medical services than all the government and organized medicine initiatives of those times combined. Almost every EMS provider who came into the field in the early 1970s distinctly remembers *Emergency!* as a positive influence. It was now sexy and exciting to work on an ambulance service or in an ED. And for the first time in the world of entertainment, the American public saw an emergency physician who was a credible doctor. They also saw a new standard of care. As Karl Mangold noted in a 1978 speech, advocating for improved emergency education,

We have a TV program that is imprinting upon many adults and certainly millions
of children what their expectations should be regarding medicine's response to those
who are acutely ill and injured. The children of today, once they achieve a position of
authority and power, will certainly not accept less than a sophisticated prehospital
and hospital emergency response program....[14]

THE EMS ACT OF 1973

It was not a mere coincidence that the EMS Act was passed by Congress in 1973, when the show *Emergency!* was becoming extremely popular with the American public. This important piece of legislation had been brewing since the National Academy of Sciences–National Research Council (NAS/NRC) report on accidental death and disability came out in 1966 (Chapter 3). Congress identified highway trauma as the priority area for injury control and passed the National Traffic and Motor Vehicle Safety Act and the Highway Safety Act of 1966. The Department of Transportation was appropriated funds to help develop regional EMS systems and standards for EMS provider training. State funding for highway safety was tied to the development of EMS. One of the first leaders to take advantage of this funding was David Boyd, M.D., a surgeon from Illinois who had a fervent interest in improving trauma care. Boyd set up a statewide trauma system in Illinois that became a model for the country. Boyd was then tapped by the federal government to head up trauma programs for the newly created Division of Trauma and Emergency Medical Services in Department of Health Education and Welfare. Like most of the surgeons who advocated for improved trauma care, Boyd did not initially appreciate any major role for emergency physicians in the provision of U.S. trauma care. But, as the congressional committee work for a new emergency medical services act gained momentum, Boyd began to confront a new, organized group of emergency physicians.

John McDade, one of the original Alexandria group physicians, was politically connected in Washington. McDade's family was from Scranton, Pennsylvania—his father was a self-made "coal baron," and his brother Joseph was elected to the U.S. House of Representatives in 1963. As John McDade watched the other "smart doctors and academics" develop ACEP and residency training in emergency medicine, he realized "we need somebody in there who's got some political savvy." McDade became ACEP's unofficial Washington insider, and helped ACEP leaders like Wiegenstein, Rupke, Hannas, and Krome negotiate the halls of Congress. McDade soon identified David Boyd as,

> ...another enemy. He was an enemy because he was convinced the only way to get the government involved in it was through a Trauma Service. He said, "Emergency physicians aren't worth the powder." He said basically something like that. Of course, it all got back to us, so the whole College got angry. We were all walking around talking about this dummy David Boyd. He finally realized that we were too much of a political group to just totally ignore us.[15]

Boyd and R. Adams Cowley, who created the Maryland statewide trauma system and is credited with defining the "Golden Hour" in acute trauma care, had visions of organized, efficient, helicopter-assisted trauma systems across the United States. For Cowley, this was a direct attempt to bring to civilian medicine what he had seen and practiced in the Army. But in their focus on trauma, the surgeons overlooked the reality of American medical practice—that trauma was just one part of emergency medical care, and that increasingly, the doctors who were practicing in hospital emergency departments were emergency physicians, not surgeons. John McDade remembers an early meeting with David Boyd,

> I said, "Do you know the most common cause of death in this country is cardiac...heart disease, heart attacks? We can do something about that." He got mad at me, which was unsurprising because I'd seen it happen before. So I said, "Look, we have a thing to go after here." When we presented all this stuff to the Congress we started out with heart disease, we started out with the fact the people were dying of heart disease that could be saved with a little bit of machinery and a...bit of speed. They bought into that. As a matter of fact we finally wound up having ourselves a set of parameters that we put together and talked to the Congress. We testified before all kinds of hearings.[15]

With this approach, McDade and other early ACEP leaders expanded the dialogue that lead up to the EMS Act to include more than trauma and injury. As the debate heated up, McDade used his brother's influence to help the cause of emergency physicians. He remembers:

> We are in Bethesda and all these speeches have gone on and we are sitting, I think it was in John Wiegenstein's suite…we were all in there talking about this and trying to figure out which way it is going to go, and we are all sitting there sucking up some booze and doing our talking. It must have been about 2 o'clock in the morning and I thought to myself—I've got a brother here that could probably help us. I don't know why I hadn't thought about it earlier. I said, "John, my brother's here and he might be able to help us with this." Two o'clock in the morning I picked up the phone and I called him. He said, "This had better be good!"[15]

It did turn out to be good. Joseph McDade agreed to meet his brother and Wiegenstein, Karl Mangold, and Carl Jelenko at 9 o'clock the next morning. The congressman listened intently as the emergency physicians went on for over an hour, making their plea for training in emergency medical services and the need for federal money for equipment and organization of EMS. When they were done, Congressman McDade said simply, "Okay, I'm with you. Where do we go from here?" Joseph McDade provided key access to Congressman Paul Rogers, who was the chair of the House Subcommittee on Health and the Environment. John McDade and other ACEP members met Rogers, and testified before his committee. Afterward, Rogers came up to McDade and said, "That is about as good testimony as I've heard for a long time. It was right on the money. You were head and shoulders above all the rest of the people."[15]

The EMS Act of 1973 started out as a far simpler idea to fund ambulances, but with the input of ACEP, trauma surgeons, and the public, it became much more than that. John McDade remembers that the position of ACEP was,

> If somebody is going to write a law we want to make sure we've got our share in it. We want to make sure it's written by people who know what they are talking about. Up to that time it was okay, but it was just an ambulance law.[15]

One thing that was debated for the EMS Act was funding to train emergency physicians in residency programs. ACEP realized that it was too early to push hard in this area. Since the American Medical Association (AMA) and other organizations had not yet officially endorsed emergency medicine residency training, and surgeons and internists were likely to oppose this, there was insufficient political capital to advance the idea.

The EMS Act did not come easily. Iterations of an EMS bill had moved through the 1971 and 1972 Congresses, but ran out of time for compromises and died. The EMS Act of 1973, championed by Senator Alan Cranston and Representative Paul Rogers was approved by Congress, but then vetoed by President Richard Nixon, who had a classic Republican view of the legislation. Nixon wrote in his veto message:

> I strongly believe the federal role should be limited…leaving States and communities to establish the full range of emergency medical services systems that best suit their varying local needs.[16]

Nixon also believed the proposed $185 million appropriation for the EMS Act was excessive, but that rural EMS should be more heavily funded. Congress took a strong stand in support of the EMS Act and came only five votes short of overriding Nixon's veto. This prompted a flurry of activity by lawmakers and the Executive Office to find a successful compromise. Gerald Ford, who would a year later succeed Nixon when he resigned after the Watergate scandal, was a strong supporter of the EMS Act. The work went fast, and the Emergency Medical Services System Act of 1973 was passed in November, just 3 months after Nixon's veto.

The EMS Act allocated funding in three main areas—planning, implementation, and operation of local and regional EMS systems, research on EMS systems, and training programs for EMS. Institutions that sought funding had to meet "15 points," which for all intents and purposes limited applicants to state or local governments or public consortiums.[17,18] Because of this, the funding, which was an impressive amount for that era, was metered out slowly, as states and regions struggled to develop the basic requirements of the 15 points. It was estimated that less than half of the EMS Act of 1973 appropriation was spent due to difficulties with eligibility, the application process, and bureaucratic problems in the Department of Health, Education and Welfare (HEW).[18]

Despite being a less sweeping program than many envisioned, the EMS Act of 1973 was an important first foray of the U.S. federal government into EMS. At a time when the impetus was on reducing government spending for social programs, it is notable that the EMS Act had enough political and popular support to be the only major new social program to receive governmental support. The federal interest and funding prompted many states to move forward with EMS programs, and thousands of para-medics and other EMS providers were trained under the EMS Act. The path contin-ued to be difficult, as President Ford's conservative fiscal policies led him to veto the HEW appropriations in 1975. Congress overturned the veto. ACEP, particularly John McDade and an ACEP-hired Washington consultant named Terry Schmidt, fought each year to keep the appropriations for the EMS Act intact. President Ford pro-claimed November 2 through 8, 1975, as Emergency Medical Services Week to direct public attention toward the need for improved emergency medical services. John McDade, John Rupke, Terry Schmidt, and others in ACEP were instrumental in encouraging the President to make this symbolic declaration.

The early ACEP leaders were not afraid to make their case in a national forum, and for some it was an exciting and awe-inspiring part of building their new specialty. Karl Mangold remembers,

> I get a call from Art Auer who is the Executive Director of ACEP at that time and says John Wiegenstein is supposed to be testifying to the Senate Appropriations Committee and he can't make it. Can you do it? You got to remember those years we paid all our own transportation, air plane fares, hotel, taxis, meals—we were doing this because we believed in it. I can't tell you how wonderfully exciting it was to be surrounded by a bunch of renegade innovators that saw the vision clearly and couldn't be deterred. It's got to be like winning the World Series. Its got to be like punch it across, 2 yards and the goal line with 30 seconds to go to put the points on the board. It was just exhilarating…([N]ext thing I know I'm sitting in front of Warren Magnuson and the Senate Appropriations Committee of the United States Congress. I'm pushing why you should spend money to train residents and emergency nurses and paramedics and prehospital. So I came out of that meeting and I called my Mom and Dad in New York and my Dad said, "This could only happen in America!"[19]

ACEP was savvy enough to ride the wave of interest in EMS. John Wiegenstein, William Haeck, and other ACEP leaders realized that the public's support for EMS was crucial to the development of the field of emergency medicine, and although they were relative neophytes in the world of media and communications, they developed a plan with Paramount Pictures to produce a movie on EMS. The film was shot primarily in Haeck's home base of Jacksonville, Florida, which was well known for its advanced EMS system. Haeck remembers,

> I scripted a motivational kind of thing and my son was the victim and Paramount sent out this whole production crew and it took a week, full-time to film that thing. It really, considering the year, was not a bad film.[13]

The movie was called "Cry for Help," and it was designed to motivate communities to develop and improve their EMS systems. The movie was viewed as quite a success, both from filmmakers and the public. Based on the popularity and effect of "Cry for Help," ACEP produced two more movies with Paramount in 1974—"Wanted Alive," another film about the benefits of good emergency medical care, and "Careers in Emergency Medicine," a film that promoted EMS jobs as occupations for students.[20]

ACEP also enhanced its visibility in the realm of EMS by forming the EMS Information Center (EMSIC). This center was conceived and developed by the

Michigan ACEP chapter, which received a grant for the project. ACEP held two workshop meetings of national organizations with an interest in EMS to develop the EMSIC concept. The center became a library and repository for EMS literature, manuals, pamphlets, newsletters, and other communications, and provided assistance to ACEP members and others who were trying to learn more about EMS. It functioned until the early 1980s.[20] By 1976, the literature in emergency medicine was substantive enough that the National Library of Medicine deemed emergency medicine a scientific entity that would be indexed.

American College of Emergency Physicians Consolidates the World of Emergency Medicine

The ACEP of the early 1970s was not much of a college in the traditional sense of that word for medical specialties. ACEP had little voice or influence in the world of academic medicine. But, led by men who were rapidly learning what it takes to have power in organized medicine, ACEP was becoming a political animal. The membership rose to around 4,000 physicians by 1973, and the "Blue Book" meeting at the AMA that year showed ACEP's ability to maneuver opinions by infiltrating and manipulating the agenda of a national meeting. ACEP had moved its offices from the basement of the Michigan State Medical Society to a bigger office space, still in the basement, of the nearby "241 Building." Art Auer quickly grew into an involved and authoritative executive director. An early ACEP staff member remembers:

> Art was a very strong personality and it was really a "cult of Art"…he was a very hands on, very temperamental in some ways, executive director. He was sort of "the guy"—into everything….[21]

Around this time ACEP adopted an approach of developing liaisons with other emergency medicine groups and in some cases forming linkages of dependency that allowed ACEP to have a strong voice in all the venues relating to emergency care. The first example, as previously described, was ACEP's provision of management services, and housing to UAEM. Barely out of its infancy, ACEP became a landlord to UAEM, and a big brother to other organizations. Although the organizations looked to the outside world like they were distinct entities, the work and administration of the organizations was interwoven in the ACEP web. Susan Dunsmore, an early ACEP staff member remembers: "You walked from one office to another and you were in another organization!"[22]

The next organization that developed a close working relationship with ACEP was the Emergency Department Nurses Association (EDNA), which later became the Emergency Nurse's Association (ENA). EDNA formed in a manner similar to ACEP, when a West Coast emergency nurses association found out about an East Coast organization, and the two groups incorporated as EDNA in late 1970.[23] ACEP and EDNA established communications in the next two years, and explored the idea of having a joint national meeting. Under the guidance of Karl Mangold, ACEP partnered with EDNA to hold a joint Scientific Assembly at the Fairmont Hotel in Dallas, Texas, in October of 1973. The meeting allowed emergency physicians and nurses to discuss the pressing issues in emergency care and politics, but what most early members of ACEP remember about the joint ACEP/EDNA Scientific Assemblies was the fraternity-/sorority-party atmosphere as young physicians and nurses went out on the town after a day's meetings. The joint ACEP/EDNA Scientific Assemblies continued until 1979. ACEP also became the organizational landlord of the Emergency Medicine Residents Association, which formed in 1974. From 1973 to 1975, ACEP provided administrative services for a regional Michigan EMS organization called the TriCounty EMS Council. Working with this group, ACEP developed and distributed training modules on "The Initial Patient Survey," "Psychological Intervention," and "Use of the Backboard."[20]

The resuscitation and critical care research community was naturally interested in emergency medicine, because the implementation of advances in cardiopulmonary resuscitation required an organized, efficient EMS system and EDs. The leader of the resuscitation movement was Peter Safar. Safar was an Austrian-born physician and scientist who came to the United States in 1949. He became interested in resuscitation through his work in anesthesiology and while at Johns Hopkins University in the 1950s became well known for his experiments on artificial ventilation. Safar recruited volunteer medical students, nurses, and laboratory assistants who agreed to let Safar sedate and paralyze them and then try various techniques for ventilating the lungs. This led to the recommendation of mouth-to-mouth ventilation as a resuscitation technique.[24] Safar later moved to the University of Pittsburgh and set up a world-famous resuscitation laboratory. He and his collaborators began to become more politically active in the late 1960s as they sought to have their resuscitation techniques put in to practice and formed the Society of Critical Care Medicine in 1970. Safar was aware of the early ACEP and UAEMS and realized that a liaison with emergency physicians would be desirable.

In 1972, ACEP, UAEMS, and the Society of Critical Care Medicine met and formed the Federation for Emergency and Critical Care Medicine. The agreement was that the Federation would consist of societies, not individual members, and that each society would appoint an officer to the Federation. The main purpose of the Federation for Emergency and Critical Care Medicine was to increase the visibility of this area of medicine in the AMA. A "federation" carried more clout, even if it was not an active coalition, and this appears to have influenced the AMA to approve a provisional section on emergency medicine in June of 1973. However, the Federation was a not a formal participant in the AMA Workshop Conference on Education of the Physician in Emergency Medicine in July of 1973—the three-member organizations were separately represented. The Federation for Emergency and Critical Care Medicine served briefly and effectively as a paper tiger, but as the critical care physicians and emergency physicians realized that a common training path for an emergency medicine–critical care physician was not likely to emerge, the groups began to drift apart. No mention is made of the Federation for Emergency and Critical Care Medicine in the ACEP board of directors meeting minutes from 1973 to 1975, and the Federation slowly dissolved and was not an entity when emergency medicine began its official quest for specialty recognition.

ACEP rapidly evolved from the staffless little group of doctors who met on overturned boxes in the basement of the Michigan State Medical Society in 1968. By 1976, ACEP had a staff of around 50 people. It moved from the 241 Building to a two-story building next to the Lansing Airport. Under the direction of Art Auer, ACEP became thorough and compulsive in its record keeping. An early ACEP staff member remembers, "the whole downstairs was this bank of file cabinets where they would keep absolutely every letter that was sent to every member."[21] The location next to the airport was convenient because documents and materials were frequently shipped to national medical organizations like the AMA in Chicago. A staff member recalls,

> *You would go to the airport, ask someone who was getting on a plane to go to Chicago if they would take this package for you and then you would run back to the office and call the docs and they would go and pick it up at the airport—before people worried about bombs.*[21]

The state chapters of ACEP were also active and effective in developing emergency medicine and EMS. The Florida chapter, which was started and run for its first few years by William Haeck, was a good example of regional success. Haeck remembers,

> *…victory started to come our way…in this state when the Florida College of Emergency Physicians was recognized as a component of the Florida Medical Association. A lot of hard work went into those things. I spent time convincing the Duval County Medical Society to have a Committee on Emergency Medicine. Those parallel activities all over the United States at the local, state and then at the national level, took a lot of time, a lot of foot work, a lot of brass and fortunately there were a lot of people willing to do that work.*[13]

Haeck went to the Florida Cabinet to plead the case for better EMS training. He remembers, "I likened the EMS story to the story of the Good Samaritan out of the bible and the donkey was the ambulance." Haeck also noted that barbers were required to have hundreds of hours of training in order to practice, but ambulance attendants' training was but a few hours. As part of the federal Regional Medical Program (originally borne out of President Johnson's Great Society Programs) the Florida Department of Health received a federal grant of over a million dollars to improve the care of heart disease and stroke patients, and tapped William Haeck to implement the grant. He was charged with setting up a basic EMS system in every county in Florida and did the job in 18 months. In 1973 Florida passed its own EMS Act to improve EMS equipment and training and establish a 911 telephone alert system.[13]

In 1973 ACEP created the Emergency Medicine Foundation (EMF) as a federal 501(c)3 nonprofit organization. EMF was a way to solicit tax-deductible contributions to ACEP for "research and education projects."[20] However, in its early years, little money was raised from members or other donors, and EMF funds were used for ACEP projects that had little to do with research or education. EMF administration costs were extremely high. John Wiegenstein remembered being bothered by this in the mid 1970s:

> ...I went before ACEP and asked them, "Here you've had this EMF for I don't know how long. You get 40 or 50 thousand a year and you spent 30 thousand for maintenance." I said, "It's doing absolutely zilch for research."[25]

Prior to the push for Board development, ACEP in 1974 produced the *Physicians Evaluation and Education Review* (PEER I). This was an examination developed for practicing emergency physicians to assess their knowledge of the core content in emergency medicine. The examination was developed under the under R. R. Hannas's Education Committee, and Richard Braen, M.D., did much of the detail work. ACEP members were charged a fee to take the examination, and were provided scores and feedback on where they stood in comparison to others who took the examination, and the areas where they needed to improve their knowledge.

Another member service that ACEP toyed with from its early existence was group professional liability insurance. Liability insurance costs for physicians increased steadily during the late 1960s. John Rupke remembers, "I still have my insurance policy someplace from Medical Protective that I got in 1964–1965, $40 for the year."[26] By the 1970s liability insurance costs had risen over a thousand percent, and a many called it a national crisis in medicine. ACEP looked at proposals from various insurance companies, and eventually selected a company called Profesco to offer its Endorsed Professional Liability Insurance Program for emergency physicians. ACEP members were required to be enrolled in this insurance program, and John Rupke believes that ACEP membership swelled after 1974 due to the liability insurance program. The vice president of Profesco, I. David Gordon, served as a valuable consultant to the ACEP leaders in the details and regulation of liability insurance. He was often seen at ACEP meetings and came to know many of the early board of directors members well. ACEP, like many large medical organizations, later offered life and disability insurance to members.[27]

ACEP published its first book in 1975, *Emergency Department Organization and Management*. A. L. Jenkins, an ACEP board of directors member from Tennessee, was largely responsible for the production and editing of the book. It sold over 20,000 copies.[20,28] The book was revised, republished, and remained ACEP's single most popular publication. ACEP then moved to publish other practice-based booklets and materials for emergency physicians.

In 8 short years, the national ACEP and its state chapters had emerged as the unquestioned leaders in emergency medicine. After being very limited in what it could provide for members in its early years, ACEP was now offering members a high-quality continuing education program; a self-assessment examination; a book and other helpful materials dealing with emergency department management; an insurance program; a research foundation; and a lobbying voice in Washington. By consolidating power, linking with other organizations, and learning the politics of organized medicine, ACEP was now the vehicle that emergency physicians could ride toward specialty recognition.

The Process of Becoming a Board

A DIFFERENT PATH

American medical boards were the result of the movement toward specialization in medicine in the first half of the twentieth century. Ophthalmology established the first medical board in 1917, followed by otolaryngology (1924), obstetrics and gynecology (1930), and dermatology and syphilology (1932). All of the other major medical fields established certifying boards by the late 1930s.[29,30] The Advisory Board for Medical Specialties was created in 1933 as an amalgam of the four original boards and the American Hospital Association, the Association of American Medical Colleges, the Federation of State Medical Boards, and the National Board of Medical Examiners. Notably missing in this group was the AMA. The AMA was preeminent as the leader in organized medicine at this time and retained an independent power in approving specialty boards through its Council on Medical Education. Therefore, a new specialty needed the approval of both the Advisory Board for Medical Specialties, as well as the AMA Council on Education in order to be officially recognized and allowed to certify practitioners.[29,31]

The board for family practice was incorporated and approved in 1969. The impetus for this "generalist" field to be granted specialty status with a certifying board came out of the great decline of general practitioners in the 1950s and 1960s. As a crisis in primary care emerged in the 1960s, full residency training for family physicians and the legitimization of this training as a medical specialty were pushed by some medical educators and the federal government. The post-Medicare/Medicaid jump in the number of patients who presented for primary care was alarming to U.S. medicine, and a certifying board in family practice was seen as one way of helping to attract physicians to primary care. Although it was not without struggle, the political pressure on the ABMS and AMA to approve the family practice board was immense, and the approval process took very little time. Family practice thus became, in 1969, the first new medical board to be approved in 20 years.

In 1970, the Advisory Board for Medical Specialties became the American Board of Medical Specialties (ABMS). The structure and process for approval of a medical specialty board did not change. The Liaison Committee for Specialty Boards (LCSB), which included representatives from the ABMS, and Council on Medical Education of the AMA did the intake work on applications for new specialty boards, and then made a recommendation for approval by the AMA and ABMS. Emergency medicine would become the LCSB's first request for a primary board since family medicine went through the process in the late 1960s. To be approved as a medical specialty, emergency medicine would need the support of the LCSB to move forward, approval from the AMA Council on Medical Education, and finally the approval of the ABMS.

The other option was to create an independent board outside of the ABMS. A number of these unofficial, "jake leg" medical boards existed, usually for smaller medical fields. For example, David Wagner, who was a practicing surgeon, remembers,

> The American Board of Abdominal Surgery got formed by a large number of surgeons, outside ABMS, and they…went for about 10 years and then withered. I think ABMS was, and still is, powerful enough that you gotta join that club to really have legitimacy.[32]

The abdominal surgeons fought an immense battle with the American Board of Surgery and the ABMS from 1957 to the late 1960s. By intermittently taking control of the Section on Surgery of the AMA, they were able to force the issue. The American Society of Abdominal Surgeons grew to 9,000 members by 1967, and put extreme pressure on the ABMS to form a new abdominal surgery board, just as it had for thoracic surgery 20 years before. However, the ABMS and American Board of Surgery were able to hold strong, and make enough concessions to appease the abdominal surgeons, and the push for a separate board eventually died.[29]

For some of the more free-spirited and antiestablishment emergency physicians, an independent board would have been acceptable, but for the leaders of organized emergency medicine, it was not. An independent board that was not approved by ABMS would have been counter to their mission. They had struggled for many years to be viewed as equals in the medical world, and they felt that an independent board would relegate them to permanent status as second-class citizens. The importance of gaining certification was increasing as emergency medicine became more established. Many of the newer converts to the field came from other disciplines where board certification was the norm. Brooks Bock, who left during the final year of his urology residency in 1973 to become a faculty member in emergency medicine with Ron Krome at Wayne State/Detroit Receiving Hospital, remembers telling his mother of his decision:

> …my mother just couldn't believe it. She said, "You're going to do what?" She said, "I thought you were going to be a real doctor?" I said, "Well, this is a real doctor, Mom." She said, "You're telling me you can't get board certified." I said, "No, there is no board certification right now, Mom—we're working on that. That's got to be something in the future, I hope." She said, "Well what if it doesn't happen?" I said, "Well, I will have made a big mistake, probably, Mom."[33]

The route to becoming an ABMS-approved specialty in emergency medicine was well known by the early emergency medicine leaders, but the path had not been traveled much in the previous decades, other than for family practice. Since R. R. Hannas had helped family practice in their rapid ascension to a specialty board, and emergency medicine was also a field of breadth, many emergency physicians assumed that the approval of a board in emergency medicine could also be accomplished in short order. However, the same political pressure that helped to push family practice to board status did not exist for emergency medicine. Although the increase in ED patients and poor state of emergency care was publically acknowledged, it was difficult for the organized medical world to conceive of emergency medicine as a true specialty. Some of the steps that were necessary for emergency medicine to reach specialty status had been delayed or blocked by the AMA and other medical fields.

The Double-Edged Sword of the American Medical Association

By the early 1970s, the AMA was beginning to pay more attention to the pesky new field that was clamoring for recognition. The AMA had been interested in emergency care since the mid-1960s, but as the field began to resemble a new specialty, with residencies forming in the early 1970s, the AMA's position on emergency medicine education was in transition. The AMA's Commission on Emergency Medical Services was established in 1966 in response to the NAC/NRC "Accidental Death and Disability…" Report. The Commission held annual conferences on emergency care starting in 1968, but these often focused on EMS and hospital ED functioning, and not as much on professional development of emergency physicians.[34,35] The AMA's Commission on EMS had representation from many medical specialty societies, the Department of Transportation, and the Department of Health Education and Welfare, but not until 1972, when ACEP gained a voting seat on the Commission, were emergency physicians represented. The Commission was interested in the upgrading and classification of hospital emergency departments and published *Categorization of Hospital Emergency Capabilities* in 1971. This booklet was a progression of the ideas of Robert Kennedy, and the American Hospital Association on how EDs could be constructed and equipped to best deliver emergency care and participate in EMS systems. No recognition or acknowledgment of a role for emergency physicians appeared in this document.[20]

The early emergency physicians were conflicted in their approach to the AMA. On one hand, they were very much aware that any progress toward specialty recognition would require working closely with and garnering approval from the AMA. On the other hand, these younger, innovative physicians did not want to be part of, as R. R. Hannas often said, "old fartsville." William Haeck remembers that

> *The example that always was pulled out was the AMA. You had to serve organized medicine for 30–40 years before you could be visible at the AMA and by that time you were in your late 60s or 70s and your big interest was the status quo.*[13]

Therefore, in the early 1970s, ACEP was like a teenager having to sit through a formal dinner with adults of the AMA—it had to be at the table, but would be frequently rolling its eyes.

The inconsistent approach of the AMA toward emergency medicine is well demonstrated by ACEP's attempt to form a Section Council on Emergency Medicine in the AMA. ACEP had pushed for a Section Council since October of 1971, but after shuffling the proposal around the organization, the AMA denied the petition in October of 1972. The primary reason given for the refusal was that the specialty society (ACEP) had not been existence for 5 years. ACEP, with John Wiegenstein leading the charge, appealed directly to the AMA House of Delegates for support. The Federation for Emergency and Critical Care Medicine also advocated for a Section Council on emergency medicine. The House of Delegates again brought the proposal to the AMA Board of Trustees. The Trustees had to create a mechanism to approve a provisional Section Council, thereby overlooking the 5-year rule. A constitutional amendment was created and passed to approve emergency medicine in May of 1973 as a provisional Section Council.[20,35] William Haeck became the first chairman of the section council. No other medical field had achieved section council status in such a short time period, but for the impatient emergency physicians, it seemed to be an unnecessarily prolonged process. The scientific sections of AMA sponsor annual educational programs for their field, and, more important, send a delegate to the AMA House of Delegates. The Section Council on Emergency Medicine presented educational sessions at the AMA annual meetings in 1974 and 1975. In 1975 the AMA approved a permanent section council on emergency medicine. R. R. Hannas remembers that an emergency medicine meeting was being held in an Atlantic City, New Jersey, hotel at the same time that the AMA House of Delegates was voting on approval of emergency medicine as a permanent Section Council. Realizing that no ACEP members were at the AMA vote, Hannas,

> *…got out and ran the whole fuckin' boardwalk between the two places and got there in time to be sure that it went through alright, and it did. You know, some of them, as such back biters, you'd never know that they didn't vote against you!*[36]

John Wiegenstein also remembers the political gamesmanship that was part of the section council approval by the AMA. At the AMA hearings for section council approval, Oscar Hampton of the American College of Surgeons, the nemesis of emergency medicine, was waiting to speak. Hampton liked to have the last word, so he would patiently wait until all others had spoken. Wiegenstein was by then familiar with Hampton's game, and recalled the meeting,

> *…we wanted to get up last so we wouldn't have to jockey for position. Oscar wanted to get up right after I got up, so I walked out of the room. I was watching outside the door…Oscar got up and gave his usual talk about how emergency medicine isn't a specialty, it's a location. It's an emergency room doctor. They work in a room. And then I came back in the room—my turn to speak—I said, "I understand what Dr. Hampton is saying, perhaps we ought to call surgeons, operating room doctors." We knew what he was going to say. It was kind of funny, Oscar…I think he was so opposed that he was more in our favor than against us. In other words he did more good for us because he was so far out there.*[25]

Karl Mangold knew Hampton through his father-in-law. Mangold remembers, "Oscar used to say to me, 'You're wasting your medical career.'" I said, "I've heard it before Oscar." It is Mangold's contention that Hampton's love for a good debate was stronger than his convictions against emergency medicine. Mangold gives credit to Hampton for making ACEP and others in emergency medicine better prepared to fight the battle for specialty status, noting that Hampton's "resistance to us made us so much better in our approach to the traditional house of medicine, ABMS and the AMA."[19]

In the end, ACEP's overall cordial relationship with the AMA and knowledge of how to work in the AMA's system produced a favorable result. John Wiegenstein remembered,

> ...[Y]ou know we were always friends with AMA. Of course we kind of padded the deck in AMA. We knew they had the Reference Committee arena and when this Section vote came up we bussed people into Chicago to line up behind the microphone and so we did stack the deck. The Reference Committee said there was a majority of opinion...for this and therefore we recommend that this happen.[25]

The favorable vote for permanent section council approval for emergency medicine was an indication that the AMA understood that it was better to engage the new field and perhaps shape it, than to ignore it and think it might go away. By the end of 1975, the AMA, while not the best friend of emergency medicine, could be considered a political ally, as it supported both emergency medicine training programs and the drive toward a specialty board.

CREATING THE INFRASTRUCTURE FOR A BOARD

ACEP leaders met with representatives from the AMA and the American Board of Medical Specialties to understand what would be needed to form a board. The process involved essentially creating a board with all the components of certification—eligibility, an examination, and a review process for residency programs—in a parallel, nonapproved world. But, the emergency medicine board would not be allowed to administer its test or certify individuals until official approval was obtained from the ABMS and AMA. Giving the examination before ABMS approval would torpedo the whole process. With this understanding, ACEP rapidly moved forward. In 1974, the Committee on Board Establishment (COBE) was formed. This committee was charged with developing the basic policies for eligibility for practicing physicians and residency graduates to sit for the board examination. By 1975 it had developed a detailed checklist and flow chart for requirements and steps needed for medical specialty recognition, and a month by month timetable for how it would be accomplished, culminating with administration of the first examination in late 1977, assuming that ABMS approval would be forthcoming.[37] A meeting was held in Palm Springs in 1975 to discuss the issues and invite comments and testimony from physicians and groups on who should be eligible for the examination and how it should be administered. Many people expressed their opinions. George Podgorny was at the 2-day meeting and remembers,

> There were people who said anybody can take the test. If they pass, they pass, if they didn't pass, they didn't pass. Somebody said no, it should only be residents and graduates. Some said only surgeons should take it. Some said only internists can take it.[38]

One of the issues the COBE had to deal with was "grandfathering"—the approval of physicians as certified based on years of practice. ACEP member statistics in 1975 indicated that at least 3,750 physicians who had no formal training in emergency medicine were practicing full-time in emergency departments in the United States.[39] In other medical fields, most predominantly in surgery in the 1930s, the initial establishment of a board had included a great deal of grandfathering of practitioners.[29] Late in 1975, the COBE recommended to the ACEP board of directors that there should be no automatic "grandfathering" of emergency physicians—everyone who wished to be certified would be required to take the examination. Those emergency physicians who were not emergency medicine residency–trained would be required to complete an internship and practice emergency medicine full time in an ED for 5 years before they could sit for the examination. The COBE also recommended that the "practice eligible" path for board certification be closed 8 years after the first test administration.[40] The issue of grandfathering would come up again a few years later when the first board of directors of the American Board of Emergency Medicine was meeting, and one member brought a motion to the table that all ABEM Directors be automatically grandfathered and certified without taking the examination. Peter Rosen was a member of the ABEM board of directors and spoke up abruptly and crudely against what he viewed as a retreat from "intellectual honesty":

> I said, okay I'll vote for that if we can change the name from "grandfather" to "motherfucker." If you're willing to be called a motherfucker then we'll mother fucker you in to emergency medicine. That got their attention.[41]

The motion was withdrawn.

The COBE began to work on plans for a certifying examination. The ABMS would have to approve the examination, but had no role in administering examinations. A special task force, run by Ron Krome and George Podgorny was assigned, and two important deficiencies were apparent as the committee began to think about developing an examination—expertise and money. The COBE members had little knowledge about how to develop an examination, and they knew that it would be expensive to do so. Estimates were that it would cost $1 million. Therefore in 1975, ACEP put out a request for proposals to develop the emergency medicine board examination. It also sent out a request to ACEP members for a "voluntary assessment" of $150 to help subsidize the cost of developing the examination. ACEP offered to accept this money in $50 installments over 3 years. The response from members was impressive. Within a year 1500 of ACEP's 8,000 members had paid the full $150 and another 1,500 had paid the first $50 installment. As an unofficial vote from members' wallets, this was an indication that board certification had become more important to emergency physicians as the field grew more established. At the end of 3 years, over 4,500 ACEP members had donated more than $830,000 to help develop the certifying examination.[20]

ACEP received bids for developing the examination from a number of organizations, including one from the National Board of Medical Examiners, but it was most impressed by a proposal from a group in its own backyard. The Michigan State University in Lansing had a progressive group of leaders in its Office of Medical Education Research and Development (OMERAD). OMERAD's ideas for an examination in emergency medicine were more innovative than the other proposals, and ACEP leaders liked Jack L. Maatsch, Ph.D., who would lead the project. Maatch was a seasoned educational scholar who was very interested in piloting and conducting prospective research on new methods of testing competency in the professions. The proximity of OMERAD in Lansing also was viewed as a plus. ACEP approved OMERAD to develop the examination in March of 1975. One of the first things OMERAD realized is that ACEP did not have enough funds to fully support their project. Maatsch worked with Ron Krome and others to submit a grant to the U.S. Department of Health, Education, and Welfare. They hit the jackpot, receiving a National Center for Health Services Research grant in excess of $1 million to develop the board examination.

One of the unique features of OMERAD's plan for the emergency medicine board examination was that it would be prepared and administered with a criterion-referenced philosophy. This meant that the knowledge and skill set would be developed for the field, questions and scenarios would be developed, and a standard for passing the examination would be set. All who passed would be certified. This differed from the board examinations in other medical fields at the time, where minimum criteria for competency were not established, and using a norm-referenced approach, a certain percentage of applicants were guaranteed to fail the examination. The comprehensive process OMERAD proposed for defining content for a medical discipline and preparing a criterion-referenced examination to test the content had never been done in American medicine.[42] OMERAD began working with ACEP, and to a lesser extent

UAEM, to define the practice of emergency medicine and from this to select the medical conditions and skills that would be tested. A survey was sent to a large sample of emergency physicians in 1975, and the data from the survey were used to develop 22 "skill and condition" categories. The task force of Ron Krome and George Podgorny developed work sheets that specified the essential knowledge, skill, and performance needed by an emergency physician for the typical disease processes and problems that would be encountered by emergency physicians. The test questions and scenarios that would eventually be developed were referenced to these content worksheets. Another differentiating factor in the early planning for the emergency medicine examination was that it would consist of a written component and oral scenarios to certify clinical competency.

ACEP formed a Certification Examination Committee, consisting of around 40 emergency physicians who developed the first test. The chair of this committee was Gus Roussi, an emergency physician who formed an early emergency medicine residency program in Akron, Ohio. Roussi was a highly respected member of ACEP and skillfully blended the more academic members of the committee with practicing physicians. The committee came to Lansing in July of 1975, paying their own travel expenses, for an intensive, 3-day session to develop basic testing content and draft questions in five skills areas: cardiorespiratory, medicine, surgery/trauma, doctor–patient/psychiatric/legal–ethical, and administration/systems. Peter Rosen remembers becoming frustrated with at least one committee member, who had already become a successful entrepreneur in emergency medicine, "but didn't know a lot of medicine."[43] After the committee's work was complete, a field test for the examination was planned for 1977.[44]

With these preparatory steps completed, and with seeming support from the AMA and ABMS, ACEP decided to formally create the American Board of Emergency Medicine (ABEM). ABEM was incorporated on March 3, 1976. Although ACEP was clearly the lead organization in forming ABEM, it realized the ABMS requirement for representation from academic organizations, therefore the initial board of directors consisted of six representatives from ACEP (James Dineen, R. R. Hannas, James Mills, Jr., George Podgorny, Peter Rosen, and John Wiegenstein), four representatives from UAEMS (Gail Anderson, Robert Dailey, Allen Klippel, and David Wagner), and two representatives from the AMA Section on Emergency Medicine (Carl Jelenko III and Ronald Krome). The ABEM board elected George Podgorny as its first president. Podgorny recalls,

> Now I must be candid and tell you, at least in part my election may not have been necessarily due to my sterling quality, but due to great fear of everybody that the endeavor would fail, and not many people were anxious to become first president of a "to fail" enterprise.[38]

One of ABEM's first actions was to formally submit an application for primary board status to the LCSB. As noted earlier, the LCSB had representation from the ABMS and AMA and was responsible for screening and initial evaluation of applications for medical specialty boards. The emergency medicine application had been prepared by ACEP's Committee on Board Establishment, but ABEM now became the leader in this process.

Sometimes a job and a person seem made for each other. Such was the case with Benson Munger and the nascent ABEM. Munger received his doctorate in research evaluation and education from Michigan State University in 1969. He then went to California to work in educational research, but also gained experience in negotiating labor contracts, acting as an arbitrator. This combination of skills and experience in educational research and negotiation was unusual and perfect for the tasks that lay ahead for ABEM. Munger met Art Auer, the ACEP executive director, on a plane around 1974, and Auer recognized that Munger had a profile that could be very valuable for ACEP. Auer offered Munger a job, but Munger turned it down. A few years later Auer recontacted Munger and told him of the progress that had been made with the Committee on Board Establishment and plans to apply for a primary board. Munger saw the potential for doing work that was a great match for his interests and signed on to be ACEP's director of education in 1976, and then became deputy executive director. His primary responsibility was ABEM, and he became the ABEM executive director when the body was officially approved. ACEP also had another Ph.D. in its workforce, Charles Maclean, who would become a key person in the quest for a board. Maclean was very involved in the development and implementation of the field test.

Approval From the Liaison Committee for Specialty Boards and the American Medical Association

The process required for approval as a certifying board was fairly tedious, but could be reduced to a number of clear steps that an aspiring specialty had to follow. Climbing these steps did not prove to be as easy as it looked on paper. R. R. Hannas remembers James Mills, Jr., describing how the course that ABEM traveled seemed to change along the way. Mills said, "Obtaining a specialty board was like being in a steeplechase where additional hurdles were thrown in the closer you got to the finish line."[42] The initial ABEM application, following the proscribed sequence, was submitted to the LCSB in March of 1976. The application included a long introductory description of what an emergency physician was and a nice review of the history of the field leading up to 1976. It demonstrated that emergency medicine arose out of a public need and the evolution of American medicine as a specialty-based medical delivery system. The LCSB met to consider the ABEM application in the late spring of 1976, and in June sent a letter to Harris Graves, the president of ACEP, requesting additional information. Apparently, the original application did not contain enough information on what emergency physicians do, how many emergency physicians were in practice in the United States, how many training programs existed in emergency medicine, or the level of interest of medical students in the field and projected output from residency programs. The LCSB also requested further information on the innovative certifying examination that was being developed by ABEM. The LCSB also noted that the proposed by-laws for ABEM were a little thin. ACEP and ABEM were pleased by this request for more information—these were relatively easy things to answer and provide. The LCSB's next action was less pleasing. In an unexpected move, the LCSB announced that it was having open hearings on the ABEM application in October of 1976 in Chicago. Representatives from other medical specialty boards and organizations would be invited to provide testimony for or against a board in emergency medicine. The LCSB sent each invited organization a list of questions to be answered about the field of emergency medicine, including such questions as: "Does emergency medical care represent a distinct and well-defined field of medical practice?" and "Will further division of medicine resulting from establishing a new specialty board be in the interest of the public by stimulating advancement in medical knowledge, practice and care?"

ABEM needed to revise its original application in time for the LCSB hearings in October. The ABEM board was in Chicago preparing for the meeting and was working on the application. Harvey Meislin was an emergency medicine resident under Peter Rosen at the University of Chicago at that time and remembers being asked to help,

> I was working that night at University of Chicago and they all came in, my gods of emergency medicine, the Dave Wagners, Krome, Rosen, and those guys and they were redoing their application and precomputers, nobody could type. Somehow, I think it was Krome, asked me if I could type, I said, "No I can't type, I think my girlfriend can." So, I called her and said, "Laurie all these guys are here and they are putting this application in tomorrow and they made some changes and they have to retype the application. Can you type?" She said, "I can type a little but my sister is really a good typist." Her sister was a schoolteacher, who came down to the University of Chicago on a Thursday evening…and literally staying there all night long, the unsung hero of emergency medicine is my sister-in-law who typed the application to the ABMS….[45]

During this process, the physician who was communicating with ACEP and UAEM and other organizations as secretary of the LCSB was Glen R. Leymaster,

M.D. Leymaster was involved with Pamela Bensen's appeal to the AMA for an emergency medicine internship at the Medical College of Pennsylvania in 1970 and 1971, and knew David Wagner, who in 1976 to 1977 was president of UAEM. Without being overt about it, Leymaster was supportive and encouraging toward emergency medicine's move for a specialty board and provided behind-the-scenes advice to the young emergency physicians. But, emergency medicine would have its day of reckoning with the open hearings in October.

The testimony in October of 1976 began with two persuasive stalwarts in emergency medicine—David Wagner represented UAEM and was followed by Ronald Krome, the president of ACEP. Wagner's remarks were particularly eloquent that day. He said in closing:

> ...emergency medicine is a reality today. It will not disappear in the future. It has definable boundaries and special skills. It has undergraduate, graduate. and continuing educational dimensions. Productive research is in progress...If we turn away, or even delay, in answer to this call for cooperative development, emergency medicine will not evaporate...The only visible loser will be traditional medicine who will appear to have self-fulfilled the so-oft stated prophecy, that we follow rather than direct and encourage the evolving course of medical care.[46]

Krome in his characteristic, forward manner chided the medical world for resisting emergency medicine development. He cited the practice of staffing emergency departments with unqualified physicians or house staff, noting,

> The medical community's guilt feelings are principally derived from the public's right to expect the finest emergency medical care and our own failure to provide it...For example, one could easily understand the anxiety of both the patient and the physician when a dermatologist is confronted with a patient with multiple injuries.[46]

Krome gave four solid reasons for a certifying board in emergency medicine, noting that:

> There is no mechanism evaluating competency and qualifications of practitioners in emergency medicine... [E]mergency medicine residency programs are increasing in both number and quality. Graduates of these programs can only be considered qualified when their competency is tested and certified. To do otherwise is not educationally sound...Certification will provide hospital medical staffs with hard evidence of physician competency... [E]ach special area of medicine has justifiably determined standards for practice, standards for education and maintained the right to certify. Emergency medicine must have the same prerogative.[46]

Predictably, the next person to give testimony before the LCSB was Oscar Hampton, M.D., representing the American College of Surgeons. Hampton gave his standard arguments against the formation of a board in emergency medicine. The LCSB minutes note that:

> The American College of Surgeons was clearly not in support of emergency medicine as a separate specialty. In their testimony, they suggested that emergency medicine was one-time care only and that they would be the only specialty without an in-hospital practice. ACS also disagreed with the manpower projections of ACEP [that] were submitted with the original application. They stated that the estimates were grossly exaggerated. They also said that the need for residencies is not well documented and that second career physicians will fill most of the future slots... Dr. Hampton also suggested that emergency medicine is for physicians who have retired from military service, are ill, or are tired of the rigors of regular practice.[46]

As Krome, Wagner, and other emergency physicians in the audience quietly seethed, Hampton went on to suggest that "the position of the ACS was for family practice to adopt emergency medicine as a subspecialty." However, when pressed on this, Hampton admitted that this was more his own personal opinion, and not the official stance of the American College of Surgeons.[46]

The next to testify were representatives from other specialty boards. The American Board of Surgery, while not as strident as Oscar Hampton, noted that "emergency care should be met in a variety of ways and not in one standard way" and that "emergency medicine does not care for the patient throughout the entire illness." The American Board of Pediatrics and American Board of Obstetrics and Gynecology were mainly in opposition because of a fear that emergency physicians would usurp pediatric and obstetrics practice, and for not being consulted on issues relating to pediatric and obstetrical care. The American Board of Anesthesiology felt "that emergency medicine did not represent a distinct body of knowledge," that "training could only be met by training in ten other specialties" and that "creation of a specialty of emergency medicine would fragment medicine by interrupting the continuity of medical care by a primary physician." The American Board of Neurological Surgery had the opinion that a board in emergency medicine would "increase the cost of emergency department care," that emergency medicine required "a body of knowledge that was too broad," and that "approval of the board would impair shifts to a second career." The American Board of Internal Medicine appeared confused about the approval process required for a new board, and needed to be "straightened out" before proceeding with testimony. ABIM did not take an official position, but seemed to tacitly approve of ABEM as long as internal medicine was part of the development of standards for emergency medicine, and provided that emergency medicine did not exclude internal medicine residents from rotating through the emergency department. The only board or association to testify in favor of the formation of a board in emergency medicine at the LCSB hearings was the American Psychiatric Association, which cited "a long standing and productive relationship" with emergency medicine.[46]

The LCSB testimony minutes note, "the surprise of the day was the appearance of the National Association of Emergency Physicians." NAEP was a splinter group of emergency physicians. As George Podgorny notes, it was a failure of "intelligence" on ACEP's part. Podgorny remembers,

> Apparently an emergency physician from Kansas City, who found out that he was ineligible to access the ABEM examination as proposed...gathered a few people together, hired a lawyer, established the National Association of Emergency Physicians, lied to AMA that they had 400 members, got some kind of a letter from AMA, unbeknownst to us that there is a screw up. And, at the hearing suddenly this lawyer appeared, nobody had ever seen him, nobody knew him, he said I am Joe Blow I am an Attorney at Law from..., and I am here to speak on behalf of National Association of Emergency Physicians. Everybody looked at me, I don't know who he is. He had a prepared statement, opposed—because American College [of Emergency Physicians] is not democratic, American College doesn't include everybody, American College is pushing for the board, board is very selective, board will eliminate competition, board will make it more difficult for the public to access emergency care, blah, blah. He never showed up again, the whole group never showed up again, we never heard of them again, all of that made us very skittish.[38]

The appearance of NAEP at the Chicago meeting was an embarrassment to ACEP and ABEM. The LCSB representatives questioned whether ACEP and ABEM truly represented all emergency physicians. However, once it became established that this was a small, splinter group in favor of lesser standards for emergency care, neither the LCSB, AMA, nor ACEP worried much about NAEP.

After the first round of LCSB hearings, ACEP and ABEM rapidly developed a response based on two main action areas. The first was to prepare a rebuttal to the major points of opposition raised in the testimony of other groups. The second was to contact representatives of all the other boards and medical societies that were not at the original hearings and ask to conduct "information sessions" for those groups. The written rebuttal testimony, given the inaccurate or poorly substantiated objections raised by other boards and societies at the October hearings, was easy for ACEP and ABEM to develop. For example, to counter the charge that emergency medicine was mainly the triage of illness and injury, statistics were cited that around 80% of emergency patients seen by emergency physicians were seen, treated, and discharged home with no triage or consultation with other physicians. To counter the claim that emergency medicine would be the only specialty without an in-hospital practice, the obvious examples of radiology and pathology were put forth. One by one, succinctly, but powerfully, the 5-page rebuttal document effectively countered each of the 15 opposition points. But, making a strong counter-argument would not be enough—the battle for ABEM would be fought in the trenches of the political world of medicine, where personal influence, contacts, money, and turf were the components of combat, and rational explanations and informed arguments were just the rhetoric of war.

A second set of LCSB hearings, this time soliciting testimony from consumer and nonphysician organizations, was held on February 26, 1977. Compared with the opposition points brought up by physician groups in the initial hearings, this day of testimony was largely a tribute to the idea of emergency medicine as a specialty. One by one, the groups explained why they supported the training and certification of emergency physicians—the Emergency Department Nurses Association; Professional Economic Services (a malpractice insurance provider); the National Association of Emergency Medical Technicians, Illinois chapter; the American Association of Trauma Specialists; the Public Safety Officers Foundation; and the Illinois Department of Public Health. All of these groups described the value of working with trained emergency physicians or the problems that arose when there was a lack of emergency physicians to provide services in their area. The American Board of Obstetrics and Gynecology appeared again to testify, softened their initial objections to ABEM, and gave "qualified support with reservation."[47]

One surprise at the second LCSB hearings was the failure of the American Hospital Association to support emergency medicine as a specialty. The AHA had long been a supporter of full-time emergency physicians in hospital EDs, and its journal had been a forum for advances in emergency care. The AHA proposed that emergency medicine should be a conjoint board, and "the Committee was quite confused by the concept of a conjoint board and why it would be an advantage in this particular situation." The ABEM sponsoring organizations, as Ron Krome remembers, "felt blind sided."[48] It appeared that the AHA leaders had been influenced by other medical organizations or individuals who were opposed to an emergency medicine board. In closing remarks at these hearings, Ron Krome as president of ACEP "in a strongly worded statement" expressed his belief that the AHA view was not shared by most hospital administrators, who "had moved very aggressively to improve emergency departments and to hire fully trained emergency physicians."[47]

The pesky National Association of Emergency Physicians made one last stand at the second LCSB hearings. An attorney, and the executive secretary of NAEP, Hank Griffin, "indicated that NAEP felt there was a great danger of inbreeding inherent in certification and that emergency physicians were not the most appropriate group to certify other emergency physicians. He said "competency should be defined by competence with competent physicians being the sole judge." As the other participants tried to figure out that statement, Harris Graves, M.D., the ACEP past president, in a clever move, asked Mr. Griffin to name the members of the NAEP executive committee. According to the minutes of the hearing "Mr. Griffin was unable to do so." With this odd and almost laughable showing, NAEP ceased to be a factor in the debate over a specialty board for emergency medicine.[47] However, the lack of unity in emergency medicine, due to the existence of NAEP, was later raised by some other boards as an argument against ABEM.[49]

The LCSB met later that day, and on March 3, 1977, Ron Krome received a letter from Glen Leymaster announcing that the LCSB had voted to recommend to the AMA and ABMS that the American Board of Emergency Medicine be approved. The recommendation had two qualifiers—that ABEM provide for representation on its board from other appropriate medical specialty boards and that the areas of competence in residency training needed to be better defined.[50] In a letter announcing the LCSB approval, Ron Krome, David Wagner, and John Wiegenstein could hardly contain their joy, noting that the field had "reached many rewarding milestones since the first official activity began back in 1968 but this announcement may be our most significant accomplishment of all."[51] The emergency medicine leaders believed that the hard part was over. All that was left to do in the process was to gain approval from the AMA Council on Education, which they felt very confident about, and the final vote of the American Board of Medical Specialties. A two-thirds majority vote was required for approval by both organizations. Since many of the specialties had already spoken at the LCSB hearings, and despite some opposition the LCSB had given its approval, it seemed there would be clear sailing to the final approval. As John Wiegenstein remembered, "We figured it was just a shoo-in."[25] As they would find out in the next few months, they were horribly wrong.

THE AGONY OF DEFEAT

In the spring of 1977, the trio of John Wiegenstein, Ron Krome, and David Wagner, working with Benson Munger and Charlie Maclean appeared before other medical boards, including the American Board of Obstetrics and Gynecology and the American Board of Pediatrics to explain the ABEM application and to answer questions. They felt that they were well received. The next vote in the ABEM approval process was before the AMA Council on Medical Education, and the procedure was less intensive and structured than the LCSB hearings and approval. The AMA Council on Medical Education held hearings in June of 1977 with the sponsoring organizations (ACEP, UAEMS, and the AMA Section Council on Emergency Medicine) and little input from other organizations. After review and consideration, the AMA announced in late July that the Council had narrowly voted in favor of the recommendation of the LCSB for approval of a board in emergency medicine. The ACEP and ABEM leaders notched another victory, and looked eagerly forward to the final vote by the ABMS in September. The ABMS member boards and six associate organizations designate voting representatives, proportionate to the number of certificates issued by the member board in the past 5 years. Therefore, the largest boards, internal medicine, surgery, and pediatrics, would have the most voting representatives. The early emergency medicine leaders perhaps did not appreciate the extent to which these voting representatives could form blocks of votes in their own fields and influence other voting representatives to do the same. Although the voting representatives were guided by their parent boards, they still cast their votes as individuals.

Warning signs were present suggesting that the ABMS vote would not be in favor of emergency medicine. In March 1977, the ABMS asked John Wiegenstein and David Wagner to attend the ABMS meeting and answer questions about the ABEM application.

ABMS noted, "that it had been particularly quiet among the other boards with four issuing negative statements."[52] Also in March, the American Board of Surgery sent a letter to the ABMS opposing ABEM. Some emergency medicine leaders were becoming a little edgy with the wait, and perhaps had a premonition that all might not go well with the ABMS. In a late July letter to ACEP President Ron Krome, Harris Graves, who was a past president and chairman of the College Issues and Planning Committee, wrote that his committee had adopted the following motion: "If the American Board of Medical Specialties does not approve the application for recognition of Emergency Medicine as a primary specialty, ACEP should consider legal action."[53] In his response, Krome noted, "Dear Harris: You have effectively made me feel the heat!"[54]

In late August, the sponsoring organizations for ABEM appeared before the Committee on Certification, Subcertification and Recertification of the American Board of Medical Specialties (COCERT). The COCERT had been charged, since 1974, with studying new applications and making a recommendation to the ABMS. Emergency medicine was the test case for COCERT. The leaders of emergency medicine made their case for ABEM to the COCERT and were asked many probing questions. In a letter to other emergency medicine leaders dated September 3, 1977, Ron Krome, Carl Jelenko (who replaced David Wagner as UAEM president), and John Wiegenstein issued a hopeful, but cautionary letter. For the first time, they openly talked about the possibility of ABMS voting down ABEM, although in the meeting they did not appreciate any major opposition. On September 15, 1977, the American Board of Medical Specialties met to consider the ABEM application. They received a recommendation from the COCERT that emergency medicine not be approved as a primary board. ABMS voting representatives then voted resoundingly, 100 to 5, to reject the application. The ABMS did acknowledge that some type of certification process for emergency medicine was necessary and that "the type of board that would be acceptable to ABMS would involve some sort of collaborative effort on the part of emergency medicine and other recognized specialty boards."[55] The emergency medicine leaders were reeling after the vote. Karl Mangold says, "I was kind of naively astounded that we didn't get it."[19] John Wiegenstein described, in retrospect, their misreading of the process,

> We never thought that this ABMS was that strong an organization. They were 50% of the vote of the Liaison Committee in respect to the boards and we thought, well if the AMA passes it obviously ABMS will pass it too. We were wrong…we were shocked. That was the primary board, and then we got some hope when their executive committee met and said maybe we should let them have a conjoint board if they can put it together so we can have a seat on their board and make sure that they don't get into our territories.[25]

The average emergency physician and ACEP member in 1977 would have been aware that ABEM was formed, that an examination was being prepared—indeed, many had contributed money to help develop the examination—and that a certifying process was on the near horizon. The average emergency physician was not aware of the laborious and politically intricate process of gaining approval from the ABMS. For many, the reaction to the negative ABMS vote was a predictable sense of frustration and fury at the medical "establishment" that was preventing emergency medicine from becoming a specialty. Harvey Meislin, then a residency program director at UCLA who had worked on the committee that was preparing the examination, remembers,

> We were angry. We were of the ilk, let's go it alone. We don't need them. We are thousands powerful, and getting bigger. We don't need them. We had the examination. It was done…so we thought, just continue onward.[45]

It was not only younger emergency physicians and residents who were furious with the ABMS. Leaders who had been there from the start were also bitter and felt that moving ahead with an independent board was the right way to go. Early academic leaders like Gail Anderson at LAC/USC Medical Center, Peter Rosen, then at Denver General Hospital, and Richard Levy at Cincinnati were fed up with the seeming arrogance of ABMS and the traditional medical specialties. Anderson remembers,

> I was one that was pushing for the attitude "well to hell with them" we'll form our own board without them…I was tired of being treated like a second-rate citizen for something I thought was very important….[56]

MOVING FORWARD WITH THE ABEM EXAMINATION

Little outcry occurred in the emergency medicine literature in the immediate aftermath of the defeat. A small column in the November *Journal of the American College of Emergency Physicians* (*JACEP*) reported on the negative ABMS vote, and noted that ABEM was going to proceed with the development and administration of the certification examination, appeal to the LCSB, and "meet with the ABMS to see if a compromise can be reached."[57] An article and set of photographs on the certification examination field test in the December issue of *JACEP* would have reinforced the feeling among ACEP members that things were on track and that maybe ABEM could just "go it alone." OMERAD and the Test Committee invited and paid travel and lodging expenses for 94 participants to take the field test for the ABEM examination in Lansing in late October 1977—just 5 weeks after the ABMS defeat. OMERAD and ABEM planned for three groups to take the examination—22 medical students, 36 second-year emergency medicine residents, and 36 practicing emergency physicians.

Half the practicing physicians were emergency medicine residency graduates. Presumably, the medical students would not do well on the examination, emergency medicine trainees would do better, and practicing emergency physicians would do the best. The test consisted of multiple-choice questions, interpretation of photographs of medical images, patient management scenarios, and simulation sessions. The simulations involved examiners providing case information and testing clinical skills as might happen in an emergency patient presentation. The simulation portion was videotaped, and all participants completed surveys on the examination content, methods, and administration (see insert, Figure 21).[58]

Richard Bukata, who was a resident at the LAC/USC Medical Center in 1977 remembers being selected, with several of his classmates, to be in the group who "tested the test." Bukata remembers,

> They took a bunch of people back to Michigan State University and stuck us in the dorms there…and over about a 3- or 4-day weekend administered about a billion test questions to us, day in day out…They were trying to determine that if a fourth-year medical student could pass this test, then there was not such a thing as a specialty of emergency medicine! So, fortunately they did miserably. They looked at the residents and they looked at some of these practice eligible doctors…and in 1980 I get a letter saying you performed well enough when you took that thing a couple of years ago that you don't have to take the examination. They allowed us to be certified based on what we did over that 3- or 4-day period.[59]

The successful run of the ABEM field test meant that ABEM was less than a year away from being able to administer its own certifying examination. Many who had been involved in the process could not understand why ABEM did not go ahead with plans to do so. The reason, as Benson Munger recalls, was, "ABMS had a very clear rule that said if you've ever given an examination you can't be an ABMS board …It was a real pure kind of virgin kind of feel to this thing…"[60]

WORKING TOWARD A CONJOINT BOARD

As ABEM and OMERAD developed the infrastructure for a certifying board in a parallel, unapproved world, the leaders of ABEM tried to interpret the cues and language that had been offered by the ABMS as part of the rejection of ABEM as a primary board. It seemed that a primary board for emergency medicine was not likely to be approved, but that ABMS had left the door open by suggesting a conjoint board. In the minds of some of the political leaders in medicine, emergency medicine had not really been turned down, just redirected. Richard Wilbur, M.D., the head of the Council of Medical Specialty Societies commented on ABEM in the *Medical World News* in 1978, saying, "It was not really denied."[61] In its report to the ABMS, the COCERT noted that a "precedent and mechanism exists which seems to best address and recognize the present status of the specialty of Emergency Medicine—the Conjoint Board."[62] In the official rejection notice to ABEM, the ABMS even offered "to review the existing definitions of primary and conjoint boards within ABMS by-laws so as to consider modifying the present definitions or increasing the options available to boards applying for approval."[63]

The ABEM leaders soon realized that a conjoint board, in its traditional structure, was not an acceptable alternative. The concept of conjoint boards dates back to British Royal Colleges of Physicians and Surgeons' approval of certain specialties with special diplomas, but this was considered a lesser standard than Royal College diplomas.[31] The concept of conjoint boards was relatively new to the ABMS. The ABMS revised its constitution and by-laws in 1970 to approve conjoint boards, and in 1971 the specialties of nuclear medicine and allergy and immunology were approved as conjoint boards. Conjoint boards operated under the auspices of other sponsoring boards, and these boards had enough seats on the conjoint board, and veto power, and could therefore control the actions and policies of the conjoint board. Certification in a conjoint board requires initial training in one of the sponsoring specialties. For example, the American Board of Allergy and Immunology is a conjoint board of the American

Board of Internal Medicine and the American Board of Pediatrics. Given how much other boards seemed to want to meddle in the affairs of emergency medicine, and the sheer number of other boards that might claim a stake in an emergency medicine conjoint board, this was unappealing to the ABEM leaders. George Podgorny, the ABEM president noted in 1977:

> ABEM has two major objections to a conjoint board…All the policies of ABEM would have to be approved by the sponsoring boards. Since this would include representatives from many, many other primary boards, we feel that this would prove to be too cumbersome. Also, a conjoint board in emergency medicine would require primary training in one of the sponsoring groups, followed by training in emergency medicine, making the educational requirements much more demanding than other primary boards.[57]

Given that many emergency medicine residencies were already established, and a certifying examination in emergency medicine was just months from implementation, the idea of a conjoint board, as originally proposed, was clearly dead in the water. No one in emergency medicine was going to agree that emergency physicians would first train in another field, say internal medicine, and then have a training period in emergency medicine before being eligible for certification in emergency medicine as a conjoint board under internal medicine. Therefore if there was to be any hope of emergency medicine becoming a board under ABMS, a grueling and unpredictable negotiating period lay before the emergency medicine leaders. At the same time, a ground swell of impatient and angry emergency physicians was calling for ABEM to spurn the ABMS and become an independent certifying board. George Podgorny remembers trying to deal with the emotions of emergency physicians at that time, "Some [we] had to console and some, had to bang their heads."[38]

THE NATURE OF THE OPPOSITION

One of tenets of war is to know your enemy, understand his or her positions, and then anticipate how he or she will act or react. It was only after the initial ABEM defeat that early emergency medicine leaders began to truly appreciate the positions and conviction of those in opposition. The reasons that other medical specialties opposed emergency medicine were a mixture of the philosophical, practical, political, and petty. Harvey Meislin, who is a long-standing emergency medicine chairman and recently became the president of ABMS, describes the currencies of the emergency medicine board controversy, "…at that level it's the adult level of sex, drugs, and rock and roll—it's money, turf and power. Boards will allow it to happen if it really doesn't really affect their money, turf and power."[45]

The easiest points to understand were the practice revenue and "turf" issues, as emergency medicine could be viewed as a legitimate threat in both of these areas. From its inception, emergency medicine was perceived as a threat to the livelihoods of other medical practitioners. James Mills and his Alexandria Plan colleagues experienced this in 1961, when concerns about patient stealing were raised by local physicians. The other long-standing fear was that private physicians would no longer be able to see their patients in EDs. By 1977 it had been demonstrated that emergency physicians did not steal patients from private practice physicians, or prevent physicians from seeing their patients in EDs. Still, surgeons expressed concern that emergency physicians, by evaluating and managing trauma or surgical cases in the ED, would delay the definitive surgical care of these patients.[64] John H. Davis, M.D., a surgeon who would later sit on ABEM as a representative of the American Board of Surgery described the feeling of surgeons in the 1970s:

> Surgeons look on the emergency department as their territory for a very simple reason…they only really care about the total body crunch that comes in. To the surgeon well, the M.I. and pregnancy problem, anybody can take care of those, and I think there is a mindset that well then, wait a minute, we're going to take this new group of people now who have no real surgical training and suddenly they are going

to be dealing with massive bleeding and legs and arms torn off and gunshot wounds, and what do they know about it? And the minute you fix your mind in to that context, you say to yourself, well I couldn't possibly allow this to happen—this is a step backward.[42]

Some ABMS members and other specialty boards voiced concern that patients were preferentially coming to EDs rather than their primary care doctors' offices because of the convenience and ability to quickly have tests and procedures done. Cost of care was often raised as a concern, without any data to support claims that emergency care was more expensive for the health care system. Ambulatory care was a hot button topic. As EDs became more sophisticated in their ability to handle ambulatory care or urgent care–type patients by creating separate sections of their ED to rapidly assess and treat these patients, primary care physicians were worried that EDs would divert many of their "bread and butter" cases. Rather than tackling the deficiencies in primary care medicine that caused this patient shift, it was easier to malign the new emergency physicians. The opponents of emergency medicine then cleverly turned this argument on its head, suggesting that if medicine changed and nonemergent or ambulatory care cases were eventually diverted from the ED, there would be less need for emergency medicine as a field.

Members of other boards were also threatened by the potential creep of emergency medicine practice into other areas of the hospital. This was first manifested as the concern of surgeons that emergency physicians would take emergency cases to the operating room. When this never materialized, other impingements were imagined— especially in critical care. This fear stemmed from the common practice in smaller hospitals of the emergency physician on duty covering the intensive care unit or medical emergencies on hospital wards. Practitioners in other medical fields did not understand that this was not a role that emergency physicians necessarily wanted to fill, but was an obligation that fell to them when they were the only physicians available in most hospitals on evenings, weekends and holidays.[49,52,64–67]

Some other specialties were concerned that if emergency medicine developed and accounted for more care of patients, there would be less need for practitioners in these areas. This concern did not account for the fact that in the mid- and late-1970s, although the overall number of physicians in the United States was increasing rapidly as a result of increased medical school enrollment and foreign medical immigrants, there was still a relative shortage of primary care physicians.[68,69] The inadequate distribution of physicians usually meant that in the communities where EDs were busiest, there was the least availability of primary care, and sometimes specialty physicians. Another concern voiced in the ABEM application process was that physicians in other fields might migrate to emergency medicine, and deplete the numbers of physicians in other specialties.[65] Because many emergency practitioners had indeed migrated from other fields, this could be a problem as long as a practice track was available for certification in emergency medicine.[65,67] It also appears that internal medicine was concerned about medical students or residents with an interest in critical care who might choose emergency medicine over internal medicine as a path to critical care fellowships and practice.

The other major battle was in the academic realm. George Podgorny believes that at that time the other specialties were thinking, "…[W]e want to control your education. If we can control your education, we control your board, we control your specialty, maybe we can be at peace with you."[38]

Henry MacIntosh, M.D., who would later serve on the ABEM board of directors as a representative from the American Board of Internal Medicine noted, "There was concern about how this specialty was going to affect my specialty…how was it going to affect my training program? There was this feeling of preserving the turf."[42]

John Davis, M.D., as a surgeon involved in education remembers,

…many of us…looked on an integral part of surgical training was for the young person to see that acute abdomen, or pain in the chest, or what have you, and…we get these experts in there, and there'll be no place left for the young, budding physician to learn. Now, it's turned out that's not what happened, but I think that was a very

real concern, that we would have no place to let people see things in a way that was frontline—this is where you see it for the first time.[42]

The same issues of practice revenue and territory that were active in the private practice world were present in academic medical centers. Since most academic EDs in the 1970s were money losers, and faculty from other departments did not usually provide billable services in the ED, other departments were not fearful of losing clinical revenue to the new emergency physicians. But if emergency medicine was to develop as an academic entity, resources like physical space, research support, administrative support, and faulty and house office salaries would have to be cut out of the large pie of the medical center or medical school. Other departments would not accept having smaller pieces of the pie unless there were other benefits derived from the new emergency medicine training programs. Although the U.S. economy battled recession during the 1970s, faculty physician salaries were increasing at a generous rate, and as Kenneth Ludmerer notes, "As medical schools grew, internal rivalries also increased. Departments, divisions, and individuals competed fiercely with each other for space and resources...."[70] Given this intense competition, it was not a good climate for the creation of new clinical departments of emergency medicine.

One of the primary concerns for other specialties and academic medical centers was the potential displacement of residents from other fields out of the emergency department as emergency medicine residents moved in. EDs were viewed as prime training grounds for interns and residents, even though the "training" consisted of unsupervised long hours in the ED. Competition for emergency cases between emergency medicine residents and surgical, internal medicine, pediatric, or obstetrics and gynecology residents was viewed as a real threat by the traditional specialties. On a higher plane, the ABMS questioned whether a physician could master all that needed to be known in emergency medicine in a 3- or 4-year residency-training period—it argued that the field was too broad. It was pointed out by Dr. Robert Petersdorf, an ABMS member and prominent academic internist, that many practicing emergency physicians in the 1970s had previous experience or training in other fields, and that physicians who completed only an emergency medicine residency might not have the same depth of knowledge and practice skills.[67] Petersdorf, as an academician, did not at that time appreciate that although some of the leaders of emergency medicine had trained in other fields, most EDs in the United States were staffed by physicians who had completed only an internship and had no formal training in emergency medicine. The lack of understanding of the nature of emergency practice by those in power in the other medical specialties and ABMS is reinforced by the other arguments that were made. A common refrain was that as a generalist, the emergency physician would need extensive training during residency in other fields. This would make the training period impractically long. The ABMS seemed to have forgotten that only 8 years before, it approved family practice as a generalist specialty with a 3-year training period with segments of training in other fields as part of the residency. The failure of these other arguments to hold much water implies that the main issue for other fields was turf—they did not want to surrender the ED as a prime training area for their residents.

The philosophical arguments were the toughest to handle. This was expressed by Oscar Hampton and others who mocked the field, saying that the only thing different was the location of the practice in an emergency room and it simply borrowed from other fields. On a more sophisticated level, leaders in other specialties and the ABMS were adamant in their beliefs that emergency medicine was not a unique medical discipline, that the knowledge and skills did not represent a distinct medical specialty, and that it should not be viewed as a new method of practice or delivery of care. In 1978, John Moxley, M.D., the dean of the medical school at the University of California at San Diego was asked to sit on a panel on "The Role of the Specialist in the Emergency Room" at the annual meeting of the American Association for the Surgery of Trauma. Moxley said,

...emergency departments, as they relate to the specialty of "emergency medicine," are really responses to a number of pressures that are outside the profession, not the

least of which is urban decay. They are not a logical professional development based on the growth of either a body of knowledge or a thoughtful advance in the organization and delivery of health care. In short, they do not have an intellectual wellspring, which causes great difficulties, at least within the academic medical center.[14]

Karl Mangold, as president of ACEP in 1978, was asked to serve on this panel. Thrown into this lion's den of surgeons, Mangold gave impassioned remarks defending the professional stature of the new field and the need for quality emergency care. However, Mangold, who had not done a residency and had few academic connections, floundered when he was asked by Moxley to describe what the training in trauma should be as part of an emergency medicine residency, saying, "I am not qualified to do that." Moxley jumped on this, saying,

I find it very difficult to accept if one of the most vocal representatives of emergency physicians can't answer a simple question, that if you want us to develop a program, just tell us what one little piece of it should be. You do it every day.[14]

Moxley went on, demonstrating the schism between the academic world and the community practice of emergency medicine, saying, "...I don't know that it is the responsibility of an educational institution to try to create a body of knowledge where it doesn't exist, in an attempt to deal with market forces."[14]

Peter Rosen was eager to engage in this intellectual battle because he strongly believed that there was a unique "biology of emergency medicine." The issue became very real for Rosen in 1977 when a new dean, Daniel C. Tosteson, came to the University of Chicago. Rosen remembers,

He interviewed the entire faculty and while I was talking to him, here's a guy who is an anatomist...starts pontificating about, well, there is no biology of emergency medicine. "When I have my heart attack I want a cardiologist to take care of me." I said, "That's all very well and good, but how do you know you had a heart attack?" "Well, I have chest pains." "And what if you don't have chest pain? What if you have nausea?" It was the first time it had ever occurred to him that maybe you couldn't run an emergency department with 47 different medical specialties...I got so pissed at him that I...I went out and wrote a paper....[41]

Tosteson had a short stay at the University of Chicago before becoming the dean at Harvard Medical College, another institution that would take a long time to warm up to the idea of emergency medicine as a specialty. The paper that Tosteson stimulated Rosen to write was called "The Biology of Emergency Medicine." It was published in *JACEP* in 1979.[71] In a rambling essay sprinkled with his typically strong opinions and wisdom, Rosen noted that the struggle of emergency medicine to define its practice was not unique, and that "the epistemological waters become very murky when trying to decide to whom to refer the facial fracture—oral, plastic surgeon, or otolaryngologist." Rosen noted that the biology of emergency medicine was not specific to an organ system or disease process, but was "defined by the level of life threat." He used one of his favorite analogies, writing that "the role of emergency medicine is to catch the climber who is falling from a precipice and return him to as much safety as can be readily achieved, but not necessarily to get him all the way back down to the valley." Later in the essay Rosen noted, "We all live on the brink of disaster and helping people on the wrong side of that brink is one of emergency medicine's biologies." Rosen pointed out that prehospital care was the proper and special domain of emergency physicians as "emergency medicine has extended the arm of the physician to the field." Rosen made strong statements in this essay that emergency faculty physicians should be responsible for training emergency medicine residents in the ED setting, and made disparaging comments about the ability of other fields to teach emergency medicine or handle emergencies. He notes, "For a number of years, I have been saying that the emergency physician must be as good as the cardiologist in running an arrest. After several recent experiences watching cardiologists in charge on an arrest, I say *they* must become as good as the emergency physician."[71]

Rosen was not the first to propose these concepts, but was the first to pen them in a journal. Rosen's philosophy and words were like a lantern for those emergency physicians who were wandering in the darkness of academic medicine. If there was a unique biology of emergency medicine, then it was proper to think of the field as a specialty and to teach these concepts and train specialists in the field. It would become imperative to conduct research in the biology of emergency medicine. Rosen's paper became a landmark reference for emergency physicians who were trying to justify their existence and standing in medicine. As John Marx, who trained under Rosen at Denver General Hospital notes, "Peter believed, and I think you and I now know this as gospel."[72]

An argument that was an obvious counter to the philosophical concerns raised by other medical specialties and the ABMS was that family practice had been approved as a primary board in 1969, and emergency medicine had much in common with family practice. The fact that emergency medicine leaders did not use this argument much highlights the interesting status of family practice in the realm of medicine in the late 1970s. Some believe that the ABMS regretted its decision to approve family medicine as a primary board. David Wagner speaking about the ABMS notes,

...they were not going to approve another primary board. They felt that with family medicine they had messed it up, they shouldn't have done that in the first place and they weren't going to do it in the second place. I think it was just a...time when there was this big movement among physicians to specialize...If you weren't involved in a specialty, it was bogus. So they were bound and determined that there would not be another mistake they way they did with family practice.[32]

One of the common refrains from members of other specialty boards, especially the American Board of Surgery, was that further "fragmentation" of medicine was undesirable.[64] This stance was a bit hypocritical, because between 1974 and 1986, the ABS allowed the creation of four subspecialty certifications in surgical disciplines.[73] Many in the medical profession and government felt that medicine was becoming over-specialized, and this left emergency medicine in a paradoxical situation. The medical establishment was saying, "Prove to us that you are a distinct medical specialty." If emergency medicine did this well, it would then hear, "Sorry, we already have too many specialties." In the end, some of the arguments put forth against emergency medicine seemed to be intellectual veils to cover the countenance of an opposition that was based not on theory or philosophy, but on turf and power in medicine. Some of those in opposition to emergency medicine realized their own deficiencies. Alexander Walt, the surgeon who hired and was the boss of Ron Krome at Wayne State/Detroit Receiving Hospital, noted in the *American College of Surgeons Bulletin* in 1979 that surgeons had created some of the problems that lead to the development of emergency medicine by having limited availability, a lack of training in trauma care, and loss of skills in trauma among practicing surgeons. However, Walt did not endorse relinquishing control to emergency physicians, noting that the department of surgery should review all surgical procedures in the emergency department, and "should have some means of exercising quality control over each individual working in the emergency room."[74]

The national mood toward medicine in the early 1970s was not always conducive to the further development of emergency medicine. As medical care advanced with the support of the federal government through Medicare and Medicaid and generous private insurance payments, U.S. health care expenditures skyrocketed from $142 per capita in 1960 to $336 per capita in 1970. The situation was repeatedly referred to as a "crisis" by the national media.[69,75] Kenneth Starr notes, "the clamor for more resources was constant, relentless and plausible."[75] Health care expenditures contributed significantly to rising inflation, and the country became edgy and uncertain about whether medical progress was worth the cost. As national health care plans in other countries were shown to be cheaper while providing equal or better care, the bell for national health care in the United States tolled once again. But, it fell on the deaf ears of the Republican Nixon administration and the AMA. Doctors' salaries had grown immensely in the 1960s and early 1970s, and there was little initiative in organized medicine to curb the cash flow in private practice. The strategy of the Nixon administration was to reduce federal expenditures for health care and to discourage new federal programs for health care (as shown before with the Nixon veto of the 1973 EMS Act).[69,75,76] Emergency departments became symbols and scapegoats of the crisis in health care. It was pointed out that ED care for patients with non-emergent problems was more expensive than going to a family doctor. There was less recognition of the fact that many ED patients were using EDs for primary care because they had no other access to care. In this way, the issue of the expense of caring for uninsured patients became entangled with the move of emergency medicine toward specialty status. A major thrust of government and society in the 1960s had been to improve quality and access to care. In the 1970s it changed to controlling costs. The creation of a new specialty of emergency medicine was viewed, without much justification, as potentially expensive and as an unwanted expansion at a time when the nation was circling its health care wagons.

FORGING A COMPROMISE

As the ABEM leaders had further discussions with Glen Leymaster of the ABMS, who was overall sympathetic to the cause of emergency physicians, it became clear that "the approval of a primary board was untenable in the foreseeable future."[77] John Wiegenstein wrote in a January 1978 letter to the sponsoring organizations,

> They strongly oppose the establishment of another primary board. They left the impression, without stating it directly, that the establishment of family practice as a primary board was considered a mistake, not to be repeated.[77]

The next steps were fairly clear for ABEM leaders—they needed to do a better job of meeting with and addressing the concerns of the other boards, and would have to find a way to make the conjoint board mechanism work for ABEM. A negotiating team of Wiegenstein, Podgorny, Wagner, Krome, and to some extent Karl Mangold (who followed Krome as ACEP president), was responsible for meeting with other boards to find common ground on a conjoint board. Wiegenstein, who was viewed by most as the founder of the field, and its elder statesman, served as the chief negotiator. David Wagner remembers frequent trips to Chicago, where many of the boards, and the ABMS were based,

> There was a time in my life when I would get up in the morning in Philadelphia, by the time I got home at night, which was usually 7 or 8 o'clock anyway, my wife wouldn't know if I went to Chicago or whether I went to work here on Henry Avenue. We were going to Chicago sometimes twice a week for daytime negotiations with the various entities.[32]

As it became clear that ABEM could not do much to address the larger philosophical concerns about overspecialization or restrictions on new primary boards, the approach of the negotiators was to allay the fears of other specialties that emergency medicine would impinge on their practice territory or the education of their residents. As George Podgorny notes,

> We had a plan that we should attack…on educational issues, not on the turf issues, because that would be very difficult. Not on political issues, not on the organizational issues or gown versus town issues, but let's talk about education.[38]

Following the ABMS dictate to involve other boards, the sponsoring organizations of ABEM hosted a meeting in Lansing in December of 1977 and invited all other medical specialty boards that claimed an interest in emergency medicine. Seven boards came to the meeting—internal medicine, pediatrics, surgery, family practice, anesthesiology, obstetrics and gynecology, and radiology. Orthopedic surgery and psychiatry/neurology were unable to attend. Some important areas of agreement were reached, including an understanding that the initial training of the emergency physician should be broad based, but that "there need not be mandatory complete training in another specialty." It was suggested that nine other boards would sit on ABEM as sponsors, that "specific decisions would not have to be referred for approval to the sponsoring boards," but that major policy changes would need to be referred. The participants realized they were creating a board structure that currently did not exist in ABMS, making it clear that ABMS by-laws would have to be changed. Glen Leymaster suggested that the proposed structure, with representation of other boards on the ABEM board, but a primary training path in emergency medicine, be called a "modified conjoint board." The ABEM negotiators quickly developed a draft of by-laws for a modified conjoint board and circulated them to the other boards, and were hopeful when initial feedback was positive.

With progress being made with the other boards, the ABEM negotiators now needed to deal with a serious problem in the ranks of emergency medicine. As noted above, a significant number of emergency physicians, both new residency graduates and older practicing physicians and academicians were pushing for ABEM to become an independent board outside of ABMS, to proceed with the certifying examination, and to offer certification in emergency medicine. The leaders of the sponsoring organizations of ABEM knew that this opposition in the rank and file of emergency medicine could not be ignored. The unrest had become organized in the fall of 1977 through activities in the ACEP Council to make resolutions for giving the examination and creating an independent board. The ACEP Council, after the 1972 revision of the ACEP constitution and by-laws, was an advisory body to the ACEP board of directors, and lacked the power to change board of director's decisions. But as John Rupke, who was council speaker at the time notes, the board of directors "couldn't get elected without the council. That was the hammer."[78] A meeting was called in January of 1978 of the sponsoring organizations of ABEM, and for the first time, the ACEP Council Steering Committee was represented in addition to the ACEP board of directors. The ACEP Council was rigid in its stance. John Rupke, as the spokesman, reported that a resolution had recently been adopted by the ACEP Council that ACEP should "adopt an official policy that only a primary board in emergency medicine will be acceptable to the College." The ACEP board of directors overrode this dissenting vote from the ACEP Council with a three-fourths majority. ACEP, along with the other sponsoring organizations, then voted to proceed with negotiations and application for a modified conjoint board.[79,80]

The new application for a modified conjoint board in emergency medicine needed to go through the same arduous approval process as the original application. The next step was to submit a revised application to the Liaison Committee for Specialty Boards. The sponsoring organizations did this in February of 1978, but then a week later asked the LCSB to delay the formal review of the revised application. The reason for this request was that many ACEP members were becoming more outspoken in their opposition to a compromise with the ABMS. Karl Mangold, ACEP president, noted in a January 1978 letter to the ACEP councilors, committee chairmen and chapter presidents, "occasionally the hue and cry from the constituency of emergency medicine borders on cacophony."[81] Mangold asked members to write him with their concerns and opinions. He received 20 letters in opposition to a modified conjoint board and 18 in support. Carl Jelenko, who was then president of UAEM sent a similar request, and found about one third of respondents were opposed. The leaders of the ABEM-sponsoring organizations did not feel they could proceed without garnering stronger support from practicing emergency physicians. In an unprecedented move, a special meeting of the ACEP Council was called on April 3, 1978, at the Innisbrook Resort in Tarpon Springs, Florida.

John Rupke presided over the tumultuous meeting. Ninety ACEP councilors from 32 states and Puerto Rico attended (see insert, Figure 22). The process for council meetings was to consider resolutions that had been submitted by ACEP Chapters. The resolutions were in the lofty language of organizational proceedings—whereas this, and whereas that, therefore be it resolved that—but the intent of some was to derail the whole ABMS approval process. The Arizona chapter, with Michael Vance, M.D., as the chief protagonist, put forward three resolutions emphasizing that ABEM should proceed with the certifying examination no matter what happened with negotiations, that

ACEP adopt an official policy that only a primary board in emergency medicine will be acceptable to the college, and no board in emergency medicine that was approved by the ABMS would be recognized by ACEP. Resolutions submitted by the Steering Committee of the ACEP Council and the Florida Chapter were more compromising—suggesting that a modified conjoint board would be acceptable if emergency physicians were the clear majority on the board, and that other boards would not have veto power over ABEM.

The leaders of the sponsoring organizations were asked to speak in front of the council at the Innisbrook meeting. John Wiegenstein, as the chief negotiator, was tapped to make a presentation before the group. Wiegenstein, who was never fond of speaking in front of large groups, was not feeling well before his presentation. He remembered,

> I had a terrible migraine headache that day and...and my head was just booming. I think it was probably caffeine withdrawal. I was up in my room and...of course I thought, it was anxiety too, and Carl Jelenko, from UAEM, he was there, and he had heard that I was not feeling well so he came up to make a house call in my hotel room. He said, "You've got a classic migraine. Bend over and I'll give you a suppository, I get those all the time." It cleared my head, I couldn't believe it, in 20 to 30 minutes I was fine.[25]

Wiegenstein, after receiving the kindly suppository from Jelenko, made his pitch to the council. Many in the audience had been openly hostile to the ideas Wiegenstein would propose. They wanted to proceed with ABEM as an independent certifying entity for emergency medicine, or wanted to sue the ABMS to force ABEM admission. The older leaders of the sponsoring organizations had begun referring to these physicians, like Michael Vance of the Arizona chapter, as the "young Turks." In many ways they admired the tenacity of these young emergency physicians, but had to convince them that the best way to advance emergency medicine was to work with ABMS. Wiegenstein remembered,

> I kept telling them from the podium that I realized it wasn't everything that we wanted but sometimes we have to take what we can get. I guarantee you that if you sue the establishment we'll never get boarded. I said this is a foot in the door and even though it isn't perfect, I said within time we will be a primary board. You just have to have faith. Let the other boards sit on our board and see how magnificent we are going to do this.[25]

Over the next 5 hours the council discussed, revised, modified, and finally voted on resolutions. Benson Munger remembers the intensity:

> People were screaming at each other...people were just livid and there were people who actually thought the college was selling out emergency medicine and people were saying we gave all this money, we did all this....[60]

William Haeck recalls "the controversy and endless discussions with a practical endpoint. Let's get the damn thing!"[13] The mood became more compromising, and eventually two resolutions were passed that paved the way for the ABEM-sponsoring organizations to continue negotiations with ABMS for a modified conjoint board with acceptable criteria to ensure that other boards could not override ABEM policies. Another component of the resolutions was that regardless of the outcome of negotiations with the ABMS, ABEM would proceed with plans to give the first certifying examination in 1978. In the final portion of the resolutions the council asserted itself by resolving that no board in emergency medicine sanctioned by the ABMS could be approved by ACEP without the approval of the ACEP Council.

In the end the seasoned emergency medicine leaders, or "wise heads," as William Haeck called them, won out. Men like Wiegenstein, Podgorny, Krome, and Wagner eventually convinced the "Young Turks," and other established emergency medicine figures like Gail Anderson, R. R. Hannas, and Peter Rosen that the modified conjoint board compromise was the best way to proceed. Richard Levy, as the new academic emergency medicine leader at Cincinnati was initially opposed to the modified conjoint board proposal. He remembers,

> I wasn't comfortable with the people who were negotiating it because they represented the practice faction of emergency medicine and I was worried that they sold out. When I looked at the details it looked to me like a good political compromise, an old fashioned political compromise, and so I subscribed to it…I went from being a doubting Thomas when it was being talked about early on to being a supporter of it… The thing that I liked about it was that even though it wasn't a prescribed pathway as they didn't say that in 2 years you'll be able to go to this, it was clearly understood that this was a way to become a full board. That's why I said to myself back then—this is a political compromise and it's not so painful that it makes it intolerable.[82]

Bruce Janiak, the first emergency medicine resident, was at the Innisbrook Special Council meeting. Although he could have been a "Young Turk," he took a more measured approach,

> At the time I was beginning to learn the necessity for compromise and the political process and that the medical political process is the same as the national political process. In that we eventually were going to win, I felt at the time, I think like a lot of us did, that it was a somewhat bitter pill to swallow to have all these other specialties on the emergency medicine board. On the other hand, we were comfortable with the fact that we held the majority and could function.[83]

Pam Bensen, who was practicing as an emergency physician in Maine at the time remembers,

> …it never bothered me that we might have to compromise because I…had no doubt that the time would come…my feeling was when you talk to people like George Podgorny who knew the politics that you just had to accept that you took a step ahead.[84]

John Rupke, who guided the Council through the contentious proceedings, says, "They got a saying down south, 'The best beach is always out of reach.' You can't get everything, you have to negotiate a little bit."[78]

The leaders of the sponsoring organizations for ABEM let out a huge sigh of relief when the ACEP Council gave its approval to move forward. The next step was to prepare by-laws for ABEM that could handle the tricky balance of having representation from other boards, but retaining some autonomy for ABEM. Over the next few months, these details were ironed out in meetings with ABMS and the other potential sponsoring boards. Benson Munger collected and analyzed the concerns of other boards, and prepared a negotiating plan. In May 1978, the sponsoring organizations for ABEM, the ABMS, and members of seven other boards met in Chicago at the O'Hare Hilton and made significant progress. Then in July 1978, the Liaison Committee for Specialty Boards hosted a meeting of the involved parties at the Oak Brook Hyatt House in Oak Brook, Illinois, and Glen Leymaster laid out the discussion topics. It was at this meeting that the type and duration of training for emergency medicine, a controversial area that all had agreed to defer, came up once again. Benson Munger remembers,

> …it was very clear that there was a lot of reluctance on the part of most of the boards in the room and it was also very clear that everybody had a stake in this that they didn't want to give up. Everybody had a kind of a finger in emergency medicine, or thought they did…John Wiegenstein, I don't know if he did this by design, or whether it was just a brilliant serendipitous event, but he said, "You know everyone around here says you've got a stake in emergency medicine. It would really help me if we could go around the table and if you were to tell me how much training in your specialty do you think a resident in emergency medicine should have?"[60]

Wiegenstein remembered,

> *Internal medicine was commenting about the fact that there is not enough internal medicine in our proposed residency program. How many months of internal medicine do you think they should take? He said about 2 years. Pediatrics said 2 years, too. Peds didn't want internal medicine to say they were more important than pediatrics and the surgeons also added a year or two. Everybody started laughing.*[25]

Charlie Maclean was at the blackboard totaling up the suggested the amount of time that an emergency medicine resident would need to train in the other fields. When all seven boards had spoken, the total was 13 years. George Podgorny remembers how this exercise broke the ice,

> *When that was added up, there was a silence and a total change of atmosphere. Suddenly all of these very intelligent, erudite people, basically good people—none of these people were bad—they recognized the absurdity of their position. ...So I said, "I think what we really need to do is approach it from the other end. We would like to tell you what we think our training should be."*[38]

Benson Munger also recalls how things seemed to ease after this discussion,

> *From that time forward the topic never came up again and we then started talking about how to solve this problem and at that meeting this idea of a conjoint board got put together in literally minutes. It was because everyone recognized, I think at that point in time it was like an "Ah hah!" Well, obviously everybody has a stake in this, but you can't take 13 years to train this person so there must be something unique about each of our specialties that needs to be included in the training, but it isn't a year of full training in each of these specialties.*[60]

The representatives of the other medical boards were powerful, experienced men. John Benson Jr., from the American Board of Internal Medicine was firm in his opposition to emergency medicine, but was also a skilled politician and negotiator who realized that some form of certifying body in emergency medicine was a necessity. John H. Davis carried the mantle of opposition for the American Board of Surgery, but is remembered by Peter Rosen as "a very, very nice man, a very bright man, and a very principled man, and I thought he brought a lot to the board."[41] Representatives from the other participating boards of family practice, obstetrics and gynecology, otolaryngology (which replaced orthopedic surgery when the orthopedic board decided it did not want to sit on ABEM), pediatrics, and psychiatry/neurology, were generally less vociferous in their opposition to emergency medicine, and psychiatry was generally viewed as supportive.

The ABEM sponsors and associated boards worked to revise ABEM by-laws and were feeling some time pressure. They were now 3 years into the process and had assuaged the young Turks, but it was an uneasy truce. If the ABEM certifying examination was not administered soon, the ACEP Board of Directors would likely be voted out and replaced by those who were in favor of going it alone or taking legal action against ABMS. The ABEM-sponsoring organizations were pointing to the March 1979, ABMS meeting as the hopeful approval date for ABEM. In the summer and fall of 1978, the ABEM-sponsoring organizations and the other sponsoring boards met to hash out the power structure of the new modified conjoint board. Henry Thiede, M.D., who represented the American Board of Obstetrics and Gynecology in the negotiations, and later served on ABEM, remembers,

> *...some of us were trying to ensure that we would have representation that would allow us to exert influence in emergency medicine and we weren't going to be put in to a position where we were outvoted.*[42]

The final agreement produced ABEM by-laws that called for 19 members (directors) of the ABEM board, with six directors to be nominated by ACEP, four by UAEM, two by the AMA Section Council on Emergency Medicine, and one each from the seven other sponsoring boards. The by-laws specify that a simple majority vote is required to pass standard issues that come before the board, but that "all issues that significantly affect training standards, evaluation standards and the establishment and amendment of by-laws shall require support by three-quarters (3/4) of the members of the board."[85] This gave emergency medicine directors a healthy 12 of 19 majority for most votes, but meant that they would need to convince three of the remaining seven directors from other sponsoring boards to vote with them in order to pass special measures. The by-laws also call for one of the two at-large members of the executive committee to be from a sponsoring board. The give and take with the representatives of other sponsoring boards was completed at a meeting in Chicago on November 6, 1978. The group then realized it would be difficult to meet the March 1979 deadline for ABMS approval since the ABMS required at least 120 days notice to place an issue on its agenda. To comply with this, all the sponsoring boards would need to sign off on the ABEM by-laws by the end of December 1978. John Wiegenstein, as the chief negotiator in this process took it upon himself to obtain the written approval of the other sponsoring boards. He recalled the process:

> I was trying my best to get everybody's signature on it in time to make it official in March and so our strategy was—we still had a lot to do—but our strategy was to get it done by the Christmas holidays so I could make a trip around to their homes when they were on Christmas holidays to get their signature. So, in 48 hours I made the trip. Benson, John Benson was in Oregon, I met him in the airport. John Davis was in Vermont. The guy who was President of ABMS was visiting his grandmother in Canada and I went to Canada…I got home totally exhausted. One hundred-twenty days before I had put an endotracheal tube down a jaundiced person and cut my finger and drew blood, and I washed it off and put a Band-aid on it. He was dying so I didn't put gloves on or anything…Anyway, I didn't think much of it at the time but after that 48 hours of an exhausting trip I became very ill. That was the '78 snow in Michigan. We were snowed in. I couldn't get the car out so my wife asked me to go get some milk and stuff. I walked through this high snow to get to the store and was bringing it back and then I kind of collapsed in the snow. All my energy was gone. I couldn't quite get home. I laid there for 10 to 15 minutes and I decided I didn't want to die there in the snow so I made my way home. I looked in the mirror and saw my yellow sclera and noticed the urine was dark and so I got an SGOT drawn and it was 6000. I was out of work for about 3 months and it was directly related, I think with the exhaustion and no sleep and that sort of thing.[25]

The long process for ABEM approval was nearing an end, but it had taken a toll as one of the key leaders lay exhausted in a Michigan snow bank, jaundiced, stricken with viral hepatitis. Wiegenstein's efforts came up 2 days short of meeting the ABMS agenda deadline. Even if he had managed to pull it off, there were still unresolved issues that prevented the American Board of Internal Medicine from endorsing the ABEM by-laws. John Benson had signed off on the proposal during Wiegenstein's sojourn, but now was hedging. Long after the other sponsoring boards had given their approval, ABIM, in a manner almost stereotypical of a cautious, methodic internist, persisted in examining the potential impact of a specialty in emergency medicine. As Benson Munger remembers, "with internal medicine it was always, just one more thing."[86] Although John Benson had given his personal support for the ABEM by-laws, there was concern about whether internal medicine residency graduates would be eligible to sit for the ABEM examination if they had enough practice hours in EDs. ABIM was also still fretting about the impact of emergency medicine on residency training of internal medicine in the ED. Concerns were also expressed about whether ABEM certification requirements by hospitals might limit the practice opportunities for internists in EDs. ABIM asked the ABEM sponsors to examine and provide written feedback on a number of these areas as "impact statements." As the process moved in to February of 1979, the emergency medicine sponsors of ABEM were becoming irritated with the hold-ups. Peter Rosen remembers losing his cool at one of the final meetings:

> *I forget what the newest obstacle they were going to place in our path, and that was the point at which I just exploded and said, "then fuck ABMS, we'll just give the examination and start certifying people. If we can't do it inside of your organization we'll do it outside—it's just going on too long!"*[41]

The plan of the ABEM-sponsoring organizations was to submit a resolution at the ABMS meeting in March whereby ABMS would approve ABEM in principle, allow ABEM to move forward in naming its directors and planning the examination, and have the official vote of approval at the next scheduled ABMS meeting in September of 1979. Internal medicine continued to move excruciatingly slow. ABIM did not officially approve the ABEM by-laws until March 13, 1979—just 2 days before the ABMS meeting. In the meantime, the ABEM-sponsoring organizations needed the official approval of its revised application by the LCSB and AMA. This was accomplished for the LCSB in February. The LCSB did not require any hearings on the revised application, and offered no significant opposition. On March 2, 1979, the AMA's Council on Medical Education met in New York City and some of the same old concerns about a specialty in emergency medicine resurfaced. George Podgorny was at the meeting and remembers,

> *When, in 1979, we went to AMA, surprisingly there was more opposition in the CME of AMA on the second go-round than there was to the first because of one man…who was a member of the Council, Chief Medical Examinationiner for the State of Maryland, a pathologist, who just got into his head there was not going to be a new specialty regardless, makes no difference, there are too many specialties already. He voted against and got some people to vote against…it was very, very touchy. Finally, we squeezed by.*[38]

The concerns were addressed to the satisfaction of the AMA Council on Education, and it approved the ABEM application.[87]

Elements of doubt and mistrust toward the ABMS still existed even as the final application received approval from the LCSB and AMA. The ABEM sponsors were fearful of being burned twice. In a February 1979 editorial in *JACEP*, George Podgorny wrote:

> *It is conceivable, but highly unlikely, that neither real support or expression of support by an adequate majority of ABMS will be shown in the March meeting. In this case, ABEM should be in a position to proceed with its own examination within an appropriate time period.*[88]

The ABMS met on March 15, 1979, and the resolution for recognition of ABEM was submitted by John Davis of the American Board of Surgery. The ABMS voted to support the resolution. The reaction of Wiegenstein, Podgorny, Wagner, Krome, and other ABEM members who had put so much effort in to the process was more relief than exultation. They also were tempered in their enthusiasm because the passage of the resolution was not the same as a final vote by all ABMS members. Announcements to ACEP members were encouraging and optimistic, but stopped short of saying it was a done deal. Over the next six months ABEM worked to develop its infrastructure, and representatives of the seven sponsoring boards were nominated and approved to sit as ABEM Directors. OMERAD and ABEM worked diligently to finalize the certifying examination.

In September, the ABEM sponsors crossed their fingers and held their breath as the vote for the approval of ABEM came before the ABMS on September 21, 1979. As Leonard Riggs remembers, "there was always that slight amount of anticipation that something disastrous could happen again."[42] Before voting on ABEM, the ABMS needed to vote to change its by-laws to allow for the new modified conjoint board. This vote was unanimous. Then, 11 years after the formation of ACEP, 5 years after

ACEP formed the Committee on Board Establishment, and 3 and ½ years after ABEM was incorporated, the American Board of Medical Specialties voted overwhelmingly to approve the American Board of Emergency Medicine as the twenty-third American medical specialty. The vote was almost an exact reversal of the 100 to five defeat in the 1977 ABMS vote. The unbelievably lengthy official title of the new board was "The American Board of Emergency Medicine, a Conjoint Board (Modified) of the American Boards of Family Practice, Internal Medicine, Obstetrics and Gynecology, Otolaryngology, Pediatrics, Psychiatry and Neurology, and Surgery, and also sponsored by the American College of Emergency Physicians, the AMA's Section on Emergency Medicine, and the University Association for Emergency Medicine." George Podgorny, in a fortuitous confluence of leadership roles, was the president of ACEP from 1978 to 1979. He was also ABEM president, and was asked to stand at the ABMS meeting when the decision was announced. At the same time, the ACEP Scientific Assembly was being held in Atlanta and many emergency medicine leaders waited there for the news. When ABMS announced its favorable vote, Podgorny seized the moment by asking the ABMS to make ABEM a voting member immediately, rather than waiting a year, as was customary. In an unprecedented move, the boards of internal medicine and plastic surgery each yielded a voting representative position to the new ABEM so it could have voting power at the next ABMS meeting. Podgorny remembers,

> I thanked them and said goodbye, got on the plane, flew to Atlanta, where everybody was sitting on pins and needles when I announced that we were now a specialty. It was a very jubilant time.[38]

John Wiegenstein, who was also at the ABMS meeting remembered, "everyone shot for the phones to call their loved ones."[25] Later at the ACEP meeting in Atlanta Podgorny would hand over the reins as ACEP president to John McDade, one of the Alexandria pioneers. McDade was very fond of Podgorny, and they "did some celebrating."[15] Buttons were handed out to elated ACEP members that read "We're Number 23!" Podgorny presided over a ceremony where the ABEM original board members were given a medallion from ACEP. On one side was inscribed, "In commemoration of the successful negotiations and efforts of those who persevered in the long effort to achieve recognition of the specialty of emergency medicine, September 21, 1979." On the other side was a quotation from Alfred North Whitehead: "the art of progress is to preserve order amid change and to preserve change amid order."[20] (see insert, Figure 23). Amid the giddy, rollicking parties and toasts in Atlanta, two other feelings predominated. One was a sense that now emergency physicians and their representative organizations could get on with their lives—as David Wagner notes, "it nailed the ceiling to the roof."[42] Resident physicians would now do their training with the opportunity through the certification process to become board certified like their colleagues in other fields. Emergency physicians in practice who had learned emergency care and committed to the field as their specialty could now declare themselves as certified emergency physicians by passing the ABEM examination. The second feeling was a realization of the immense amount of work that lay ahead for the young, yet now legitimate, specialty.

Wiegenstein believes that the cause of emergency medicine was so just, that it was inevitable that the field would become a specialty. In summarizing the ABEM approval process, he said,

> Emergency medicine was right for the country, it was right for the public, and it was sort of like motherhood and apple pie. I didn't see how anyone could turn us down. I didn't know much about politics, but I learned very quickly that it doesn't always happen that way. I was very naïve, but in the long run I think that's proven to be true, that politics can throw up roadblocks and interfere for a short length of time, but time always wins if it's right.[42]

It appears that many of the representatives of other boards who worked with the ABEM-sponsoring organizations to develop the modified conjoint board proposal also came to feel that certification in emergency medicine was the right thing for the country. Some, like the surgeon John Davis, were initially strongly opposed to a board in emergency medicine, but in a manner analogous to the Stockholm syndrome, where hostages become sympathetic to the cause of their captors, the members of other boards came to be advocates rather than opponents. Speaking of Davis, John Wiegenstein said, "We made a convert of him."[25] As Benson Munger remembers, some of the participating boards "sent people that just adamantly opposed the idea totally, and everyone of those individuals eventually became one of the strongest supporters of emergency medicine."[60] These representatives played a crucial role in convincing their boards and the voting representatives in ABMS to support ABEM.

Looking back at the choice that was made to stay the course, accept a modified conjoint board and work toward official ABMS approval, the other option now looks like it would have been foolish. If the ABEM-sponsoring organizations had decided to spurn the ABMS after the initial 1977 defeat, give a certifying examination, and establish an independent board, this would clearly have infuriated the medical establishment. However, referring to an independent course, Peter Rosen says that the ABEM "would have been recognized 5 years sooner if we had done that earlier."[89] Others who were involved in the negotiations disagree that working outside of ABMS would have forced ABMS to recognize emergency medicine. George Podgorny notes,

> I am 98% sure if we would have gone on our own ABMS would not have embraced us…I think we would not have been absorbed and if we would have been absorbed in some manner or form, I think the best we could have hoped for would have been a parallel to hand surgery or critical care, being a subboard of several boards.[38]

Harvey Meislin, who saw the process as a young emergency medicine faculty member, and now sits as the ABMS president, notes,

> The ABMS, I would say in the [19]70s and into the [19]80s, was a more elitist old boys club than it is today…They responded to political pressure…they would bend but they wouldn't break…I think had they gone alone, I think the same result actually would have happened. I think, you can't be outside the house of medicine and still want to be in medical schools and still want to be part of the ACGME, you just couldn't do it, at some point you would come in. I think we were better off doing it this way. It took us a couple more years. It took us a structure we weren't happy with, this conjoint modified rather than initial primary board …The issue had been—get in. That was the wisdom. That was real wisdom.[45]

When compared to the length of time it took other U.S. medical specialties to be granted board specialty status, emergency medicine was actually quite expedient. Other fields of medicine took years longer to develop and organize. Emergency medicine was probably asked to jump through more hoops than the traditional medical fields, but given the move in the 1970s to put the brake on further specialization in medicine, the three and a half year time period from incorporation of ABEM to approval by ABMS now seems brief. The modified conjoint board designation still stuck in the craw of many in emergency medicine who had wanted primary board status for the field. But, in almost all respects except the long official name, ABEM would function like a primary board within ABMS. To those more peripheral observers, September of 1979 was the point of credibility for emergency medicine—it was now a full-fledged specialty. Newspapers, magazines, television news programs, and other media announced the approval of ABEM in optimistic terms. To the lay public this meant that the care of emergency patients might be improved, and apart from all the political maneuverings and controversy in approving the new specialty, this was what really mattered.

CERTIFYING EMERGENCY PHYSICIANS

When ACEP first formed the Committee on Board Establishment, and OMERAD was contracted to do the work, there was a vision that the emergency medicine certification process needed to be both different and better than what existed in other medical fields. After the 1979 approval of the modified conjoint board in emergency medicine this feeling persisted. Benson Munger recalls,

> The goal was to get to be a primary board still. There was some understanding…that downstream emergency medicine would come back and demonstrate that they had evolved to a point where it should be a primary board. So, we knew that we had to be better than anybody right off the bat. We didn't have the luxury of things taking 5 years to figure this out. It had to be right from the very beginning and I think the board did make a commitment to do that. Everything they did, certainly the examination, but just the quality of the decision making, quality of the process just kind of captured the imagination of the people that were involved….[60]

The comprehensive, scientific, and methodic process that OMERAD and ABEM went through to develop the test had never been done in another medical field. Other fields had defined content, but none had scientifically weighted their test questions to practice patterns, or validated their test questions with a field test that was administered to subjects with different levels of training. The planned method of a written examination followed by simulated practice scenarios in an oral examination was also new. Other boards had oral examinations, but they were not real-time, simulated case scenarios or multiple case encounters. By 1980 many other boards were dropping their oral examination component.[90] The involvement of Jack Maatsch and the other medical education and testing experts at OMERAD, who were using emergency medicine as a fast-moving research vehicle in new testing methodologies, created a forward-thinking, innovative spirit as the ABEM examination was developed. Even before the first ABEM examination was administered, ABEM had reaped the benefits of its careful preparation. Henry MacIntosh, M.D., who was an ABEM member representing the American Board of Internal Medicine remembers,

> The message that we had to sell back to internal medicine was very easy to sell because of the remarkable job the American Board of Emergency Medicine did in developing its test mechanism. This I think was really one of the high points, and if I would identify any one thing that was responsible for making the house of…academic medicine stand up and take notice, and say this is a group we need to think about working with and to bring in as partners in to what we are trying to do, it was because of the careful, methodical way in which you developed the test process.[42]

The newly approved ABEM was under a great deal of pressure to rapidly administer the first certifying examination. The examination would be in two parts, the written examination, followed by the more logistically difficult oral examination. George Podgorny and the other ABEM directors set a date for early 1980 for the first written examination. In short order, Benson Munger was officially named as the executive director of ABEM. Munger, who had used his negotiation skills to assist ABEM's passage in the ABMS now focused his educational knowledge and organizational skills on finishing the written examination. David Wagner remembers how important Munger was to the process:

> Without question Ben Munger was absolutely the genius behind this whole original examination development; as a matter of fact the whole growth of the board…He established the process by which a legitimate…examination that had credibility was established.[32]

As the written examination questions were finalized, it was noted that although the clinical content and questions were well worked out, some basic science knowledge should be tested on the examination. As more "academic" members of ABEM, Peter Rosen and David Wagner were charged with coming up with some basic medical science questions to insert as trial questions. They became aware of a service that provided a package of these types of questions, and inserted them at the end of the first written ABEM examination. Wagner recalls,

We were so insistent that this examination not be seen as a "piece of cake" …that we bought a set of basic science questions that had been validated and that were legitimate basic science questions. They were awful. I mean in terms of trying to pass them. Of course they didn't count. People didn't realize that we weren't really counting them, but…oh boy did that create a firestorm!

In February of 1980, over 600 emergency physicians came to Chicago for the first ABEM written examination. They were a mixture of emergency physicians who had met the eligibility requirements through the practice path, and those who had completed emergency medicine residencies. The first part of the written examination was standard multiple-choice questions, the second part was pictorial multiple-choice questions. Images of electrocardiograms, radiographs, and photos of disease pathology were provided in the test booklet. Pamela Bensen, one of Wagner's protégés, remembers sitting for the 1-day examination,

It was horrendous. It was the basic science that was horrible. I mean we just couldn't believe you would put this thing on this board…At about 11 o'clock in the morning the entire room burst out laughing. We must have all hit the same bunch of questions because it was ludicrous. How many molecules of ATP are used when…and we are like what, what, does this have to do with emergency medicine?[84]

Peter Rosen remembers, "There was one question about testicular hormones that particularly infuriated the people taking that examination. I truly thought I was going to get lynched in Los Angeles."[42] George Podgorny took the brunt of the complaints about the first written examination.

I was in Chicago—I was the chief examiner. Actually, it did pretty good, the examination itself. Nothing happened during the examination…After the examination was over—tremendous number of complaints about questions on the examination…There wasn't a single question that probably was not criticized. Probably most criticism was directed toward certain questions that could be classified as basic medical science…These questions were not to be a part of the score. They were to be evaluated for future examinations. Of course, people didn't understand this. Oh, letters I got, phone calls I got, threats and what have you.[38]

Even with the basic medical science questions excluded, the test was not easy. Some of the emergency physicians who took the test may have approached it more as a formality, and did not appreciate how diligently ABEM and OMERAD had worked to make the written examination reflective of emergency practice. The criterion-based process meant that a part 1 (written examination) score of 75% or more correct answers was required to pass the examination. This meant that an examinee's score and likelihood of passing was not at all dependent on the cohort with which he or she took the examination. A significant number of emergency physicians did not pass the test. Peter Rosen remembers the response,

Well, I thought we set the examination level at a pretty fair basis, that no student would pass and not every resident would pass automatically. Well, the fall out was that there was about a 65% flunk rate for practice eligible people including two of the board members. I was summoned to the ACEP board to explain to these guys why they had failed…I didn't mind going and making nice saying, "You're not bad people and it's not unfair and this is how we set the criterion for pass/fail and it doesn't mean that you are a bad doctor or bad person just take the examination again," (but I didn't add— and study this time!) I think that we did it the honest way. That was something that I was very willing to be strong about at the board meetings, we simply had to have intellectual honesty and that if the board examination was going to mean anything then everybody should take it.[41]

Ironically, some of the leaders who were most instrumental in developing the examination never sat for the ABEM examination or were unable to pass the examination.

One of the rules for ABEM directors and others who were integrally involved with the examination process was that they would have to be totally out of ABEM activities for 2 years before taking the examination. For some, like George Podgorny, who was previously board certified in surgery, and served as ABEM president, chief examiner, and was then involved in writing the written and oral examination, nearly a decade passed before he could have sat for the examination he helped to create.[38]

The next step was to administer the oral examination. The method of examination called for an examiner to present a simulated emergency case, or a multiple-case encounter, to the examinee and then "play" out the case over 20 minutes by allowing the examinee to ask questions and receive further information. Examinees were then graded on several criteria—data acquisition, problem solving, patient management, health care provided, patient relations, and comprehension of pathology—and were assessed an overall clinical competence score. The criterion for part II was an average of 5.75 on all cases (five or six cases were administered, along with one or two field test cases) or a minimum of 5.0 or more on every problem. For each oral examination case, a separate ABEM examiner reviewed the performance of the examiner. This was done to try to ensure internal consistency since no inter-rater reliability for examiners had been established at this point.

Some examiners relished acting out the plight of sick patients during the oral examination. David Wagner says, "We'd get so carried away in these scenarios…and there were just curtains and you practically would hear the person going next door to you because there weren't separate rooms."[32] In subsequent years, the ABEM reserved floors of a hotel, and the part II oral examination was administered in individual hotel rooms that were set up for testing. At one of the early oral examinations John Rupke was an examiner, and John Wiegenstein was the observer or "verifier" in the room— the "two Johns" were still working together. Wiegenstein remembered,

> This young man came in, he was pale, had a growth of beard, looked like he slept in his clothes, he was sick and he had a book in his hand as he was coming through the door and studying up to the last minute…John starts a case and he was doing okay until John got to the point where this guy was supposed to put a nasogastric tube down, he wasn't doing it, so John started retching and carrying out his act, like we used to. This guy went "Oh!" and clapped his hands over his mouth and ran to the bathroom and then we heard real heaving in the bathroom. We looked at each other and said, "Oh my God, what are we going to do?" Pretty soon we decided we'd help him into the bed, we were in a hotel room, so there was a bed, laid him down, put a cold cloth on his forehead and he was just too weak to get up off the bed. Times up. So, we had to get him to another room because the next candidate was there, so John gets on one side of him and I get on the other and kind of drag him out of this room and just outside the room was this young lady who was the next candidate. Her eyes got big![25]

Despite some early foibles, the ABEM certification examination became recognized by other medical specialties as a state-of-the-art method for certifying physicians. Other boards asked Benson Munger for input on their examinations, and Jack Maatsch and his co-workers at OMERAD published the research that was conducted as part of the ABEM development process.[91] The ABEM examination was a source of pride. Emergency medicine did not have the clinical clout, research activity, or power in medical schools enjoyed by the traditional medical specialties, but it did have a highly respected certification process. Under Benson Munger's leadership, ABEM came to be regarded as a clean, efficient, extremely professional organization. Many emergency physicians, those in community and those in academic practice, sought to be part of ABEM as test question developers, examiners, or leaders.

ABEM, as a modified conjoint board in its first 10 years, benefited greatly from the senior expertise of the directors from other boards who sat on ABEM. George Podgorny, speaking about these directors, notes,

> Both in terms of internal business of the board, because all of them were members of their own boards and many of them were members or presidents of the board

for years, they had a lot of experience that we did not have, plus of course they could give us a lot of advice about dealing with other boards. So, in fact, after the initial concern that there will be within us seven other people whom we do not know and are not emergency physicians, practically after our first meeting that all dissipated and…those people who were appointed for all practical reasons became members of our board. In no way either hassled us, and in fact became our advocates.[38]

For those who would lead ABEM in its first decade, the modified conjoint board, which was such a contentious, undesirable compromise when first proposed, turned out to be a blessing for the young specialty. The path was now clear for the development of emergency medicine in the 1980s. Certainly impediments, old prejudices, and conflicts would await, but no longer could anyone question emergency medicine's place as a specialty. The field had paid its dues and now was a card-carrying member of medicine in America.

In the summer of 1975, R. R. Hannas was asked to be one of six honored speakers at his Harvard Medical School twenty-fifth year reunion. Because of his work in helping to bring family medicine to specialty status, and his efforts to do the same in emergency medicine, Hannas's talk was titled "Spreading the Specialty Spectrum." As his second wife, Kay, and his son listened, Hannas delivered an address that likely raised the eyebrows of the reserved New England audience. He remembers,

The first story I told to open it up was, (this is one of my problems), this guy brought this gal into a bar, and somebody noticed that there was something different about her…Of course, this has application to what we are talking about. They finally got up close to her and they noticed that her breasts were pinned together with a great big safety pin. They said, "What the hell is going on?" The guy said, "It is very simple. If you can't lick them join them." Of course that is exactly what we were doing there. That was the first one. That went over pretty good. So I closed it with another one that was maybe too much of a shocker. I said you know it wasn't easy to get things done. I said there was a lot of turmoil and we had a lot of conflict and I said it reminded me very much of what the hurricane said to the palm trees. What was that? Well, "Okay fellows, better get ready, this is going to be the biggest blow job you've ever had!" You know afterward, Kay was in the audience, as was my boy Andrew who was a third-year medical student there at the time, so I said to Kay, "Babe, you know I got pretty good laughs on that last one." She said, "Laughs hell, those were gasps!"[36]

The *Harvard Alumni Bulletin* for July/August 1975 notes that the theme of Hannas's presentation "could be summed up by the aphorism, 'if you can't lick 'em, join 'em'."[92] The *Bulletin* did not further describe Hannas's attempts at humor. While the salty stories of this former Marine made some people cringe, his aphorism for how to get ahead in medical politics was undeniably on target. Emergency medicine became viable and put itself in a position to flourish, only after it surrendered its insolence, and decided to seek the assistance and adopt the habits of the medical establishment.

7 The Blooming of Emergency Medicine

The flower simile that Robert Dailey used to describe emergency medicine resonated with the early physicians in the field. To this, Peter Rosen added the concept of a unique biology of emergency medicine—a science could evolve to study this flower. The grit of men like R. R. Hannas and Ron Krome provided the stability and substance for the specialty to grow. And men like John Wiegenstein, George Podgorny, and David Wagner can be viewed as the gardeners, tending to the details, monitoring the environment as the specialty moved forward. The climate of the late 1970s and 1980s was not always hospitable to emergency medicine, and the inclement moods of the traditional specialties and prestigious academic medical centers would nip more than one program or department in the bud. By 1978, five emergency medicine residencies had started and then disbanded. Three of these programs lost their institutional support after having a Liaison Residency Endorsement Committee (LREC) visit that did not recommend endorsement. In one case, a residency dissolved because it could not retain its residents. The residents were lured away by the attractive salaries in local community hospitals, which were happy to hire anyone interested in emergency medicine as a full-time emergency physician.[1] Despite these failures, the overall picture after the approval of the American Board of Emergency Medicine (ABEM) by the American Board of Medical Specialties (ABMS) in 1979 was positive, and the emphasis changed abruptly from fighting for recognition to doing the work of a new specialty.

The Residency Review Process

Before ABEM approval, emergency medicine residency programs could not be officially approved by the Accreditation Council for Graduate Medical Education (ACGME). The American Medical Association (AMA) approved the first residencies, but no substantial review process was involved. As noted in Chapter 5, the LREC was formed out of ACEP in 1975 with representation from the newly incorporated ABEM and University Association of Emergency Medical Services (UAEMS). The LREC reviewed existing programs, and by 1975 18 residency programs were approved, but nearly that many were awaiting review. The number of newly forming programs was outpacing the ability of the LREC to do timely reviews. Although many of the existing emergency medicine programs were credible, the LREC found some that were of dubious quality. Peter Rosen remembers doing a review with Bob Dailey at Oklahoma City, where

> ...they had started a residency with a group of guys, most of whom, as I remember, were osteopaths and that was the sum total of their program. They didn't have a single faculty, they had no relations with any other departments, they had no rotations outside of the emergency department, they basically were just there taking care of all the patients in the emergency department for a resident salary. So we voted withdrawal, which was done, and overnight they hired all those residents as faculty and resubmitted an application. I think that shocked me.[2]

The situation for the LREC also changed in 1977 after the initial defeat of the ABEM application to the ABMS. The ABMS and AMA were now more closely scrutinizing emergency medicine, and these organizations became aware that the LREC was "approving" residency programs in emergency medicine. In ABMS-approved specialties, the approval of residency programs by that specialty's Residency Review Commission (RRC) [part of the Accreditation Council on Graduate Medical Education (ACGME)] is required before the residency is able to recruit its first class. Because it was approving existing programs in emergency medicine, the LREC was viewed by the ABMS as an illegitimate certifying body. The ABMS began to exert pressure on George Podgorny, who was president of ABEM, to halt the LREC reviews. Podgorny remembers, "I was told in no uncertain terms by AMA, ACGME, and ABMS if we continue doing our reviews outside of ACGME that was going to be very problematic."[3] Some troubling issues within the LREC were also threatening the process.

The procedure the LREC used to certify programs was to approve all new programs with "provisional endorsement." If an approved program developed the residency and corrected any deficits from the initial site visit, it was approved with "full endorsement" by the LREC. Programs that were just starting were given a cursory review and then had "permission to recruit" their first residency class, with a pending LREC visit. Dailey and his LREC colleagues often struggled with how to handle substandard programs. As Dailey wrote in 1978, "No program satisfies all the essentials and guidelines."[4] When deficient programs were judged, Dailey wondered, "Does it benefit a weak program more to deny endorsement than to endorse it with strong reservations?"[4] The emergency medicine leaders were very concerned that the new emergency medicine residencies would not be perceived as legitimate, high-quality training programs by the rest of the medical world. They were cognizant of the poor reputation for educational quality that family practice residency programs had in the academic world and were determined not to follow in that path.[4,5]

Judith Tintinalli, who was residency program director at the Wayne State/Detroit Receiving Hospital emergency medicine program, succeeded Robert Dailey as the chair of the LREC in 1979. Up to that point, according to Tintinalli, "it had been sort of a sleepy LREC and then suddenly we had had the greatest upsurge in residency programs ever."[6] Twenty-two new program applications were received over a 6-month period in 1977/1978.[4] In its first few years, the LREC review process had been somewhat informal. Sometimes it too much resembled a social visit and lacked the professional qualities that would be expected by the ACGME. Podgorny remembers one LREC reviewer who put up a poster recruiting for physicians for his own program while he was doing a site visit.[3] This is not to say that the LREC reviewers were compromising in their basic principles. Peter Rosen, in particular could be a challenging reviewer. George Podgorny remembers, "That was very taxing experience…going with Rosen to inspect the program."[3] As the new LREC chair, Tintinalli tried to provide a tighter organizational structure for the LREC, and to "get a bit more impersonal."[6] The LREC began applying its criteria more tightly, and some programs did not measure up. Some in the LREC believed that many existing programs were not in compliance with LREC requirements and should be disapproved or censured. Peter Rosen as one of the most exacting of the LREC members demanded at meetings that the LREC uphold its standards. George Podgorny remembers,

> …there was a big problem with Rosen on LREC. They wanted to do away with half of the then existing programs. I came to the meeting and told them I will dissolve the LREC, and Rosen stormed out.[3]

The LREC had to make a tough decision with the emergency medicine program at Hershey Medical Center in Pennsylvania. The program was run by Arnold Muller, a very well-liked and respected ACEP leader who had put together a residency at the small, rural medical college set in the mountains of central Pennsylvania. Muller's problem was a low patient volume of only around 15,000 emergency visits per year. The LREC reviewed the program and decided that it did not have adequate volume or enough faculty to train emergency medicine residents. The program was denied approval. Tintinalli recalls, "I had a lot of difficult decisions that really had to pave the way for the future and people felt, well, if you don't have the basic requirements, you won't…get approved."[6]

Around this same time, another more famous Pennsylvania program came under scrutiny during its LREC review. David Wagner's program at the Medical College of Pennsylvania (MCP) was the first program to send residents to another hospital for emergency medicine training. Wagner's emergency medicine residents did part of their emergency department (ED) training at Frankfort Hospital, where they sometimes worked with a faculty member during the day, but were unsupervised at night. He notes that "it was…a clinical resource…but it was mainly an economic resource." Wagner developed a moonlighting contract with Frankfort Hospital for the resident's independent work, and then used the money to support his financially strapped program at MCP. While supportive of the concept of emergency medicine, the hospital and medical school administration at MCP had provided almost no financial support for the new program. Wagner notes the importance of the Frankfort contract: "We were scrapping by on minimal, marginal faculty salaries as it were, but we didn't have any other support for the program other than that."[7] Wagner also used some of the revenues from his pediatric surgery practice to support the developing emergency medicine program.

Although Wagner's arrangement was legal at the time, the lack of faculty supervision was cited as a problem by the LREC, particularly Dailey and Rosen, who were good friends of Wagner. The LREC voted not to approve the MCP program. The LREC members agonized over this decision, as Wagner was a much loved and respected colleague. Bob Dailey remembers,

> We all knew that Dave was a good warrior, fighting a tough fight at MCP because the institution didn't have a pot to piss in…the poor guy was between the devil and the deep blue sea…Either his residency program was not going to be able to be maintained at the University or he was going to have to do this.[8]

Many sympathized with how he had creatively managed to build a successful program. Tintinalli remembers, "He was very innovative. He had no money, built that out of nothing and went to…these community EDs."[6] The decision not to approve MCP was controversial and produced some rancor in the group. Wagner was predictably upset, pleading his case, and recalls "we had a head-on clash."[7] After what Dailey remembers as "sort of a stunned silence for about a week" there was immediate political fall out from the denial of the MCP program.[8] Wagner had just completed a term as president of the UAEM, which was housed in ACEP, and the word soon got out in ACEP and ABEM. George Podgorny, who had already been receiving negative feedback about the LREC from the ABMS and ACGME, told Ben Munger to deliver a letter to Dailey. Dailey remembers,

> Good old Ben, toddled up to me and handed me a letter that indicated that I thought well okay I've been fired…as the residency committee chief, it's okay. That wasn't what it said. It just said that there has been a moratorium declared on its decisions. I think it was a very political and a very good way to kind of say, "Okay, wait a minute here. Let's stop and see where we are going. Let's catch our breath." And so at that time there was a moratorium on decisions.[8]

Judith Tintinalli remembers being very unhappy with the decision. She remembers "big fights with George Podgorny…he was just shouting from the back of the room."[6] Even in its unofficial capacity, the LREC was viewed as a credible certifying body by most in emergency medicine, and the halt on reviews was unsettling. Many programs had been in existence for years without being formally reviewed. Others were starting and needed approval to garner institutional support. Now, the process was on hold until the negotiations for a modified conjoint board were finalized and ABMS reconsidered the application. However, some, including Bob Dailey, felt that the LREC was becoming obsolete and new people and a new structure were needed:

> …we were approaching the time of specialty recognition and we were transitioning from a residency endorsement, informal, if you will, process, to a residency review process. And so we were graduating from ad hoc into the big time. And also, we were

becoming part of the true medical establishment with all of the organizational and regulatory features that other specialties had. So, I think that it was right and appropriate that the kinds of people that were—I should say more naturally politically attuned, and who would work more comfortably within the structures of the medical establishment—that such people would gradually come into control of process.[8]

The transition to an official RRC of the ACGME occurred from 1980 to 1982, and George Podgorny, in addition to serving as ABEM president for the first year, became the chair of the RRC for emergency medicine and served in this capacity for 6 years. Dailey, Rosen, Tintinalli, and other LREC members were not asked to serve on the RRC. Rosen had resigned from the LREC around the time that the moratorium was imposed. In an ironic twist of fate, David Wagner, whose program was not approved by the LREC, went on to serve as chairman of the RRC for emergency medicine from 1991 to 1994. The RRC adopted most of the requirements for an emergency medicine residency that were originally developed by Bob Dailey and the other early LREC members, but the methods and review process became much more standardized and efficient. A separate staff devoted to the process was now available to assist with the paperwork and reviews. Once it was officially in the ACGME with an established RRC, emergency medicine could participate in the National Residency Match Program (NRMP). In 1982/1983, 33 residency programs submitted 190 positions in the NRMP. Emergency medicine programs that started at the PGY-2 level (around 30 programs at this time) did not submit positions through the NRMP and held their own special match.[9]

One aspect of the RRC formation caused some organizational controversy in emergency medicine. RRCs in other specialties were typically sponsored by the certifying board in that field, the AMA section for that field, and for half of the RRCs, the specialty organization in that field. In the case of emergency medicine, ACEP was the primary specialty organization recognized by the AMA and the ABMS and had given birth to ABEM. Therefore when the application for an RRC was filed by ABEM, it was a *fait accompli* that ACEP would be invited to be a sponsoring organization, and UAEM, the academic specialty society, was excluded. This was particularly hurtful to UAEM, because it had played a big role in the development of the LREC and had spent a good portion of its meager budget supporting the LREC. On the other hand, UAEM, due to its struggle to define itself as an academic organization when it was initially dominated by academic surgeons, had missed its earlier opportunity to become a leading voice in academic and organizational emergency medicine. The failure of UAEMS to strongly endorse residency training in emergency medicine in the early 1970s left a bad taste in the mouths of the ACEP leaders. ACEP's power move in controlling the RRC seats was in part due to a lingering suspicion that the academics would not be faithful to the roots of the specialty.[10] The ill will generated over the RRC formation was an early divot in what would eventually become a more significant rift between ACEP and UAEM in the 1980s and 1990s.

NUMBERS AND FUNDING FOR EMERGENCY MEDICINE RESIDENCIES

The number of approved emergency residency programs progressed at a relatively constant rate of around 20 new programs per 5-year interval between 1975 and 1990. In 1980 there were 43 approved programs, by the end of 1990 there were 81, and by 1995 there were 108.[11] The failure rate for programs was around 10%. One of the factors that contributed to the increase in the number of emergency medicine residencies in the late 1970s was federal funding. The EMS Act of 1973 (Chapter 6) and the National Health Planning and Resources Development Act of 1974 provided for funding for emergency medical services (EMS) systems and improving the allocation of health resources, but not for residency training of emergency physicians.[12] The only emergency medicine program to start with federal aid prior to 1977 was the Los Angeles County (LAC)/University of Southern California Medical Center (USC) program, where a customized federal grant had been obtained by Gail Anderson's predecessor, most likely with the help of some political connections in Washington. In 1976, President Ford, who was viewed as a friend of emergency medical services development, signed an amendment to the EMS Act. ACEP had aggressively lobbied for money to train emergency physicians, and under the Health Professions Educational Assistance Act of 1976, $10 million per year was designated "to train physicians in emergency medicine" in 1977 to 1979, although the actual appropriations by Congress during this time of economic recession were less than this.[13] Harvey Meislin remembers,

> ...in the mid-[19]70s when the Title Twelve EMS Act had money—the first part of the EMS act was monies to set up the 911 system and a significant number of those systems in the country were set up from that—the second half of the Title Twelve Act, which was about [19]76–[19]77 allowed for physicians to be trained with federal money. A lot of residency program started with those monies...When I went to UCLA [University of California at Los Angeles], we started that program with those monies."[14]

The federal grant money also played a role in determining where the new residencies would be created. Since medical schools and large teaching institutions were more experienced and usually more adept at obtaining grants, they were more likely to be interested and successful in applying for federal funding. In Los Angeles, the grant also influenced how residencies developed. Meislin initially tried to partner with UCLA Harbor Medical Center to develop a residency shared between the two institutions. When the issue of how the generous federal indirect costs would be distributed between Harbor and the Westwood campus came up, the plans for a combined residency evaporated, and the institutions submitted separate grants. Meislin received a grant of over $800,000. He recalls, "I was flush. I was in the money. I couldn't spend the money fast enough. I was hiring faculty, I was building offices..."[14] Many of the emergency medicine programs which were started in the late 1970s and early 1980s used the lucrative appeal of federal funding to warm up their institutions to the idea of emergency medicine and were able to create a more solid infrastructure for their programs than the early, poorly funded and resourced emergency medicine programs.

Private foundation funding also had a small, but significant impact on emergency medicine. As described later in this chapter, the Robert Wood Johnson Foundation in 1974 funded the development of the Johns Hopkins University emergency medicine residency, and provided a similar grant to the University of California, San Francisco to train and support emergency medicine faculty.[15]

CINCINNATI BECOMES MORE THAN JUST FIRST

When Richard Levy became the acting director of emergency medicine at the University of Cincinnati program in 1977, he was inheriting a poorly resourced enterprise with a spotty record of educating resident physicians. Much of the residents' time was spent on other services, and the ED continued to be busy, but dreadfully disorganized. Although fresh out of residency himself, Levy did not function like a neophyte (see insert, Figure 24). As he assumed his new role, he developed a list of goals for the department, including how to improve the emergency department, the residency, research activities, and prehospital care. Early on, Levy also hand wrote a list with the title: "How to Survive—Axioms for Survival." Levy's 25 axioms show that he was very in tune with how to achieve success, both in the sense of traditional values and the more covert uses of power. Some of Levy's noble axioms for his emergency medicine division were: "Become indispensable; Work harder than anyone else—80 hours; Create group harmony; Stand above any fray." Some of the more astute and cunning, given that this was Levy's first foray as a leader were: "Control the money; Avoid conflict—they can't hit you if they can't see you; Form alliances—a rigged election wins close votes; Pick a battle you can win—hit them on the snout; Never bet the farm—your farm; Stay out of the limelight—light bulb(s) kill butterflies; Develop an external power base—local and/or national."[16]

Levy became the director of the division of emergency medicine in 1978. He hoped to be granted an academic department from the start, but the powerful department chairs in medicine and surgery squelched this idea. Instead, Levy sought to have the least interference possible from other departments and he successfully petitioned the dean to form an independent division of emergency medicine under the dean's office. This approach was also used by other early emergency medicine programs. Levy realized that to have equal standing with the departments in the traditional medical specialties, he had to build strong educational, research and financial components in his division. He recalls,

> I understood to be successful in an academic world it came down to two things. And that is space and money. Those were the two tracers and it's like one of those games...whoever had the most space and money that's who wins the game. Especially where you have a lot of competing interests, usually the heads of those departments that are there for long periods of time who can manage to accomplish more space, more money are the ones who win.[17]

Levy was advised by medical school administrators not to aggressively seek departmental status until he had an enterprise that looked like a department. He remembers them citing the case of family practice, where a state mandate required the medical school to have an academic department. However, family practice did not build a solid academic infrastructure and was viewed as a weak department in the institution.

Levy was perhaps an ideal person to play the money and space game at the Cincinnati medical school. Recalling his heritage, where a peddler or rag merchant begot a storeowner, who begot a professional man, Levy says, "Down deep...I'm a rag guy that's just what I am—I like to deal."[17] Most medical schools in the late 1970s took a hands-off approach to their clinical departments, and Levy remembers, "How you made money is your business." Nearly all of the money coming to the division of emergency medicine was paid by the hospital in exchange for providing emergency services. The Cincinnati General Hospital's indigent patient care was funded by a large county tax levy. Levy developed a contract with the hospital and medical school and found that he was "probably a natural born negotiator."

> ...if you put me in a room with others who were in a negotiating setting, I tend to get a good deal, even though I'm not a person who I think is seen as doing that... I think I got us good deals in emergency medicine and also anytime that we would pick up a gig along the way, a gig meaning training programs, or, if we had money that would come in for various research activities or any consulting work, I always took that money and put it aside in hidden accounts. Those dollars were always around. Those were the ways that we got a decent amount of money early on."[17]

Levy was also cunning in finding and concealing other revenue sources. The EMS contracts for training and services in Cincinnati were lucrative, and Levy negotiated with the local EMS organizations for contracts. But, it became something of a shell game. He recalls, "One party thought that the other party was getting the money, and the other party thought that the first party was getting the money, and in reality we were getting the money."[17] In this manner, Levy was able to build up a stash of money to build his division. He notes,

> So I was always interested in trying to create an enterprise that paid people well and gave them decent working environment in terms of space and also gave them the ability to do things that typically took some additional dollars, whether it was assistance or it was supplies or whatever it took.[17]

Levy's financial success allowed him to recruit some of the best and brightest graduates of the residency program as faculty members to Cincinnati. Daniel Storer, who had been a part-time faculty member was put in charge of EMS and became the EMS leader in Cincinnati for more than two decades. Alexander Trott was a residency classmate of Levy's who had previously worked in community EDs, was a talented teacher, and was hired by Levy. Levy recognized that a bright and ambitious resident, William Barsan, would make a strong faculty member and convinced him to stay and join the faculty. Another graduate, Edward (Mel) Otten, the former Vietnam medic, who was a renowned bedside clinician, was retained on the faculty. He later became board-certified in toxicology.

After securing this local talent, Levy called up David Wagner to find out who were his most promising graduates. Wagner told Levy about Jerris Hedges, a stellar resident who had recently graduated. Hedges had initially looked at a faculty job at Hershey Medical Center, but this was located near the Three Mile Island nuclear facility, which had a calamitous accident in March of 1979. After he made a verbal commitment to join the faculty at Hershey, Hedges's wife became worried about "turning radioactive," and said, "You get on the phone and tell them I'm not moving there."[18] Hedges then returned to his home state of Washington where he settled into the community practice of emergency medicine. Levy contacted Hedges and paid the expenses for him and his wife to visit Cincinnati. This was an uncommon practice at the time. Hedges, who had become disenchanted with the business side of community emergency medicine and wanted to return to academics and do research, remembers, "There was a lot of excitement about building something."[18] He was hired as the research director and became the key figure in creating a viable basic science and clinical research program in Cincinnati. Around this time, Levy drew in another MCP graduate, James Roberts, who had trained in toxicology, and with Hedges, wrote an excellent book on procedures in emergency medicine. In short order, Levy also hired Steven Dronen, who had trained at the Henry Ford Hospital residency and then served in the military, and another MCP graduate, James Amsterdam. By the early 1980s, Levy had built a stable of faculty who were strong clinicians, teachers, and researchers. Levy's ability to creatively manage departmental finances gave him an advantage over some other academic programs because he was able to pay faculty salaries that were more in line with private emergency practice.

The Cincinnati program had previously been notable only because it was the first emergency medicine training site. By the 1980s, it was regarded as one of the best places to train (see insert, Figure 25). The residents were an interesting collection of personalities whose experiences produced some memorable stories. Kenneth Iserson remembers the Beverly Hills Supper Club fire in the spring of 1977. Just across the river in Northern Kentucky, this popular nightspot could hold thousands of guests. When a raging fire broke out on a Saturday night, all physicians and nurses were called into Cincinnati General Hospital, the closest trauma and burn center. Iserson recalls,

I got there and there was kind of pandemonium, no patients, but kind of pandemonium…right from…the ambulance entrance, you could see the flames. This is 20 miles away. You could see the flames obviously, shooting up into the sky. Very shortly thereafter they bundled me, a surgery resident, and an attending surgeon into the back of a police car…and off we went…Any way we get there…I make my way up to what obviously has got to be an area for a Command Post, and Dan Storer was standing there with the Fire Chief…He has a little white hat…and so he briefs me on what is going on, which is that they have already pulled out about 100 or so bodies. I look over there and there they are just lined up on the ground, no sheets covering them because we don't have sheets, they are about my age, they are all dressed up, not a mark on them and they are all dead. They'd already tried to defibrillate all of them as the one thing that they might be able to do. They didn't save any…I said, "okay, what happened to the other ones? Some ambulances already left. Did they go to the Burn Center?" Cincinnati was the only Burn Center. He said, "I don't know but I think they went to these little local hospitals." I said, "Okay, tell you what I will do. I'll take this whole bevy of ambulances. We will go from hospital to hospital, we will pick up all the bad burn patients, bring them back to University." That is what I did. At that point I collected all these ambulance people, gave them their orders and off we went. We went to all these little hospitals, and said you know, "Where are the bad burn patients?" Some of them were parked in the middle of the hall or in a back hall or who knows where. We loaded them up and brought them back to the university. We did save some because of that. Some were really seriously burned…All the way back, we could see the flames still just burning out of control. The interesting thing is that the surgery attending and the surgery resident ended up carrying stretchers, because they didn't know what else to do. It was emergency medicine people who really shined.

*People recognized that. They recognized that, "Hey this is a different breed of people."
Also the next Monday or Tuesday, for the first time ever…there was a debriefing. What
we call a PTSD debriefing now, run by psych to a whole auditorium full of people.
I didn't realize it at the time, but I certainly needed it, because of all the things that
have ever happened to me in emergency medicine, it was the only one that I had night-
mares about for quite awhile afterwards.[19]*

Another incident led to Iserson's first publication. Iserson and William Barsan were
participating in an advanced cardial life support (ACLS) course at Cincinnati. After
lunch, as they came back into the room before the teaching exercises resumed, Barsan
walked up to the resuscitation manikins and playfully grabbed the defibrillator. He
assumed that this was a "dummy" defibrillator, and was not charged. Barsan said,
"Look, I'm going to defibrillate my brain," and proceeded to do just that. The current
arced around his glasses, but delivered a substantial shock that rendered Barsan
unconscious. He was taken to the ED where he regained consciousness, but was still
a bit addled. Iserson remembers, "We released him to his wife and she said he basically just sat in the chair for 3 days and she fed him."[19] Iserson was encouraged by
others to write up this interesting case report, and Barsan, who was a good sport,
became a co-author. The paper, "Accidental 'cranial' defibrillation" was accepted by
Ron Krome for publication in the *Journal of the American College of Emergency
Physicians* in 1979.

As he achieved academic success in the early 1980s, Richard Levy's goal was to
become an academic department, but he had unwavering opposition from the outspoken and volatile chair of surgery, Josef E. Fischer. Levy felt that Fischer, "instinc-
tively and deep in his gut didn't like emergency medicine."[17] The approach Levy
used to get around Fischer's opposition was to "build those markers [that] made us
look like other clinical departments and also to isolate him so that his vote was simply
a vote as opposed to being the powerful chairman of surgery who would veto something." By forging alliances Levy was able to secure enough votes so that in 1984 the
department of emergency medicine was established at the University of Cincinnati.
A couple years later, Levy decided to have some fun with his new status. He had just
turned 40 and had seen advertisements in magazines for Jockey underwear. The ads
initially featured baseball pitcher Jim Palmer, but then Jockey started to include in
these ads "normal guys" in their work environment but wearing only their Jockey
underwear. Levy recalls,

*I thought I could do that, why not…? So I called up Jockey, and I was eventually
connected to the head of marketing, and I said, "Do you need a model? I'm a doctor
and I could be a model for you." We met a couple of times 'cause he wanted to make
sure I wasn't a total nut case. Actually he said come to New York, so I never told anybody, including my wife.[17]*

Levy had a successful shoot and was featured in an advertisement in *People* maga-
zine, posing in his white Jockey briefs by a locker where his white coat is hanging.
He and his wife were flying to China where Levy was to be giving some lectures.
Levy notes,

*I knew that the first set of ads were coming out and so I went to the newsstand and
I handed a couple of these magazines to Beth, and I said I have to go to the bathroom
but there is a really interesting article on page 83…I came back and she was sitting
on the floor and she said, "We can't ever go back to Cincinnati! …We are dead—
you've just lost your job! This is the dumbest thing you have ever done in your life,
and how am I ever going to be able to face anybody?"[17]*

The ads were more than a 40-year-old man having some fun with his wife and
friends. As Levy notes, after years of being put down by the other academic chairs at
Cincinnati, he was saying, "…in your face, and I was saying you can't touch me now,
and I'm having a good time and here I am!"[17] But Levy was never a person to do
anything without fully understanding the consequences, and he had made plans

for this. When he returned to Cincinnati, as his wife had predicted, many in the medical school were upset. But when Levy met with the acting dean, he told him, "Any money I make out of these ads they go to the Medical School, they are your money." This softened the dean's displeasure with Levy, but several chairs, lead by Fischer, "came to the dean and they said we want that guy out of here. He has been blasphemous to what we represent, and this is a degenerate, and this is Cincinnati, Ohio, he's out of here!"[17] The dean told the group that the medical school was receiving funds from the ads and that no punishment would be forthcoming for Levy. Thus, Levy was successful in thumbing his nose at the establishment. At the year-end residents' roast, Levy was treated to a slide show featuring each of the male members of his faculty posing in Jockey underwear.

By the mid-1980s, the Cincinnati emergency medicine program was a breeding ground for academic faculty. Men like Hedges, Barsan, Roberts, and Dronen moved to other locations where they built programs in the Cincinnati mold. Residency graduates from Cincinnati became sprinkled around the nation's academic centers as junior faculty who were versed in how to achieve success in an academic environment.

MEDICAL COLLEGE OF PENNSYLVANIA MOVES FORWARD

The formula that Richard Levy used for success in Cincinnati would not work in all medical centers, but others found their own routes to success. At the MCP, David Wagner had been threatened with the loss of his program due to using outside contracts to support his academic activities. But, once he was able to get some support to hire full-time attending physician coverage at the outside EDs, these outside contracts became fine teaching environments and were the chief source of revenue for the MCP program. One of Wagner's early residents was Steven Davidson, a native of Philadelphia who went to Temple Medical School and then did the MCP acute care internship, which had been pioneered by Pam Bensen. Davidson did his emergency medicine residency at MCP from 1976 to 1978. He remembers the MCP ED as still operating out of separate tracks for medicine, surgical and pediatric patients, with emergency medicine residents assigned to different sections of the ED. Davidson best liked the rotations at Frankfort Hospital, the community ED training site, as these allowed for the most interaction between emergency medicine residents. He remembers, as a senior resident assigned with junior residents, they were all "busy teaching each other and depending on each other."[20] Davidson remembers being surrounded by gifted physicians. One of the residents in the class behind Davidson was Lawrence J. Carley, who had done medical school at MCP, and was the first male student body president of the previously all-female school. According to Davidson, Carley had an almost preternatural ability to recognize sick patients, and when his co-residents needed help,

> ...he would just, almost Superman-like...he'd just sort of levitate, fly over everything, and be there at the bedside when you needed another pair of hands. He could slide in a femoral line, starting from 30 feet away, he'd just know you needed access on that patient and in one smooth, fluid motion you'd have a Carley line, he was just spectacular like that."[20]

Davidson and the other residents revered David Wagner and were cognizant of the sacrifices Wagner had to make to keep the program running at MCP. Wagner engendered fierce loyalty from his trainees. It was an easy decision for Davidson to stay on the faculty when he finished residency, and he functioned as the residency director. Davidson remembers that each year the quality of the residents increased. He refers to the period from 1978 to 1990 as a "golden age" of residency recruitment. For him and other faculty it was sometimes a bit unnerving to see how bright and talented the new residents were, and to figure out how, as young physicians themselves, they could teach them. Davidson remembers,

> I'd go to work and I'd know that there were kids that I was working with who were smarter than me, were more driven than me, were reading more medicine than I was

at that moment, and I think as a young guy…I was still struggling to find my own place…but I was presenting abstracts, I was moderating sessions, I was…doing what passed for academic emergency medicine in the first part of the [19]80s. At the time, shit, I was a scared guy in my early thirties, didn't have a freakin' clue how I was going to deal with these real smart heads.[20]

As emergency medicine residencies matured, the quality of emergency medicine residents, as measured by medical school performance, improved. Residency directors found themselves recruiting more academically gifted residency candidates who were interviewing around the country and had a better understanding of the field. The percentage of entering residents who came straight out of medical school increased dramatically between 1975 and 1985. Fewer and fewer "retreads," or physicians who were in practice or in other residency programs were accepted into emergency medicine residencies. Even from the early years, emergency medicine was able to attract primarily U.S. medical school graduates, and did not rely on a high percentage of foreign medical graduates (FMGs) to fill residency positions. A 1978 survey of emergency medicine residency programs at 35 medical centers found that 7.4% of emergency medicine residents were FMGs compared with 9.6% in internal medicine and 12.3% in surgery.[21] Other specialties noticed that emergency medicine was attracting better and better residents, and part of their resistance to a board in emergency medicine stemmed from a fear that they would lose potential residents to this inviting new field.

EMERGENCY MEDICINE MOTORS IN DETROIT

Other strong emergency medicine residencies developed in the late 1970s. In Detroit, where there was never a shortage of sick or injured patients, the Wayne State/Detroit Receiving Hospital residency began in 1978 after Ron Krome had secured a stable position for emergency medicine underneath his old mentor in surgery, Alex Walt. The Detroit Receiving Hospital ED was one of the busiest in the country, and setting up a training program in that environment, as it had been at Los Angeles County/USC, was very challenging. John McDade, one of the original Alexandria four remembers a visit to Detroit Receiving Hospital in the 1970s to see the ED:

…the first time I ever went to Krome's hospital at Wayne State I couldn't believe my goddamn eyes. He had a room filled with stretchers, with gurneys and they didn't have enough handcuffs to keep these guys on the stretchers. They had one guy's hand and one guy's foot connected on these stretchers. I said, "Krome, you wouldn't find this in the Dark Ages." He said, "I know, but that is the way it is."[22]

Krome remembers the time when Carl Levin, currently a U.S. Senator, asked to visit:

Senator Levin, when he was a city councilman taking the quadrennial annual tour of Receiving for City Council—they had to do it before election time…He was walking through the middle hall through the ER…Levin was standing next to me…and we had a psychotic in leather straps and he kind of pointed at Levin and said, "Come over here." I said, "Please don't do this!" He said, "He may be one of my constituents." I said, "Don't do this, please, don't do this." He said, "I have to." So he (the patient) said, "You motherfucker, get your ass out of here." I said, "I told you, Mr. Levin, not to do this."[23]

Despite the tough surroundings, Krome was able to assemble a solid faculty in a short time by pulling from local talent. Hal Jayne, Brooks Bock, and Judith Tintinalli were all members of the Wayne State Medical School class of 1969 and knew Ron Krome when he was a surgical resident and then the new ED director at Detroit Receiving Hospital. Bock remembers that Krome took him through his first surgical case as medical student—a lymph node biopsy. Tintinalli had what she calls a "life molding moment" when as a third-year medical student rotating on trauma surgery she encountered,

…this hairy guy back in the ER and he says, "Hey, you can fix that. I'll show you how to do it." It was a guy that had gone through a plate glass window and had

*partially lacerated his Achilles tendon. I'm like, if he says I can do it, I can do it,
so I sewed up his Achilles, sewed up his skin, put him in a posterior mold…I'm like,
"this is pretty cool."*[6]

The "hairy guy" who showed Tintinalli how to suture was Ron Krome (see insert,
Figure 26). Jayne, Tintinalli, and Bock did their internships at Detroit Receiving
Hospital and became friends. Tintinalli was a native Detroiter and would go on to be
named "Michiganian of the Year." After internship, she had a child and then worked
part time in the ED for Krome. She then went on to do a residency in internal medicine from 1971 to 1974 at the University of Michigan. Tintinalli considered quitting
her internal medicine residency, but when she called Ron Krome he encouraged her
to finish. When she did finish, Krome offered her a spot on his faculty. By then, Hal
Jayne had been recruited by Krome to help run the ED. Krome had also signed up
Brooks Bock, who was a senior urology resident, to help develop an emergency medicine residency. Bock had done moonlighting in EDs as a resident and found that he
liked emergency medicine practice more than urology. He remembers, "I think it was
about at that point in time that I was learning to do TURPs, and that was a very
common procedure in urology, and I thought, is this what I want to do all my life?"[24]
To this group of young faculty Krome added Blaine White. White had trained in internal medicine and had excellent previous research experience. Krome saw the potential for developing a research program with White as the leader of this effort.

Although he desperately needed the manpower, Krome took a long-term approach
to developing an emergency medicine residency. He knew it would be foolhardy to try
to establish a residency without the support of other departments, and he and Bock
spent the better part of 3 years meeting, negotiating, and gaining approval from the
other Wayne State medical school and Detroit Receiving Hospital departmental leaders for a residency in emergency medicine. Finally they started a program in 1976 with
two residents. The program soon grew into a respectable residency, and White's
research enterprise became the one of the first successful and funded program of its
kind in emergency medicine. The chaotic atmosphere at Wayne State/Detroit
Receiving Hospital had its downside, but it provided the freedom to try new
approaches to clinical practice and teaching. Tintinalli describes it as,

> *Wild! I have never had so much fun in my whole life as a Wayne State. There were
> no rules. There was no decorum. You could do whatever you wanted. There was no
> CQI, there was no risk management. It was just so much fun.*[6]

In time, Krome's magic trio of Jayne, Bock and Tintinalli would each go on to
become leaders in academic and organizational emergency medicine. Both Bock and
Tintinnali would become presidents of the American Board of Emergency Medicine,
and Bock joined several of the early leaders in the field in becoming president of both
ABEM and ACEP. The remarkable development of the Wayne State emergency medicine faculty as nonemergency medicine trained physicians who became true believers
and leading advocates for the field was paralleled in other academic centers across the
country. Most emergency medicine faculty groups had one or two members whose
start in emergency medicine was too early to have done residency training. They
became board certified through the practice track and were as fervent in their desire
to advance the field as the early leaders who came before, and the emergency medicine residency trained faculty who would follow them.

Just a few miles away from Detroit Receiving Hospital, emergency physicians were
also busy at Henry Ford Hospital. Richard Nowak, M.D., and Michael Tomlanovich, M.D.,
who was in Peter Rosen's first full class of emergency medicine residents at the
University of Chicago, started their emergency medicine residency at Henry Ford
Hospital in 1976, the same year as the Wayne State/Detroit Receiving Hospital
program. Although it did not have a medical school, Henry Ford Hospital was historically a strong academic institution and had a faculty group practice dating back to the
early 1900s. It was a very good environment for the development of a strong emergency medicine program. But, it was not easy. Nowak and Tomlanovich paid their
dues, as Tomlanovich recalls,

My first 5 years here were incredibly difficult. We had a limited number of faculty and we had a 45-hour clinical week mandate. That was our mandate. That was a culture here. Every fourth week I worked seven midnights in a row, so I had a 63-hour clinical work every fourth week for 5 years. At the same time we were developing and implementing a residency program and Richard and I starting do research together.[25]

Their effort paid off as they built a strong residency program and strong clinical research programs studying asthma, resuscitation, and stroke. The Ford residency spawned many academic emergency leaders. Detroit was maligned because of its violence and urban blight but by 1980 the city had, in the Henry Ford Hospital and Detroit Receiving Hospital programs, arguably the best pair of emergency medicine residencies in the nation.

ROSEN AGAIN HEADS WEST: EMERGENCY MEDICINE IN DENVER

Peter Rosen left the University of Chicago when he and his wife Ann decided they had enough of the angst and rancor that Rosen's position seemed to generate in that highly political medical school. As Rosen notes, the University of Chicago

…had unanimously agreed to develop emergency medicine, and then unanimously did everything possible to kill it. So, what we rote in Chicago was by dent of blood bath and I was ready to leave that, it just wasn't any fun anymore.[2]

Paradoxically, the University of Chicago even made it difficult for Rosen to leave. When he interviewed for the director of emergency medicine at the UCLA, Rosen thought he had a verbal agreement and had invited Harvey Meislin, one of his star residents at the University of Chicago, to come with him and be the residency director for a new residency program. Rosen remembers,

They told me that I looked good and that I should just submit a letter with what I needed and the job was mine. So, I submitted a letter and I never heard another word from them. Never—and I finally heard that the chairman of surgery at the University of Chicago had written a really nasty letter to the dean at UCLA about me and that was probably why they decided not hire me. So, we were feeling kind of depressed about being able to escape Chicago….[2]

Rosen had interviewed at the University of Michigan and Ohio State University, but these positions or locations were not as appealing. He and Ann decided to give the University of Chicago one more try, but a convolution of fate would not keep them there. Rosen was asked to give a lecture at Denver General Hospital, and while there was told that James Brill, the current director of emergency medicine was leaving to return to California. Brill was negotiating with the UCLA program where Rosen had just been shunned. Brill suggested that Rosen should take his job in Denver. When Rosen phoned Ann to discuss it, she had the response of a woman who was ready to get out of Chicago. As Rosen remembers, "I…said I've been offered the job in Denver and she said if you don't take it I'll leave you."[2] Rosen knew that the situation in Denver was not necessarily much better than in Chicago, and found that the University of Colorado "was not very hospitable to emergency medicine." But the mountains and lure of the West brought him and his family to Denver in 1977.

Rosen inherited an emergency medicine residency, and his reputation as a leader and teacher, along with Denver's choice location for outdoor-minded emergency medicine applicants, almost immediately attracted high-quality residents. Rosen's problem was in securing position and power in the faculty structure at Denver General Hospital (DGH) and the University of Colorado. Like the other early academic leaders in emergency medicine he found "there is a finite pie—anybody new coming in is going to take somebody's space, positions, and money." The clinical service director of DGH was, according to Rosen, a Machiavellian figure who had previously abolished the position of chief of emergency medicine. Rosen would have to be assigned as a director under another department. The chair of surgery, Ben Eiseman, who was a leader in the movement to improve trauma care (see Chapter 3), had refused to allow Rosen to be appointed in the department of surgery and was in the process of leaving. Likewise, the department of internal medicine chairman was refusing to accommodate Rosen in his fold. Rosen remembers that Eiseman, still relished a good battle before he departed.

> *He was only there for another month. My first week at Denver General I issued a memo that consults couldn't be called by nurses, they could only be called by senior residents or the attending. He came to my office and started screaming at me that this was unreasonable because the nurses used to call the surgeons when they heard there was a trauma coming in. I said, "Well look at it this way, Dr. Eiseman, you are in the middle of a gastric resection and all of a sudden one of the internists appears and starts doing a cardiac evaluation on your patient because the nurse called him. What would you do?" He said, "I'd cut her head off." I said, "Well how is it any different?" "Because you're emergency physicians." I said, "Well, that's not going to cut it. Doctors talk to doctors, nurses don't call consults. We're not doing surgery in the emergency department, but we will decide when we need a surgical consult." He said, "The only thing you've brought to Denver General is the manners of the garment district." I said, "It takes one to know one," and the fight was on. It was such a stupid thing for me to do because he was leaving anyway. He says "You are a rude prick, get your legs off your desk." I had a bad knee and I had my leg elevated on my desk. I said "It's my office, if you don't like the way I sit in my office get the fuck out." You know it was just childish and stupid but I never had very good temper control and I don't like to be bullied. Actually, I realized after he left that it was a stupid mistake, so I went up and apologized to him in front of the department of surgery head at a department M&M [mortality and morbidity]. He said, "You are a fucking idiot, and as long as I draw a living breath you will never have a faculty appointment at the University of Colorado."[2]

Although Rosen was content to function as an independent entity without a departmental home base at the DGH and University of Colorado School of Medicine, it was partly due to his and Bob Dailey's LREC stipulations that he eventually had to resort to a creative method to secure university appointments for him and his faculty. The LREC had issued a requirement that residency faculty should have a university appointment. When Rosen's attempts at DGH and the University of Colorado were unsuccessful, he was in jeopardy of losing his residency. Also, Rosen notes that he had the personal incentive that his TIAA/CREF retirement savings from the University of Chicago would become taxable if he did not find a university appointment. At the time, emergency medicine residents from the Oregon Health Sciences University (OHSU) were rotating at DGH for supplemental trauma experience. Because Rosen and his faculty were teaching these residents, he called the director at OHSU and asked if they could receive faculty appointments from OHSU. This was arranged, and for many years, the DGH emergency medicine residents were taught by faculty who were technically appointed at another university. Rosen became professor of emergency medicine at the University of Oregon and he recalls, "Colorado thought I was the devil."[2] John Marx, M.D., who started his residency 1 year after Rosen came to Colorado and then joined the faculty notes, "I had never set foot in Oregon in my life but I rose to the level of clinical or adjunct associate professor at the University of Oregon."[26]

Marx came to emergency medicine residency straight out of medical school, but more than 40% of first-year emergency medicine residents in 1977/1978 decided on emergency medicine after they had left medical school and were pursuing training or practicing in other fields.[27] Marx remembers,

> *We had, I guess, eight residents and I was the only kid. The other seven had come from surgery and medicine and private practice. These were people who were all older than I was—who had all trained more than I had. I only had the internship.*

> *Every single other person was well ahead of me and in the first week of orientation that became pretty clear and I wasn't too crazy about it. I mean, it made me a little nervous and made me realize I didn't know one lick about toxicology. I didn't know anything about trauma. I didn't know anything about OB [obstetrics]. I was really, I felt like I was a first- or second-year medical student.[26]*

Rosen brought Vince Markovchick, one of his former residents from the University of Chicago, into be the residency director. The Denver program came into shape rapidly and began attracting high-quality residents (see insert, Figure 27). But, daily battles were fought as the emergency medicine faculty and residents tried to carve out their niche in an environment where they had little political might. Rosen was the constant force. His residents gave him a plaque that said "Not always right, never in doubt."[28] Marx remembers Rosen at the M&M conference.

> *Peter's presence probably was greatest at M&M and some of the other didactic sessions. He did well in the clinical arena—he would typically be out there for something significant. But at M&M Peter would sit in the front row. Peter's got that kind of hunched over, rounded shoulder look, and when he's thinking about something he's got his head down a little bit. Once you get to know him and you know his posture you're pretty sure you know what's coming when, but there were moments in retrospect I'm sure were instrumental in helping me appreciate what the field was trying to do, led by people like himself. So for example, we had a patient who was having a hypertensive emergency, clearly malignant hypertension, pressure of 250 or 260. This would have been in 1981 or [198]2 so we put him on a Nipride drip, not an art line, and either we lacked equipment or who knows what, get him up in the elevator, by the time he gets upstairs his pressure has dropped some, nothing scary, the guys not ischemic, the guy isn't dying, we present the case at M&M. So, a chief resident in internal medicine at the back of the room pronounces somewhat in a condescending fashion that it is probably more appropriate that we not be permitted to use drugs as powerful as Nipride in the emergency department. We should simply admit people with hypertensive emergency to the hospital and let the "really smart" people upstairs figure out how to dose it and put in lines and that kind of stuff. Well, that was not one where Peter had to sit then and think much. He was out of his chair in a heartbeat. He turned, he basically described emergency medicine to this guy and to the audience and said, "This is what we do. This is what we are about. We know how to use this just as well, if not better than you do. We see this more than you do. We're better on managing this than you are. If we don't have all the equipment we need or the personnel to go up in the elevator, that's a problem we have to deal with. But, the suggestion that we're not going to give that medication is absolutely horse shit." And he probably said something far stronger than that. Silence—there was no reply. Whoever it was who offered this bad recommendation in the first place either dissolved or shrank into a little pool and slid back under the other side of the door. I saw him [Peter] do that a number of times. Peter owns as good an extemporaneous speaking ability as probably anyone I've ever known. When you get into a situation like that, he knows the fights to pick and he knows how to represent the specialty and he would simply…say, "That's just not the way you do it." As a kid I'm in there watching, that's good, this is funny, this guy's getting his ass kicked. But, truly in those spots, those…10 or…20 years later when you're a chair and you are in exactly the same kind of situation, it is then when the words of Peter ring true and ring loud and allow me to know exactly how I should behave in that kind of situation.[26]*

A New Generation of Emergency Medicine Program: The University of Pittsburgh

After Ronald Stewart had personally trained almost every paramedic in Los Angeles County, he was looking to help develop a smaller system and become more involved in emergency medicine in an academic medical center. He remembers that he "had become identified with EMS to the exclusion of other things." The city of Pittsburgh had a struggling EMS system that "was killing people in the streets." At the University of Pittsburgh School of Medicine, Peter Safar the "great guru of resuscitation" was developing a very strong research and clinical program in critical care, but he did not want to become heavily involved in EMS or the emergency department. A new mayor who wanted change and the continued disarray in EMS and emergency medicine prompted an associate dean at the University of Pittsburgh to call a friend in Los Angeles and ask if he knew anyone who could head up the ED and direct the Pittsburgh EMS system. Ronald Stewart was an obvious choice. Stewart was initially reluctant, but recalls he "was standing on my boat…warm and sunny and everything" when Peter Safar called and convinced Stewart to come to Pittsburgh to interview. He "discovered the city was entirely different than I ever imagined it to be" and in 1978 was hired as director of the ED and City of Pittsburgh EMS system. Stewart arrived as "the only trained emergency physician in the city, trained by residency."[29] He had the help of a surgeon, William Robinson, who was a proponent of emergency medicine. Stewart quickly made connections in the departments of internal medicine and surgery at the University of Pittsburgh, and then, only 3 weeks after he arrived, came his first test as the medical director of the EMS system. A construction worker suffered a severe crush injury to his lower legs while he was working on the demolition of a bridge 150 feet above the river. His legs were trapped in the unstable structure. As a huge crowd gathered, and local and national news programs carried the story live for over 2 hours, Stewart rushed to the scene, bringing with him the chief surgical resident from the hospital. He was put up a ladder to evaluate the patient. He recalls,

> I'm marching up this railing thinking I'm going up the stairs, and then suddenly there is no more railing and I'm a hundred and some feet in the air and I suddenly fall flat on the ladder grabbing the rungs every so slowly and trying not to look down. Anyway, I got up there and there was no way we were going to get him out but we did manage to get one leg loose by cutting with the torch a bigger hole, but the other leg was impinged by the vertical strut holding the bridge up, and in dislodging this leg the bridge shifted 3 inches…I remember looking down and the transportation officials were standing there under an umbrella because it was beginning to rain, and calculating with some sort of a thing that the bridge had shifted.[29]

Stewart decided that the worker's leg must be amputated,

> I had the chief surgical resident bring the saw down and we did some local anesthetic and we did some morphine…The surgical resident did the actual disarticulation of his knee. We gained more notoriety in a very positive way for the EMS system, for there being a Medical director who got in and got his hands dirty and almost fell off the ladder in the process, that it was the clincher, we got the "Award of Courage" or something for it. We got all these wonderful things which I appreciate very much, but I was more thinking of this is good—this man's leg has not been lost in vain as far as I was concerned, because I was going to use that to get a proper emergency department and emergency medicine program and that is the legacy of that guy….[29]

Stewart quickly seized on the notoriety that this incident gave him. He was thinking beyond his own hospital. He wanted to set up a Center for Emergency Medicine in Pittsburgh with 14 hospitals contributing to a program which would run an emergency medicine residency, educate practicing emergency physicians and collaborate on research projects and practice improvements. Stewart remembers using a gimmick to make his point.

> I went down to the variety store…and I bought…one of these big plastic keys that look like a key to the city or something, and I took it and made an appointment for all 14 CEOs [chief executive officers] of the hospitals and I would take the key out and I would put it on his desk. I would say, see that key, that is the key to your emergency department, and I'd put it in my pocket. I said don't you want to have your hand on

that key? I can't give you the key but make sure your hand is on that key...I would like to form a consortium to make sure that there is no favoritism, that we have a balance...I just said that I think we are all in this is as a public utility kind of thing and would you like to sit around the table and be part of the decision-making process?[29]

Thirteen of the 14 institutions signed on to Stewart's plan. He then needed to find some space for his center. He found out that the vice chancellor of the University of Pittsburgh had praised emergency care in a speech. Stewart went unannounced to the office of the vice chancellor and requested that they visit some office space that had been occupied by accountants. Stewart thought this space would make a good home for his center. Stewart remembers,

I had gone in the night before with some paramedic friends and we had put some very formal looking names on the door—Division of Education, Division of Transport, and such—with nothing in them, nothing in the rooms, nothing, and I toured him around.[29]

By November 1978, just 6 months after Ron Stewart arrived from Los Angeles, the Center for Emergency Medicine was inaugurated, with the mayor of Pittsburgh cutting the ribbon. Stewart recruited an energetic and talented physician, Paul Paris, who had done an emergency medicine fellowship at Cedar Sinai Hospital in Los Angeles. Paris was home in Pittsburgh visiting his sick grandfather when he saw the large new sign for the Center for Emergency Medicine. He soon joined Stewart and the two became a dynamic duo, building a strong and popular residency and research programs at the University of Pittsburgh, with a special emphasis on EMS. Stewart approached this job with his typical, obsessed style, and remembers often falling asleep in a chair, "because I was monitoring the radio 24 hours a day with an earpiece."[29]

Stewart took his skills at organizing to a national level in EMS by banding with other EMS leaders around the country to form the National Association for Emergency Medical Service Physicians (NAEMSP) in 1985. Emergency physician leadership in EMS in the early 1980s, despite the obvious connection, was still in a primitive state. UAEM offered to host the organizational meeting for NAEMSP at its annual meeting. Stewart remembers how easily he rose to the presidency of the new organization:

I as well as several others were ...alarmed at the fact there was no consistency of medical directorships in the cities around the United States. People were being hired ...for their billing number or their license and then the medics would just do what they wanted or what they were told to do by fire or police or whatever. We thought this was bad. We had evidence that it was not working well. So, about eight of us got together in a room at Hilton Head and talked...and we said we have to do something. So we said let's have an organization, at which point I had to go to the washroom, I had to go pee. I came out and I had been elected president—so it's often called the "bladder Presidency." I remained president for 3 years but I actually wasn't doing as much as a lot of other people were doing.[29]

EMERGENCY MEDICINE IN THE IVORY TOWERS

As was noted in Chapter 5, emergency medicine residencies proliferated in the 1970s at many medical centers, but not at the prominent medical schools. At highly ranked places like Johns Hopkins University, Harvard University, Duke University, Stanford University, the University of California–San Francisco, the University of Washington, University of Michigan, and Washington University, the academic battles for space, money, and prestige were so fierce that a new department, whether it be emergency medicine, family medicine, or another field, had little chance of succeeding. Only if a calamitous event occurred in the ED or other higher political forces like municipal or state governments or a board of trustees or regents insisted would an emergency medicine program get off the ground. Even those who were given approval to start were often shaded out like weak saplings by the towering canopy of the traditional departments. This was seen at the University of Chicago, where Rosen had an ongoing battle within his own department and with other departments. An emergency medicine program at Stanford University folded soon after it began. Other institutions did not even consider letting emergency medicine in the door. Speaking of the University of Michigan, one long-time Detroit academic leader notes, "Internal medicine and surgery could agree on only one thing—that emergency medicine would not happen there."[30]

One of the biggest deficiencies in the academic realm for emergency medicine in its first decade was the lack of senior, experienced leaders. The men who helped the field get started and nurtured it in the political and organizational world of medicine were not well connected in the academic world. Many of them did not have residency training and were uncomfortable around the well-educated, research-oriented academic physicians. Even though John Wiegenstein went to medical school at the University of Michigan and R. R. Hannas went to Harvard, neither of these men had strong ties that could be used to leverage emergency medicine as an academic discipline at their alma maters. It was left to academic emergency physicians who were relative rookies in the academic world to contest the seasoned veterans in other fields in the game of medical school politics.

While the real reasons for the suppression of emergency medicine in the traditional academic medical schools were political and financial, the argument usually put forward by opponents was that emergency medicine lacked a true scientific core. Ben Eiseman, the surgeon and nemesis of Peter Rosen at Denver General Hospital, expressed this view in a 1978 commentary. After hearing arguments from Ron Krome and David Wagner on why emergency medicine should be a specialty and have academic departments in universities, Eiseman wrote:

> ...the emergency room is a busy money-making place that serves an important clinical service. To me, this clearly qualifies it for hospital departmental status. But this does not equate with a university or medical school department...Housekeeping and food service serve a hospital function, but scarcely qualifies the guards, cooks, and dietitians for a professional chair or a place on the medical school curriculum committee.[31]

Eiseman then wrote that emergency medicine needed to define its "body of basic knowledge," expertise in comparison to other specialists in handling emergencies, its research realm, and educational role in a medical school. He called emergency physicians "20-minute experts," citing that "they have to be effective until help from the specialist arrives." Eiseman then described his personal thoughts in the event of an emergency:

> When I get hit by a car or mugged by an antagonist, I certainly want a skilled (and well paid) emergency service physician and his team directing the ambulance that picks me up and cares for me during the first few minutes after I arrive in the emergency room. But I couldn't care less whether these doctors who may save my life hold academic tenure or professorial chairs.[31]

As Eiseman intimated, the key to power in a university or medical school is academic departmental status. When the early residency programs at University of Southern California and University of Louisville were granted academic department status at their inception, this may have caused early academicians to think that departmental status would become commonplace for developing emergency medicine programs. However, after this pair of successes, things dramatically slowed down. In 1976, there were three academic departments of emergency medicine in U.S. medical schools, but 5 years later there were only five, and only 12 had been created by 1986 (Table 7.1). For every three emergency medicine residencies formed during this time, only one new academic department was formed.

Although many academic medical centers were eager to create emergency medicine residencies to help solve the clinical service dilemma in their increasingly busy emergency departments, departmental status was a privilege not easily granted. Most of the

TABLE 7.1   Academic Departments of Emergency Medicine in U.S. Allopathic Medical Schools Established from 1971 to 1990

University of Southern California, 1971
University of Louisville, 1971
University of Missouri-Kansas City, 1972
Brody School of Medicine at East Carolina University, 1980
Wright State University, 1980
University of Kentucky, 1983
George Washington University, 1984
Loma Linda University, 1984
Medical College of Pennsylvania, 1984
University of Cincinnati, 1984
Albany Medical Center, 1986
Summa Health System/Northeastern Ohio Universities, 1986
Wake Forest University, 1989
State University of New York, Buffalo, 1989
Texas Tech University, 1989
Ohio State University, 1990
State University of New York, Stony Brook, 1990
Wayne State University, 1990

From the Society for Academic Emergency Medicine Website. Available at www.saem.org. Date accessed: October 20, 2004.

early residency programs were tucked away as divisions of internal medicine or surgery. They were treated like stepchildren, who were "fulfilling a service function for university hospitals."[32] In terms of personal development, emergency medicine faculty members were generally not on career paths that could result in promotion with tenure. By the early 1980s, this was creating both consternation and despair in academic emergency medicine leaders. In an editorial, Harvey Meislin called it "trouble in paradise."[32] In some cases, for example at the University of Cincinnati, medical schools and their emergency medicine programs creatively formed new entities in the dean's office. This type of arrangement allowed for some autonomy for emergency medicine programs, but kept them from having a seat at the table in the important meetings of department chairs. In order for emergency medicine to become an equal on the local medical school scene and nationally, it needed to win academic departmental status at a significant portion of the 125 U.S. medical schools. And, until it cracked the glass ceiling at the oldest and most renowned medical schools, emergency medicine would remain an interesting second-class citizen in the world of academic medicine.

EMERGENCY MEDICINE AT JOHNS HOPKINS UNIVERSITY MEDICAL SCHOOL

Johns Hopkins University School of Medicine is perhaps the most venerable of American institutions of medical education. The first medical school developed after the Flexner report, it became the model for how to integrate scientific discovery and clinical medicine. All of its major academic departments boasted faculty who were leaders in their field. But the medical school that dismissed Lewis Goldfrank because of his liberal views and support of civil rights was rooted in tradition and was not paying much attention to emergency medicine in the 1970s. Hopkins did, however, pay close attention to funding opportunities. Starting around 1973, before the federal government started making funding available for emergency medicine residencies, the Robert Wood Johnson (RWJ) Foundation announced that it would accept proposals to help promote education in emergency medicine. Donald S. Gann, M.D., a junior surgeon who was put in charge of emergency services, submitted a grant to the RWJ Foundation and was rewarded with a $750,000, 4-year grant.[33] This allowed him to start an emergency medicine residency in 1974, but Gann still had almost no faculty and little institutional support and spent most of his time in research. By 1978, Gann had handed over the reins to Hubert Gurley, M.D., an internist who was not well connected with UAEM or other emergency medicine organizations. Gurley received an additional 4-year, $700,000 grant from the RWJ Foundation to train faculty in emergency medicine. Gabor Kelen, M.D., came from Toronto, Canada in 1982, after completing an internship and internal medicine residency, to train in emergency medicine at Johns Hopkins Hospital because it was the only "big name" institution on the East Coast that had a residency. Kelen remembers,

> The surgeons and the medical people here were pretty tough individuals, and many of the trainees back then, by the time they graduated, were what I call almost "broken" people, psychologically. In our own clinical space, initially the department was divided into five areas, medical, surgical, psych, an ortho area, and a GYN area.[34]

The emergency medicine residents were "outmanned" by the medical and surgical residents—at any one time, up to 18 residents were assigned to the various sections of the ED. While stationed on the medicine side of the department, Kelen remembers working 27 days straight followed by 3 days off. The surgical side had a 24 hours on/24 hours off rotation, and Kelen and his residents, "tended to look at the bright side as—I've got every other day off!" The emergency medicine residents at Hopkins were "tolerated on the other services," and in the emergency department it was a battle of wills among the residents to see who would manage critical cases. Kelen notes,

> For me the training was just superb, I loved it. I loved the free-for-all. I loved it—you had to do whatever you had to do for yourself. In trauma we had lots of fights with the surgeons, but at least most the time they were residents who got to do what, who got to control what. There was really nobody to appeal to as to whether something was fair or not…It was by force of personality as to what you did or not.[34]

There were at the most three or four "emergency medicine" faculty, and Kelen remembers that they were remarkably detached from resident training,

> I would say…there might have been a faculty wandering out in the area 2 to 4 hours out of that 365 days. Not per day, but for the entire time. In the midst of the arrest rooms and trauma rooms, critical care rooms…what the faculty would typically do is—the administrative offices…were adjacent to the main ED. They'd hear the code thing go off, then they'd look behind this glass to see what we were all doing, but they'd never come in the room, they'd never interject, no matter how ugly the fights got, no matter what we were doing wrong. They never laid hands on anybody and they never taught at the bedside…They'd come in in the morning, all go down for breakfast and they'd come back and read the paper and they'd all go to lunch, they'd come in the afternoon maybe…go to a meeting or something and then leave. That was their life.[34]

For the next decade, the emergency medicine program at Johns Hopkins University remained alive, but its growth was stunted. Other early programs like Cincinnati, MCP, LAC/USC, UCLA, Louisville, Hennepin County in Minneapolis, Wayne State/Detroit Receiving, and Henry Ford Hospital rapidly developed strong residencies and gained some status in their institutions. At Hopkins, emergency medicine remained a "forgotten, back water, poor cousin, division of surgery."[34] A new ED director was appointed in 1984. Heath Sivertson had graduated from the Hopkins emergency medicine residency the year before and practiced for a year on the Maryland Eastern shore. Sivertson was allowed to hire faculty, and Gabe Kelen joined the faculty and became the research director, and then in 1986 the residency director. For the first time, in 1984/1985, the Johns Hopkins Hospital ED had emergency medicine faculty who actually supervised care. As Kelen remembers,

> It was really awkward because we started initially that first year working Monday through Friday, 8 AM to midnight, supervising residents who weren't use to being supervised, particularly in medicine and surgery. Some of the surgeons were like fifth- and sixth-year surgeons who would come down to consult and this and that, who were around even before some of us were interns. It was hard to supervise some of them….[34]

Although it was not an ideal situation, Kelen and the other emergency medicine faculty at Hopkins remained there because the program did have at least a foothold in the world of big-time academic medicine. Kelen remembers that at the time,

> *Harvard didn't have a program yet, Yale didn't, Stanford folded along the way and then got rejuvenated. Vanderbilt didn't have one, Emory didn't have one. We really felt we were sort of a beacon as it were. For me is was fulfilling to be part of this history and looking at it back then I did not envision that we would be an academic department within my life time there. Things were moving but the politics were so against it, I just didn't see it happening. Then the dam broke very, very quickly.[34]*

Kelen began doing research, and when the HIV epidemic arose in the late 1980s, he became well known and well funded as he and his colleagues at Hopkins documented the high incidence of HIV infection in urban emergency patients. Emergency medicine gained credibility at Hopkins, and nationally, due to this work. Then in 1991, Sivertson left and Kelen became the acting director. Kelen decided to act boldly. He remembers,

> *I felt like I had almost nothing to lose...I could to go back to Canada, so I made a series of what I thought were relatively bold moves for the day and all these things that we feared would come to pass, like the place would blow up, didn't happen. Though as soon as I took over one of the first things I did was I eliminated this medical/surgical/ortho/GYN, all this nonsense and I said we are going to be an integrated department in July. The medicine chief jumped up and down and the chief of surgery jumped up and down and said no, it's not good for their training, and I said fine if it's not good for training, pull out your people and send them wherever you think it is. I guess somehow we proved the emperor had no clothes because they finally agreed to have their people see undifferentiated patients and then we instituted that the attending has to see every patient one way or another and sign every chart and we started billing...and so we started bringing in a real amount of money. The institution changed presidents at that time...and changed schemes at the medical school, so there was a new era and they held a committee to determine what should even be done with us. It wasn't even a search committee initially, it was just a committee—should we make emergency medicine a department, keep it a division, or just do away with it altogether? That committee deliberated for something like 6 months to a year and after a very heated debate at the committee level recommended that we be an academic department unto our own.[34]*

The recommendation needed to be approved by the Johns Hopkins Medical School Board of Trustees, and at this point a little academic competition helped to cement the deal. Kelen was approached by the University of Pennsylvania Health System as a potential candidate for chairman of their new academic department of emergency medicine. William Kelly, M.D., the chief executive officer, and dean of the School of Medicine at the University of Pennsylvania, who had previously been an ardent opponent of academic emergency medicine while the chair of internal medicine at the University of Michigan, had an interesting way of recruiting. He typically visited the home institution of those people he was considering for chairmanships at Penn. Kelly spent a day at Johns Hopkins, and the fact that this prominent academic leader was paying attention to emergency medicine and wooing Kelen, made an impression on the Hopkins leaders. Soon after, the Johns Hopkins medical school board met, and Kelen was allowed to present his case. He wisely invoked the name of William Osler, remarking that many years before, Osler had proposed the idea of postgraduate medical training at Johns Hopkins, and that it was initially rebuked. Kelen made the same argument for emergency medicine. He remembers,

> *...that very few people at the table believed in academic emergency medicine, but given all the potential for this new field, would Hopkins want someone else to define it...or would they like us to have a real opportunity at leading this whole new specialty? I think they kind of liked that, they had such a great respect for Osler that if you mention his name properly in anything you say, it sort of rings a bell.[34]*

Johns Hopkins University officially established an academic department of emergency medicine in 1993. In the 1990s, emergency medicine began to break the glass ceiling at other major academic medical institutions. University of Pennsylvania, Emory, Yale, Harvard, Michigan, and Washington University all developed emergency medicine residency programs and academic divisions or departments. These programs had some difficulty in shedding their institutions' anti–emergency medicine image, but the lure of these major centers soon allowed most to compete successfully for high-quality residents. However, the problem of inadequate status and representation for emergency medicine at medical schools persisted. In 1994, only 38, or about 30%, of U.S. medical schools had academic departments of emergency medicine.

TAKING ITS TIME: EMERGENCY MEDICINE AT THE UNIVERSITY OF MICHIGAN MEDICAL SCHOOL

The University of Michigan in Ann Arbor might have been good place for the academic side of emergency medicine to develop. ACEP had formed just an hour's drive to the west in Lansing, and southeast Michigan had many practicing emergency physicians and by the late 1970s, strong residency programs at Wayne State/Detroit Receiving Hospital and Henry Ford Hospital. The first annual UA/EMS meeting had been hosted by surgeon, Charles Frey, at the University of Michigan in 1971. But despite being in the middle of a hotbed of emergency medicine activity, the University of Michigan Medical School took its cues from the traditional academic medical centers of the East. Charles Frey, after having an intense interest in emergency care, went back to being an academic surgeon. He was succeeded as ED director by James McKenzie, an early UAEMS member and academic surgeon who was originally from Canada. McKenzie was an active voice in UAEMS—his acerbic critiques of scientific presentations at the UAEM meetings were so notorious that the McKenzie Award was established and presented for many years to the faculty member who provided the most obnoxious commentary during scientific presentations. During the 1970s and 1980s, the small ED of the University of Michigan Hospital was on the fourth floor and was staffed by one medical and one surgical resident with no faculty supervision. Judith Tintinalli, who did her internal medicine residency at the University of Michigan from 1971 to 1974, did a few rotations as the resident physician in charge on the medical side of the ED. She notes,

> *I remember having no instruction, and that's one of the things that really kept me going to do emergency medicine, because it was so disgusting. You know, a major medical center, 24-hour shifts, I didn't know any faculty, didn't know any protocols. I mean, I remember calling all these famous people to find out what to do for this or that or whatever. I just called whatever attending was head of the service to find out what shall I do if this is a PE [pulmonary embolism] or what should I do with this hemophiliac?[6]*

As emergency medicine developed at other midwestern medical centers, the University of Michigan stuck to its old model. The strong chairmen of surgery and internal medicine battled for control of the ED, with surgery ultimately winning, but many internists were used to staff the "medicine" side of the ED. Because of its suburban location, the University of Michigan ED did not have a large bump in its patient volume until the 1990s. The idea for an emergency medicine residency at the University of Michigan never gained enough momentum to emerge as a reality until some local competition came into play. In 1991, a strong emergency medicine group at neighboring St. Joseph Mercy Hospital prepared an application for an emergency medicine residency and inquired about residents doing some off-service rotations at the University of Michigan Hospital. The university, with a combination of academic arrogance and a fear of lost clinical revenue, felt that if an emergency medicine residency was to exist in Ann Arbor, it should be based at the University of Michigan. A national search was conducted for someone to lead emergency medicine at Michigan, and William Barsan, M.D., who had recovered from his accidental cranial defibrillation to become a very successful residency director, researcher, and eventually second in command to Richard Levy at the University of Cincinnati, took the job. Emergency medicine remained a section under the department of surgery, but was well supported, nurtured, and protected by the chairman of surgery, Lazar Greenfield, M.D., the famous vascular surgeon. Once the infrastructure for an academic department of emergency medicine was in place, Greenfield gave his blessing, and the University of Michigan Medical School in 1998, nearly 30 years after academicians had started the process, approved an academic department of emergency medicine.

PARADOX IN THE NORTHWEST: EMERGENCY MEDICINE AT THE UNIVERSITY OF WASHINGTON

The city of Seattle had one of the first emergency medicine practice groups, which started at Ballard Hospital in 1966. The Northwest region of the United States was also advanced in implementing ambulance and EMS services in the late 1960s and early 1970s. Leonard Cobb, M.D., started the Medic One program at Harborview Medical Center and the University of Washington Medical Center to train firefighters in cardiopulmonary resuscitation (CPR) in 1970. Mickey Eisenberg, M.D., who a few years later would become a major contributor in EMS and cardiac resuscitation, remembers that from the start Cobb insisted that the EMS system be designed so that it could "study each event...collect data...and try and improve the outcomes."[35] Within a few years, the Seattle Fire Department EMS system became fully trained with an advanced cardiac life support (ACLS) emphasis, and was a model for the rest of the country.

Mickey Eisenberg did his internal medicine residency at the University of Washington, and then trained as an epidemiologist, eventually getting his doctorate. Eisenberg had a long-standing fascination with cardiac resuscitation. He remembers in high school,

> We dissected frogs, live frogs...we must have chloroformed them and then dissected them. I remember asking the teacher if I could take home the heart, which was still beating. Amazingly enough it kept beating for several days. I must admit I was blown away by that.[35]

When Eisenberg was an internal medicine resident, he trained under Robert Petersdorf, M.D., who would become a major icon in the field. He remembers Petersdorf as a "very remarkable individual but very intimidating to house staff and students."[35] Eisenberg did a Robert Wood Johnson Clinical Scholar fellowship and during this became involved in a project on sudden death and EMS. He joined the internal medicine faculty at the University of Washington and soon learned from Petersdorf that he would be in charge of the emergency department at Harborview Medical Center. Eisenberg and Michael Copas, M.D., supervised resident physicians in the traditional split medical/surgical ED, but their main passion was out-of-hospital cardiac resuscitation. Eisenberg extended the Medic One concept to the entire Kings County area around Seattle and used the system to test whether ACLS made a difference. Eisenberg and his colleagues became the leading research team in the United States in studying EMS and cardiac resuscitation.[36]

It would seem that the ground-breaking EMS work done by Eisenberg and others at the University of Washington (UW) would have naturally extended to the development of a strong emergency medicine presence in the institution, but this was not the case. Eisenberg remembers, "the context of UW was that emergency medicine was not embraced at any level of the organization."[36] The very strong internal medicine and surgery presence at Harborview Medical Center ED prevented the development of emergency medicine as an academic discipline. Robert Petersdorf was very skeptical about the ability of emergency medicine to become a viable academic entity, and he opposed any efforts to hire true emergency physicians in the Harborview ED. Petersdorf eventually softened his opposition and became supportive of emergency medicine when he was the president of the Association of American Medical Colleges

(AAMC), but his opposition at the University of Washington was perpetuated by Petersdorf's followers well into the 1990s.[37]

As an internist who practiced in the ED, Eisenberg could have sat for the ABEM examination and become certified in emergency medicine, but he notes he "was getting too many gray hairs" by that time, although he was only 35 when the ABEM exam was first offered. Eisenberg, as an academician, was working only part time in the ED and as a successful, funded researcher did not need ABEM certification to advance his career. In fact, it may have been viewed by his peers as a somewhat traitorous act. Eisenberg was not plugged into the national academic organizations in emergency medicine. Those in emergency medicine who were also doing research in cardiac resuscitation interacted with Eisenberg in this realm, but this did not extend to developing emergency medicine as an academic discipline in Seattle.

As the rest of the country began to accept emergency medicine, Eisenberg and others at the UW realized "that these guys were out there and they were going to become a reality, and you couldn't wish them away, they were going to happen" (36). The requirements for faculty to work in the Harborview ED gradually changed from board certification in internal medicine to the acceptance of the first faculty member who was dual-boarded in internal medicine. Then in the 1990s, emergency medicine board certification was required. A residency in emergency medicine, almost a laughable concept at UW in the 1980s, was eventually started in the middle 1990s. An alternative to the UW starting its own program came about when UW and Harborview linked with the military emergency medicine residency at the nearby Madigan Army base and added four civilian residents per year to this program.

A NEW LEVEL OF SUPERVISION

As has been demonstrated from the accounts of early emergency medicine residents, faculty supervision of residents was at best minimal, and typically, the more "academic" the institution, the worse was the supervision. This situation was not unique to emergency medicine. Almost all postgraduate training in medicine in the 1970s and early 1980s consisted of resident-run services or departments with part-time supervision by faculty. By the late 1970s, some emergency medicine residencies had a consistent faculty presence during the day, and sometimes even into the early evening. True case-by-case supervision and direct teaching of residents by faculty was more common in emergency medicine than in most other fields. But, on nights, weekends, and holidays, faculty physicians were rarely present in teaching hospitals except for the occasional on-call attending anesthesiologist or operating surgeon. Some in emergency medicine began to discuss providing a more consistent teaching presence in the late 1970s and early 1980s. Unlike other services, the ED was often busiest in the evening and night, and emergency attending physicians were often leaving for the day just as the ED was heating up. In emergency medicine, residents were taking care of critically ill patients, making important diagnostic and treatment decisions, and seeing many more patients per day than their nonemergency medicine counterparts in other residencies. The benefits of 24-hour faculty coverage were obvious. Residents would receive instruction and guidance throughout their shifts, mistakes might be prevented, and patient care might be improved.

At community teaching hospitals where the ED was staffed by an emergency medicine group that billed for its services, 24-hour attending physician coverage was common, and resident physicians were treated as an addition to the mix. For example, the Henry Ford Hospital emergency physician group had 24-hour attending physician coverage for at least 2 years before the residency was started in 1976.[25] The situation was different in the traditional university and urban teaching hospitals, where faculty typically did not bill patients for their services and had barely enough members to cover the ED during the day. These faculty members felt they would be overworked if they were required to provide around-the-clock coverage, and did not relish the thought of spending their nights, weekends, or holidays in the ED. Paradoxically, a mandate to provide 24-hour teaching coverage was viewed as antiacademic by some because the additional clinical supervision time required of faculty members would limit their time to conduct research and write papers and books.[38] The situation created a strange inversion in the early to mid-1980s, where many practicing physicians and the ACEP board of directors called for 24-hour faculty coverage in emergency medicine residency programs and many in the academic world opposed it.

The issue arose out of discussions at the national level by the Graduate Medical Education Advisory Committee (GMEAC) of the AMA and the ACGME. It was brought to the forefront by the 1984 Libby Zion case described in the last section of this chapter. The idea for mandatory 24-hour attending physician coverage in emergency medicine training was advanced in the RRC for Emergency Medicine in 1985 in its revision of the special requirements for emergency medicine residencies. An immediate outcry was heard from some emergency medicine residency faculty around the country. Brooks Bock, who was on the RRC at the time, remembers, "People were very angry…at the RRC. I can remember folks…writing about this and saying you'll close down our program."[24] The Society for Teachers of Emergency Medicine and the ACEP Academic Affairs Committee formally opposed the requirement for 24-hour faculty coverage. The ACEP board of directors overruled its committee by coming out in favor of the requirement, and many academicians spoke resentfully about ACEP overstepping its "proper role" and delving into these academic matters (39). UAEM remained officially silent on the matter. Markedly contentious editorials appeared in the emergency medicine journals, with some residency leaders claiming that a requirement for 24-hour coverage would cause their residencies to collapse.[39,40] Brooks Bock recalls,

> They didn't believe that their institutions would provide the financial support and I also think quite candidly they didn't want to work the night shifts…Nobody would say that one up on top of the table. You know, the RRC did what I think is the right thing—ten people who took a bold step together and said we don't really care that there are a lot of our colleagues who say this is wrong, we are going to support this.[24]

Some academicians did support 24-hour coverage. Peter Rosen and Vince Markovchick wrote a strong essay supporting around-the-clock faculty coverage in EDs and noted, "Emergency medicine has an unparalleled opportunity to provide a new kind of education and patient service…Let us not sacrifice our opportunity for leadership for convenience of lifestyle."[41,42] They noted that the requirement could be used by emergency medicine chairman and directors to appeal to their institutions for money to hire more faculty. This, in fact, happened at several traditional medical school teaching hospitals, including Gabor Kelen's program at Johns Hopkins University.[34] Twenty-four–hour attending physician coverage in emergency medicine residencies was discussed and debated for more than 2 years in the RRC, ACGME, and AMA. The opposition was strong enough to prevent any definitive action. Finally, in 1989 the ACGME mandated that all RRCs must change their special requirements to address resident working hours and supervision. The RRC in Emergency Medicine, with ACGME approval, required 24-hour faculty supervision of emergency medicine residents, effective July 1, 1989.[43,44] Emergency medicine thus became the first medical specialty to mandate this level of supervision, and this had many indirect repercussions. The emergency medicine attending physician became the only attending physician in the hospital after midnight at most teaching hospitals, and medical students and resident physicians from other fields saw that emergency medicine residents were receiving direct, hands-on supervision of their work, rather than *ex post facto* review during daily attending rounds. The educational high road that emergency medicine took in this case helped to build the academic credibility of the young specialty.

SETTING TRENDS IN POSTGRADUATE MEDICAL EDUCATION

The emergency medicine residency programs of the middle 1980s were extremely different from the pioneer programs of the early 1970s. In just over a decade, the educational quality improved markedly, and it can be argued that emergency medicine became a leader in how to train residents. Although postgraduate medical education in traditional medical specialties continued to follow the old paradigm of resident-run teaching services and once-a-day attending rounds, emergency medicine had full-time faculty supervision and real-time, direct bedside teaching. Standards for attending emergency physicians on supervision, teaching, publications, and research were proposed by James Pointer and Robert Dailey in 1984.[45] Emergency medicine was also making strides in other areas of resident education. The refinement and standardization of off-service rotations by the RRC helped emergency medicine residents to learn and experience from other specialties those things that were crucial for emergency care, and to avoid servitude that had little educational value. As emergency medicine faculty became more experienced as teachers, didactic programs and curricula were developed to teach the core content defined by ACEP and ABEM. The plan was for each resident to receive formal instruction in all elements of the core content by the end of residency.[46]

Some programs became creative by offering unique away rotations for their emergency medicine residents. The University of Maryland Shock/Trauma Unit welcomed visiting emergency medicine residents, and several programs that lacked a busy trauma volume sent their residents to shock/trauma for a trauma rotation. At the Henry Ford Hospital emergency medicine residency program, residents have the opportunity to do a visiting ED rotation in Hawaii, working in a hospital ED that was run by a former residency graduate. Emergency medicine residencies in the 1980s also began to train their residents in emergency medical services—the realm that was truly unique to the field. The University of Pittsburgh program run by Ronald Stewart and Paul Paris was probably the most advanced in this regard, as residents dashed about the city in small trucks, meeting ambulances at the scene of cardiac arrests and accidents.[47]

Many of the military surgeons from the Vietnam War were excited about the potential for implementing civilian emergency medical helicopter services. The Maryland Shock–Trauma Program began using helicopters in the early 1970s, and by the middle 1980s, helicopter ambulance services were springing up at many large private medical centers.[48] Physicians became part of some medical helicopter teams and once emergency medicine residents were plentiful enough to be used in this capacity, they were asked to fly. By the end of 1987, there were 145 emergency aeromedical transport programs, and around 20 of these regularly flew physicians on the helicopter team.[49] Safety became a major concern as hospital-based aeromedical programs experienced a high rate of crashes and events. Between 1975 and 1986 42 people were killed in 15 medical transport helicopter crashes. The aeromedical program at Loma Linda University in California had two crashes, with nine fatalities, before it was terminated in 1981. An emergency medicine resident physician was killed in a crash while flying as part of the medical team on the St. Vincent's Hospital Life Flight program in Toledo, Ohio, in 1985.[50] Given this poor safety record, some emergency medicine residents, particularly those with spouses and children, were not enthusiastic about being on aeromedical teams, but most liked the idea of flying.[51] Residency programs usually allowed residents to choose whether they would fly, and aeromedical programs became a recruiting tool for emergency medicine residencies. The fact that emergency medicine residents were flying to the scene of medical emergencies and accidents and intubating patients, placing chest tubes, and managing critically ill patients—all before the patient arrived at the hospital—added to the allure of the field for many medical students. EMS and aeromedical experiences were two distinguishing features of emergency medicine training. While residents in other fields could, as part of their training, work in EDs, handle critical medical or surgical cases, and might do elective rotations like emergency medicine residents, they did not have EMS training as part of their residency. Turf issues were always present inside the hospital, but no other residents could legitimately claim that EMS was not the domain of emergency medicine resident.

The first emergency medicine residencies were 2-year training programs after an internship year. From its start, ABEM required 36 months of postgraduate training, 24 months of which had to be in an emergency medicine residency, to sit for the board examinations. The Medical College of Pennsylvania program became the first to incorporate the internship into a 3-year emergency medicine residency. The advantages of a 3-year integrated program were that medical students could match straight out of residency into an emergency medicine residency, without the uncertainty of applying to a residency during internship, and the added educational material that could be presented in a 3-year emergency medicine curriculum. Other programs followed MCP's lead and adopted a postgraduate year (PGY) 1,2,3 format, so that by 1985 about half of emergency medicine residencies were PGY 1,2, or 3 and half had an internship followed by PGY 2 and 3.

In 1984 ABEM mandated that beginning in 1987, 36 months of emergency medicine training would be required to sit for the board examination.[52] Some resistance was voiced, but it was hard for anyone in emergency medicine to argue that in this broad field, which also encompassed critical care, that the duration of training should be less than what was required in family practice and internal medicine. ABEM stopped short of requiring that all PGY 2,3 programs become PGY 1,2,3 programs, therefore many PGY 2,3 programs simply added another 12 months of training to become PGY 2,3,4 programs. By 1988, of the 68 U.S. emergency medicine residencies, 62% were PGY 1,2,3 programs, and 27% were PGY 2,3,4 programs. The remaining 11% (eight programs) represented a new breed of emergency medicine residency program—the PGY 1,2,3,4 programs.

It was a natural progression that the creation of PGY 2,3,4 programs would stimulate some academicians in emergency medicine to consider a 4-year residency program that included the internship. Richard Levy who was director of emergency medicine at Cincinnati and William Barsan, his former resident who had become the residency director, wrote an article in *Annals of Emergency Medicine* in 1982 that touted the benefits of a 4-year residency.[53] They cited that residents would be able to learn more in the clinical setting and in didactic programs and there would be more opportunities for elective off-service and critical care rotations. Surprisingly, they did not mention research experience or development as an educator as other advantages. From the emergency medicine faculty member's standpoint, having a group of PGY 4 residents around who could help to supervise junior residents and medical students in the ED was highly desirable. The first PGY 1,2,3,4 residency program in emergency medicine started in Cincinnati in 1983, where 13 years earlier Bruce Janiak had been the first emergency medicine resident. By 1987, eight emergency medicine programs had followed Cincinnati's lead and offered 4-year, integrated residencies.

A lively debate developed, which exists to this day, over whether all emergency medicine residencies should go to a 4-year format. The arguments advanced by Barsan and Levy in 1982 are viewed by many as still valid. The question is posed: if it takes 4 years to train a pathologist or radiologist, how can 3 years of training be adequate for a specialist who must acquire a huge bank of medical knowledge and learn how to apply that knowledge in emergency situations? The advocates of a 3-year emergency medicine training program point out that it has never been proven that 4-year residency graduates make superior clinicians or academicians on completion of residency and that those 3-year graduates who wish to further their education can do so with fellowship experiences.[54] The economics of medicine crept into this debate starting in 1986, when caps were established on federal funding for residency training, limiting the payments for additional years beyond the standard training period.[55] The debate has created an odd, static state at the level of the RRC, such that emergency medicine remains the only medical specialty where training programs of different durations are permitted. (Some surgical and surgical subspecialty fields have embedded research years in their residencies, but these are in addition to the RRC-mandated clinical training requirements.)

Resident physicians have historically supplemented their meager salaries by moonlighting at other medical institutions, and this work has often been in emergency departments. Many smaller hospitals have relied on resident moonlighters to cover their EDs on nights and weekends. Karl Mangold started his emergency medicine business as a resident moonlighter and sustained it for many years in the Bay area of California by hiring other resident moonlighters. In most states, a physician license could be obtained after 1 or 2 years of postgraduate training, and this was all that was required by most hospitals for a young physician to be hired as an ED moonlighter.

For other medical fields, allowing incompletely trained, unsupervised physicians to work in an ED is risky and inappropriate, but for emergency medicine it is also hypocritical. The mantra of academic emergency medicine and ABEM was that emergency medicine should be practiced by ABEM-certified, emergency medicine residency trained or practice-eligible physicians. From the early days of emergency medicine, resident physicians were wooed by smaller regional hospitals to moonlight in their EDs. In many cases, an incompletely trained emergency medicine resident could practice at higher level than the "regular" emergency physicians employed by that hospital. Emergency medicine residency program directors and faculty generally looked the other way, rationalizing that this work was adding to the resident's clinical experience. Only when residents began to look worn out from their extracurricular moonlighting activities, or began driving better cars than their faculty, were they reined in. Some resident moonlighters could double their income through outside ED work and some received additional income by functioning as physician staffing brokers or managers of other residents. The moonlighting issue was occasionally challenged by those who had fought to sanctify emergency medicine. Ron Krome wrote in a 1986 editorial,

> It seems schizophrenic to me that, on one hand, we insist that physicians complete a 3-year training program before we allow them to be let loose on the public, and on the other hand, we allow them to practice independently prior to completion of the training program under the guise of growth and experience.[56]

Despite these cautions, emergency medicine residents in most programs continued to moonlight with impunity. It was not until 3 years ago that SAEM came out with a policy against resident moonlighting, referring to the practice as "unsupervised emergency department care."[57]

CREATING THE ACADEMIC TRAPPINGS OF A NEW SPECIALTY

When emergency medicine was approved as a specialty in 1979, it had a single journal, only one textbook with an emergency physician editor, little role in medical school education, and almost no research base. Because no one had taken on the task of describing, in a scholarly way, the realm of emergency medicine, critics could effectively argue that emergency medicine lacked a defined, distinct core body of knowledge. The great breadth that made the field so much fun to practice—an old man with a heart attack one minute, a child with a cut finger the next—made it difficult for early academic leaders to proclaim areas of expertise. In the eyes of the medical world and public, the cardiologist was the expert in heart attacks, the hand surgeon in wounds of the hand, and the emergency physician was a curious new figure in the mix. The handful of emergency medicine academicians who were expert in their areas of research or medical education had not yet gained national notoriety.

TEXTBOOKS

Few of the early leaders of emergency medicine had the academic training or position to be able to embark on a textbook of emergency medicine, and their time was consumed with fighting the political battles for specialty recognition. The first textbooks of emergency medicine following the establishment of independent emergency practice were not written primarily by emergency physicians. As was noted in Chapter 2, Thomas Flint wrote the first modern U.S. textbook of emergency medicine in 1954. In 1967, Charles Eckert, M.D., the chairman of the department of surgery at Albany Medical College in New York published a textbook called *Emergency-Room Care*. This book featured chapters on medical emergencies organized by body system or disease process, written by 24 faculty members at Albany Medical College. The book describes the academic ED at Albany Medical Center Hospital, but treats each emergency condition as a specialist's problem, rather than describing the approach an emergency physician would need to take.[58]

The first emergency physician to edit a textbook of emergency medicine was George Schwartz, who had as co-editors, David Wagner, Peter Safar, Patrick Storey, and John Stone. *Principles and Practice of Emergency Medicine* was published in 1978 after about 6 years of planning and writing. Schwartz was an emergency physician who had worked in the community, then joined Wagner's program at MCP as one of the first faculty. Wagner speaking of Schwartz, remembers,

> He was always a prethinker and thinking on the edge, but you knew that you needed—if you are going to have a specialty—you need a textbook. You need your body of knowledge. Your body of knowledge is what comes together. The first one came together just as the specialty did, by individuals from traditional specialties.[7]

Schwartz and Wagner used experts like Peter Safar, the anesthesiologist from Pittsburgh, to write about cardiopulmonary resuscitation and John Stone, the cardiologist and poet from Emory University, to write about myocardial infarction and other topics. The book was quite successful, but probably not more so than other emergency medicine textbooks that came out around this time, which were written by nonemergency physicians. Earle W. Wilkins, Jr., who was a surgeon at Harvard, and the chief of emergency services at Massachusetts General Hospital teamed with James Dineen, who had run the MGH Fellowship in Emergency Medicine for many years, and an MGH surgeon named Ashby Moncure to edit the *MGH Textbook of Emergency Medicine*, also published in 1978. The first textbooks published after the advent of residency training for emergency physicians were not much different from prior textbooks on emergency care. They lacked a cohesive feel and ended up being a cobbling of separate chapters, by separate experts, who often wrote little about the practical emergency diagnosis and care of their topics. Peter Rosen remembers submitting a chapter on shock for the Schwartz text as a rough draft. Rosen never heard back about the chapter, and it was published in this draft form without being edited.[2]

Rosen felt the need for a textbook from his early academic days, and perusing what was available in the late 1970s left him thinking that he should undertake a big task. He remembers thinking that some of the nonemergency medicine writers in the Schwartz book were "incredibly arrogant" and condescending regarding the capabilities of emergency physicians. In Rosen's view, a true emergency medicine textbook needed to be written exclusively by emergency physicians.[2] David Wagner also felt this way, noting that he dissociated himself from the Schwartz text,

> I bowed off after the second edition because I thought the time was right, and of course Peter was very right in doing this, and that was to get your textbook done and get it edited by emergency physicians and we have had this as a philosophy…and that is: Emergency medicine is taught by emergency physicians.[7]

Rosen recruited as co-editors other academic leaders in emergency medicine who he thought had the editing and organizational skills to pull together a comprehensive text. He called on his friend Bob Dailey, Frank Baker, who succeeded Rosen as director of emergency medicine at the University of Chicago, Richard Braen, who was chair of emergency medicine at the University of Kentucky, and Richard Levy from Cincinnati for the effort. Rosen had been having a dialogue with Thomas Manning, a representative from C.V. Mosby Publishers, who was a former paramedic, and wanted to get Mosby involved in the emergency medicine market. Manning made two important suggestions. The first was that the textbook should be referenced in the text. Previous emergency medicine textbooks, and most medical texts of the times, consisted of chapters written by experts, who dispensed dogma, but did not provide in-text references to support their recommendations or conclusions. A well-referenced textbook would take a year longer to produce, but Manning convinced Rosen and his associate editors that this was the future of medical textbooks, and they would have added credibility if they used this approach. As the editors considered how to organize the book, Rosen remembers that Manning also came up with the suggestion to split the book into two major sections, one on trauma, and the other on nontraumatic disorders and diseases. These first-time textbook editors did not attempt to cover every aspect of emergency medicine. They intentionally left out chapters on ED administration, preferring to focus on the science of the field.

The next step was to recruit emergency medicine authors for the chapters in the book. At this time, there were only a handful of emergency medicine academicians who could be considered expert educators or researchers in specific areas of emergency medicine. For example, no emergency physician of those times was considered to be an expert on abdominal trauma. The editors were faced with the paradox that a textbook written by only emergency medicine authors would mean that most of the chapters would be authored by physicians who were not expert in the topic matter. Rosen and the associate editors recruited or consigned physicians from their programs and around the country to write chapters. John Marx, was a junior resident in the Denver program in 1979. He remembers Rosen approaching him,

> He comes up to me and says, "Say, Marx, want to write a chapter on abdominal trauma?" Of course we needed a textbook that we would write—we emergency physicians would write...Peter just corralled a bunch of people, who believe me, were not necessarily the least bit skilled in writing and, that sure as hell includes me, who were not necessarily expert in the subject....[26]

The authors sometimes consulted with local experts to increase their knowledge in the topic area, but the chapters were often a solitary endeavor. For example, for his abdominal trauma chapter, Marx says, "I didn't ask anyone for help. I pulled every article I could find in the world, scattered them around me and started."[59] Peter Rosen remembers the final stages of preparing the textbook:

> I read the galleys, forwards for content and backwards for typos. Because when you are concentrating on meaning you can't see typos. I finally got a copy of the bound book and I opened it up and the first word I came to was a typo. I decided that words were like radioactive isotopes, that they were all right in galley but they decayed in the final version.[2]

Some important topics were not covered. Rosen remembers that they inadvertently did not include a chapter or discussion on child abuse, each associate editor thinking that the other had covered the topic. The end product, *Emergency Medicine: Concepts and Clinical Practice,* was the first, well-referenced, comprehensive textbook of emergency medicine by and for emergency physicians. The book was long, and not easily used as a quick reference guide in the ED, but it became very popular and respected as an authoritative text by both academicians and practicing emergency physicians. In subsequent editions, produced regularly every 4 to 5 years, "Rosen's" was refined and became the standard by which emergency medicine texts were judged. As John Marx notes,

> ...and now after five iterations we do in our field have the people who own the expertise through research and writing and other manners, who belong as the authors of a highly recognized chapter in a well-recognized book.[26]

Apparently, many other authors and publishers recognized the need, and market, for textbooks of emergency medicine once there was a board in emergency medicine and as residency programs proliferated. Within a year of the publication of Rosen's text, at least three other new textbooks of emergency medicine were rolled out. Thomas Kravis, M.D., chair of the department of emergency care at Mercy Hospital in San Diego, California, edited, with Carmen G. Warner, R.N., the first West coast–produced textbook of emergency medicine in 1983.[60] Two other new texts published at this time were not written by emergency physicians and repeated the old pattern of physicians in other specialties attempting to define and describe the field of emergency medicine and prescribing how emergency medicine should be practiced.[61,62] George Schwartz continued to produce his textbook and in later editions began to use more emergency physician authors. Ann Harwood-Nuss, M.D., who was an early emergency medicine residency director at Butterworth Hospital in Grand Rapids, Michigan, and then became chair of emergency medicine at University Hospital in Jacksonville, Florida, edited a popular, practice-oriented emergency medicine text, *The Clinical Practice of Emergency Medicine*, first published in 1991. Niche textbooks began to appear in emergency medicine, with a procedures textbook edited by Robert Simon, M.D., first published in 1982.[63] Roberts and Hedges *Clinical Procedures in Emergency Medicine*, published in 1985, became the definitive book on emergency procedures.[64] Soon to follow were books on emergency pharmacology, toxicology, emergency radiology, and atlases of emergency medicine. A predictable flood of handbooks and quick guides to be used while practicing in the emergency department then appeared.

While the large textbooks were the repositories for the core knowledge in the field, emergency physicians in practice, and emergency medicine residency graduates who were pointing toward the ABEM certifying examination needed a useful review text or study guide. This need was answered by Judith Tintinalli, M.D., who at the time was a young faculty member for Ron Krome at the Wayne State, Detroit Receiving Hospital program. Tintinalli remembers,

> At that time Peter Rosen, Bob Dailey, a guy named Gus Roussi…they were writing these worksheets, which were the basis for the questions on the board exam…for what they determined was the scope of what we needed to know in emergency medicine. So, at the end of their work, they had questions for the board exam and…a room full of papers. So, ACEP said what are we going to tell people to study for this exam? They said we need to write a book. I knew what the worksheets looked like and I thought, I've written for JACEP, I can do this…Well, like so many things in my life, I just said I can do it…So I called them and they said, "You're on!"[6]

Tintinalli traveled back and forth to Lansing, Michigan to peruse the mountains of papers and began to organize the material into sections and chapters that would provide condensed, essential information for the board exam. She wrote "85%" of the initial text and solicited others to write the pediatrics and toxicology sections (see insert, Figure 28). The initial book was published by ACEP in 1979 as a loose-leaf binder, and Tintinalli's intent was to provide a continual upgrade to the information. When she realized that she did not have the time to do this, the *Study Guide* became a book that was updated every few years, published first by McGraw-Hill in 1983. The *Study Guide* became an immediate success as a preparatory text for the boards, but also as a bedside practice guide at a time when the only reference works were the large text-books of emergency medicine. The *Study Guide* had the basics of disease presentation, diagnosis, and management in a few simple pages and was viewed as being more clinically useful than Rosen's and other textbooks. It also seemed to better fit the short attention span of the average emergency physician. The book became quite famous both in the United States and worldwide. Tintinalli always intended the book to be a guide, but saw that the book came to be viewed as the "world of information" in emergency medicine. She became unexpectedly well known for the book, and notes,

> My husband laughs. He says you are like a rock star, no shit…I was in Mexico on a vacation, it was not medicine…some ER doc found out I was there, before I know it there was a cocktail party in my honor…and then the next day they call me up 10 o'clock, "We are taking you on a tour of our EMS Training School." I mean this happens everywhere.[6]

After a slow start, emergency physicians, with medical publishers, had a very productive decade. By 1990, emergency medicine was as well supplied with quality textbooks, subspecialty books, and handbooks as any of the traditional medical specialties. Importantly for the field, the emergency medicine textbooks and other emergency care–related books produced by the late 1980s were edited and written by emergency physicians, not by physicians in other specialties.

JOURNALS

The early emergency medicine textbooks cited the existing scientific literature on emergency care, but that literature remained very sparse. As part of their membership in ACEP, emergency physicians received the *Journal of the American College of Emergency Physicians* (*JACEP*). *JACEP* served its purpose as a symbol of a credible journal, and a forum for keeping emergency physicians informed in the 1970s, but it did not compare favorably to established peer-reviewed journals in other medical fields. Lewis Goldfrank says, "I remember reading *JACEP* and really being discouraged entirely. I had been brought up on the *Annals of Internal Medicine* which is pretty rigorous and looking at this—what were we talking about—nothing."[65]

Emergency physicians of that era were as likely to consult and read *Emergency Medicine*, a proprietary, "throw away" journal (see Chapter 4), as they were *JACEP*, and the scientific content was not much different between the two journals. *Emergency Medicine* was published in New York City by Fischer-Murray, Inc., and had a colorful, lightly scientific approach of presenting discussions or reviews of clinical topics in emergency medicine by physician "experts" who often did not work in EDs. As a marketing-driven magazine, it was packed with dynamic medical advertisements that helped the emergency physician feel good about his or her practice. The magazine was extremely popular and widely read.

It was not until the late 1970s that original research manuscripts were regularly published in *JACEP* and the usual allotment was no more than one or two per issue. Most of the articles in *JACEP* were reviews or opinion pieces on aspects of emergency practice. The journal had a problem in that there were few emergency medicine researchers who could produce scientific manuscripts and those who did would be unlikely to want their research published in a weak, unheralded emergency medicine journal. John van de Leuv guided *JACEP* in its first year, and then handed the editorship over to Stanley Gold, who served until 1974 when Ron Krome was appointed editor. Krome was the first editor who was an academician and understood that *JACEP* had a long way to go before it would be considered a true scientific specialty journal.

One source of continuing friction regarding the journal was the role of UAEM and the desire of some in UAEM to form a separate journal. The academicians in UAEM were obviously not impressed with *JACEP* and believed that it was too heavily controlled by ACEP. They lobbied for an associate editor from UAEM to be appointed to the journal. When they threatened to form their own journal, ACEP, which was still linked to UAEM through its administrative service contract, appeased UAEM by making the journal "a joint venture" of ACEP and UAEM. In reality, UAEM did not have the financial resources to start its own journal at that time. One of UAEM's suggestions was that the journal name should drop the ACEP designation and be changed to *Annals of Emergency Medicine*. This issue had been tied up in legal proceedings since the early 1970s with the publishers of *Emergency Medicine*, who claimed that they owned the name. By 1980 this issue had been resolved so that ACEP was allowed to use the name "emergency medicine" in its journal.

When *JACEP* became the *Annals of Emergency Medicine* in 1980, Ron Krome, who was ideally situated in the ACEP and UAEM realms, made strong efforts to improve the organization and credibility of the journal. The journal began to have at least one or two original scientific manuscripts per issue. Scientific articles were aggressively solicited—presenters at the ACEP and UAEM scientific meetings were required to submit their papers to *Annals of Emergency Medicine*, which had right of first refusal for these manuscripts.[66] Krome eliminated the "blue pages," which consisted of ACEP news and reports, and gradually *Annals of Emergency Medicine* began to resemble the peer-reviewed journals in other fields. The manuscript rejection rate was about 40% in 1980, and the editorial board found that it increasingly had better quality manuscripts to review. Timeliness in the review process was a problem, and many authors complained about this. Krome ruled in a stern, but fair manner, and insisted on editorial independence for the journal, with ACEP and UAEM having no role in editorial content.[23]

Other emergency medicine journals sprang up in the 1980s. Peter Rosen got into the act in 1983 as the founding editor of the *Journal of Emergency Medicine*. His incentive came from the fact that he and other emergency physicians had articles rejected from *Annals of Emergency Medicine*, and then accepted for publication in other journals. This made Rosen think that there was room for another journal in emergency medicine. Rosen's journal was very clinically based, with many case reports and reviews of existing literature, and fewer original research manuscripts. The *Journal of Emergency Medicine* also provided Rosen with a ready platform from which to dispense his views and opinions. He wrote many influential editorials over the next decade on clinical practice and education in emergency medicine. These essays became, as David Wagner notes, somewhat of a "moral compass" for the specialty as it matured.[67]

The *American Journal of Emergency Medicine* was also started in 1983 with J. Douglas White, M.D., as the editor. This bimonthly journal published both laboratory and clinical research from its inception, and the scientific quality of manuscripts was as good as what appeared in *Annals of Emergency Medicine*. Some academic emergency physicians who were displeased with ACEP in the 1980s appear to have intentionally supported *American Journal of Emergency Medicine* and *Journal of Emergency Medicine* over *Annals of Emergency Medicine* because the latter journal was seen as run by ACEP. The few credible emergency physician scientists in the 1980s who were conducting high-quality laboratory or clinical research were quite loyal to the emergency medicine journals as venues for their scientific work. Some researchers, like Blaine White and James Niemann, could have published more extensively in other, more prestigious medical journals, but sent many of their manuscripts to emergency medicine journals for review and publication.

DEVELOPING RESEARCH IN EMERGENCY MEDICINE

In the late 1970s and early 1980s, emergency medicine developed, at least in a rudimentary manner, all the elements of a valid medical specialty. But in the area of scientific investigation emergency medicine had made little impact. Although the importance of research in an emerging field was stressed by R. R. Hannas and other early leaders from the very first ACEP meeting in 1968, there were many factors working against the development of research in emergency medicine. Most people who were initially attracted to the field found it fun and exciting to practice clinical emergency medicine and were less interested in focusing on scientific exploration. For those who had interest in research, the path was muddy. The traditional medical specialties had a tried-and-true development process for producing successful researchers. Young physicians did a research fellowship or training period under a well-funded mentor. Those physicians then wrote for smaller grants, then larger [usually NIH (National Institutes of Health)–funded] grants, and when successful would advance to become independent investigators. This formula was not appreciated by most early leaders in emergency medicine, who seemed to assume that some academicians and resident physicians would become interested in research and would independently learn how to do it right. The recognition that researchers were developed, not hatched, did not sink in for the field of emergency medicine until the 1990s. Another reason for the slow development of research in emergency medicine was a lack of skill and experience in obtaining funding. The NIH had large coffers for physician scientists who could identify the correct areas to study and write compelling grant applications, but few emergency physicians had mentors who could teach them how to do this and provide the connections at the NIH that might help. The most successful physician scientists were at the leading research-based medical schools, and emergency medicine had almost no presence at these institutions in the 1970s and 1980s. Mickey Eisenberg notes that emergency medicine investigators had some wide-open areas to claim as their own:

> ...the best bets at the time were resuscitation, overdose, prehospital, because no other specialty really cared that much about those things. So if you look at the original investigators in the field they were...trained outside the field of emergency medicine. A lot of them were cardiologists, others were internists, they wound up doing emergency medicine type research.[36]

It was often difficult for early academic emergency physicians to liaison with or model themselves after the leading investigators in other fields. Compounding this problem was the attitude of some emergency physicians. The battles for turf and respectability in the clinical realm created negative feelings between emergency medicine and other fields, making it unlikely that research relationships would develop. A final issue was lack of funding for emergency research. The only emergency medicine based funding source was the ACEP Emergency Medicine Foundation (EMF), which did not have a large enough endowment to make a significant impact. EMF was also viewed in a negative light by academicians in the late 1970s and 1980s. Jerris Hedges remembers his impression was that "EMF had been taking in lots of money from corporate sponsors and putting out almost nothing in terms of grants for researchers."[18] EMF was indeed using donor contributions to support its administrative costs. Brooks Bock, who was ACEP president in 1983/1983, heard these criticisms and decided to act on them. When he was past president and on the EMF board, he was instrumental in restructuring the foundation to include representation from UAEM, but ensured that ACEP paid the administrative overhead so that all money raised for the foundation actually went to support research.[24] Bock worked with James Niemann, a pioneer in emergency medicine research who was the chair of the ACEP research committee, to develop research fellowships and career development grants to support young investigators in emergency medicine. For the first time, emergency medicine was able to provide substantial funding to help develop the careers of young investigators.[68] Even with these changes, some academic physicians were disappointed that ACEP sometimes used its influence with EMF to siphon off money to pay for workforce or practice management studies. This reduced the amount of funding going to support original research by emergency physicians. As the only foundation to exclusively support emergency medicine investigators, EMF was an important symbol of what emergency medicine could do, but far more funding and fellowships would be needed to propel emergency medicine research to a level seen in other medical fields.

In the realm of research, as in residency training, emergency medicine in its early days tried *not* to follow in the footsteps of its predecessor, family practice. After it was approved as a specialty board in 1979, family practice emphasized clinical care, community medicine, and public health over research. This hindered the academic development of the field, especially at the major medical centers. Mickey Eisenberg notes that at the University of Washington in Seattle one of the arguments against establishing an emergency medicine presence was,

> *...that family medicine had become a specialty before emergency medicine and the argument was, well family medicine really hasn't been that academically productive, and maybe emergency medicine will also be unproductive.[35]*

In emergency medicine, the early academic leaders, although they were not researchers themselves, wrote about the importance of establishing credible research programs in academic emergency medicine.[69] Many early emergency physicians were enthusiastic about research and were constantly primed with research questions from their clinical emergency department work. Few therapies had been explored or fully investigated in the emergency setting, and new ideas for diagnosis and treatment popped up on almost a daily basis. But, like a child in a candy store, it was hard for the early emergency medicine faculty to focus their research efforts. Most were drawn to the field because of the great variety in clinical care, and they also liked variety in their research. It was not uncommon to have a faculty member dabble in one study in cardiac care or resuscitation and then shift to another in toxicology or infectious disease, or in some cases, to be simultaneously conducting multiple studies in different areas. This small-scale, hodgepodge research helped to inform many of the diagnostic and treatment dilemmas of early emergency practice, but it was not a way to establish successful research programs or careers. As James Niemann notes, in other academic disciplines,

> *...success was characterized by a research career that was more or less focused in an area of expertise in which you eventually gained national and international notoriety for your contributions. You can't do that by studying ten different things. You have no demonstrated expertise in any one of them.[70]*

The emergency medicine residents of the late 1970s and early 1980s were often more academically oriented than their teachers. Niemann believes

> ...they did not have a lot of direction from department chairmen. So the people who were heading departments of emergency medicine did not come up through a traditional academic track. They got their position because they were one of the first to be boarded in emergency medicine and they needed people that were boarded and they needed people who have some administrative skills. Those individuals don't serve well as mentors for research.[70]

Like parents of a gifted child, faculty encouraged their emergency medicine residents to become involved in research, but they usually could not provide proper mentors or tutors. Many emergency medicine programs tried to build their research programs off resident projects. Rebecca Anwar and David Wagner wrote in 1980 that, "Residents in emergency medicine offer a potential source of expertise that could be utilized in the development of...research activities."[71] Indeed, some of Wagner's residents—Michael Greenberg , Jerris Hedges, and William Spivey—developed into credible academic researchers. But using resident physicians to drive the research program of a developing academic emergency medicine program was laden with problems. Residents did not have the experience, training, or time to conduct meaningful, sustained research. A common result was small, nonfunded, underpowered research studies that often did not make it to publication. In coordinating or attempting to supervise resident research, faculty members were diverted from their own research interests and projects.

This shifting of the responsibility for research down the ladder was also seen in emergency medicine faculty groups. Emergency medicine academic departments in the 1980s, unlike most other medical specialties, often appointed a faculty member to be a research director. It was not uncommon for residents who had done some research during their training to be hired by academic programs and made research directors straight out of residency. At precisely the point in their careers where these young investigators should have been provided support and worked under the guidance of an experienced mentor, they were asked to administer research and mentor others. This smothered many promising young researchers in the field, who became too busy and fragmented to develop their own research careers. James Niemann notes,

> It continues to boggle my mind that there are people who are directing research who have probably two book chapters and a case report yet have the responsibility viewed by title only, to direct the research efforts of a residency training program, which is probably totally inappropriate.[70]

The problem of the inexperienced leading the inexperienced persists. A survey of emergency medicine research directors from 1995 found that 42% lacked fellowship training or a research degree and over half were at an assistant professor level or below.[72]

For many early emergency medicine faculty physicians, research pursuits were limited because of a lack of research infrastructure or departmental support. Expensive laboratory equipment was very hard to obtain. At the Cincinnati program, Mel Otten notes,

> I remember doing research as a junior faculty member here in my office—I had a centrifuge on my desk, big old refrigerator in my office where we kept all the blood specimens and we would spin them down on the centrifuge and we would borrow equipment from different labs around the city...Bill Barsan...and I went over and borrowed the physiograph and some other stuff from Jewish Hospital...We went over there because they were closing down...the lab and they had all this great machinery...and stuff that we wanted to do research, animal research with, so Bill and I went over there and got the stuff and the cardiology department here had lent us a space in their animal lab where we could set up our equipment, and did all our dog research and stuff. That's how we did it. All with borrowed equipment and no money.[73]

The old Hewlett-Packard physiograph that Otten and Barsan "borrowed" from Jewish Hospital was used by a generation of residents and faculty who did large-animal research in borrowed laboratory space at the University of Cincinnati.

Fortunately for emergency medicine, a few research-oriented physicians carved their niches and had some success in research. One of the first was Blaine White, M.D., who was hired by Ron Krome at Wayne State/Detroit Receiving Hospital. Krome calls White, in the same breath, "a fantastic hire," and "a true eccentric." The department of surgery provided laboratory space and enough money for animals and equipment for White to set up a laboratory to study global cerebral ischemia and the biomolecular changes seen in the brain following cardiac arrest and ischemia. For all of his quirks, White, who often smoked a pipe in his nonsmoking lab as he planned new research ideas and experiments and, according to Krome "used to resign once a month," became a funded investigator.[74] A few months after *JACEP* became the *Annals of Emergency Medicine* in 1980, the lead article was authored by White and his colleagues. The title, "Mitochondrial O_2 use and ATP synthesis: kinetic effects of Ca^{++} and HPO_4^{-2} modulated by glucocorticoids," was probably a bit foreign to the clinically oriented emergency physician readership.[75] But at the same time they applauded the fact that a fellow emergency physician was conducting basic science research.

David Wagner was also determined to create a research program at the Medical College of Pennsylvania. His early residency graduates were the most precocious of the early emergency physicians in terms of research productivity. Michael Greenberg, M.D., and James Roberts, M.D., became well known for their work on administering resuscitative drugs through an endotracheal tube rather than by the intravenous route or intracardiac route. Wagner remembers that this work was "a practical application of something that was just the right thing at the right time—to discover that you could give these medicines without puncturing the heart and it would work just as well."[7] The early work was done in dog models at MCP and then progressed quickly to experiments in humans. In 1979, Greenberg and Roberts authored two papers in the December issue of *JACEP*—one describing the use of endotracheal epinephrine in a dog model of anaphylactic shock and the other using endotracheal epinephrine in patients with cardiorespiratory collapse.[76,77]

David Wagner was also the first person to begin researching the epidemiology and demographics of emergency medicine and residency training. He hired a young doctor of philosophy, Rebecca Anwar, who was interested in social and health services research. Anwar secured grant funding from the National Center for Health Services Research and developed several studies on the professional and social characteristics of residents in training. Her papers documented the growth of emergency medicine in its first decade and the reasons for this growth. As an independent investigator who was not tied to ACEP or UAEM, Anwar's work helped to provide a scholarly chronicle of how the field was developing.[78,79]

The emergency medicine program at the University of California Los Angeles, and the UCLA–Harbor program became the west coast leaders in emergency medicine research. James Niemann, M.D. was a faculty member in emergency medicine, who like Blaine White, had previous training in internal medicine. During his residency, Niemann began to do cardiac resuscitation research with Michael Criley, M.D., who was a cardiologist but also a key faculty member in the emergency department. Niemann discovered that his research interests and clinical interests merged,

> ...*everything just sort of fell into place at the right time. It was a perfect storm as you will, and then I was completing my training in internal medicine and came to the realization that my greatest satisfaction was caring for the most acutely ill and that my major area of interest happened to be acute cardiovascular physiology so everything happened at the same time.*[70]

Niemann joined the new emergency medicine program at UCLA–Harbor in 1979 as an assistant professor. Unlike most emergency medicine faculty who were interested in research, Niemann followed the traditional approach of mentoring under and collaborating with other investigators at UCLA and at other institutions. He struggled as did all emergency medicine investigators with research space, supplies, and funding, but he slowly built one of the most successful research programs in emergency medicine. Finally, in 1988, Niemann was rewarded with his own, independent laboratory space at UCLA–Harbor.

Niemann remembers the excitement of meeting other emergency medicine researchers, in particular Blaine White, at a UAEM meeting in 1981. Niemann says, "We sort of looked around and said, boy there is a lot of surgeons here but not too many emergency physicians."[70] Niemann's interests in cardiac resuscitation and White's in brain resuscitation were different, but they shared the same passion and commitment to advancing research in their new field.

Given the limited research backgrounds of most early academic emergency physicians, it is not surprising that physicians with nonemergency medicine backgrounds played the biggest role in stimulating and advancing research in the field. Both Blaine White and James Niemann trained in the research traditions of internal medicine before they came to emergency medicine. Mickey Eisenberg similarly became one of the most important EMS and resuscitation researchers out of an internal medicine home base. One of most visible and controversial proponents of research in emergency medicine was trauma surgeon Kenneth Mattox. Mattox, who was an early member of UAEM, stayed in the organization as he watched many of his surgical colleagues leave. As someone who was heavily involved in EMS and trauma care in Houston, Texas, Mattox saw that emergency physicians were not going away, so he made it his mission to critique and cajole emergency medicine to do the hard work required for academic advancement. Mary Ann Schropp who worked with Mattox when he was UAEM president remembers "…he was real loud, he just loved to fight…He wanted to be devil's advocate on everything…and he pushed research very early, much earlier than the rest of the people in emergency medicine did."[80] James Niemann distinctly remembers Mattox's role in UAEM.

> Ken was sort of a provocateur by choice—tended to be fairly radical. He would make these…broad statements criticizing and critiquing current medical practice, which on the surface could be interpreted as being either self-serving or totally off the wall, but he really lived for what he was talking about. He was pretty much right on.[70]

Although not well liked by many academic emergency physicians, Mattox was a very effective grain of sand in the oyster of academic emergency medicine. He seemed to hope that his irritating presence would help to form a quality research pearl. In numerous essays, speeches, and editorials, Mattox implored emergency medicine to investigate in a sound scientific manner the many untested, unproven therapies in resuscitation, toxicology, and trauma.[81,82] While president of UAEM in 1979, Mattox trumpeted the organization for having membership requirements of academic standing and interests and for having the only scientific meeting where original research was presented and critiqued.

Other emergency medicine investigators began to establish credible research programs in emergency medicine. Charles Brown at the Ohio State University program also conducted cardiac resuscitation research, built a strong laboratory program, and trained emergency medicine fellows. James Niemann helped to train two bright and talented research fellows, Charles Cairns and James Manning, who would go on to establish research laboratories at other institutions. Niemann in particular became a strong advocate for fellowship training in emergency medicine.[68] Blaine White established a hatchery for emergency medicine investigators in his Wayne State laboratory, producing several investigators who went on to become funded, independent investigators in emergency medicine. By the end of the 1980s, high-quality emergency medicine research programs had also developed at Henry Ford Hospital, the University of Pittsburgh, and Johns Hopkins University. This handful of programs was starting to resemble the strong research programs in other medical disciplines, with a focused research approach, federal grant support, fellowship training, and a willingness to collaborate with investigators from other fields.

THE ROLE OF EMERGENCY MEDICINE IN MEDICAL EDUCATION

Emergency medicine became popular as a career choice for a small proportion of medical students within a few years of the beginning of emergency medicine residencies. Those students who did electives in EDs where there were successful emergency medicine training programs usually found it fun and invigorating to see undifferentiated patients, make a diagnosis, and initiate treatment. Few other medical school experiences allowed them to function "like a real doctor." By 1976, about 75% of U.S. medical schools offered electives in emergency medicine, but medical student supervision in the ED was typically as bad as it was for residents.[83] Since most academic teaching center EDs in the 1970s and 1980s were divided into separate sections for medical, surgical, pediatrics, and psychiatric patients, there was little chance for the average medical student to understand how a well-functioning ED might work. They also did not see emergency physicians in action, because faculty members were frequently not present in the ED, and the few emergency medicine residents were not always distinguishable in these busy environments.

The increased specialization of medicine and increased role for specialists in educating medical students meant less time for basic education in emergency care, and few emergency medicine faculty existed to champion education in their realm. However, a number of people were developing training programs in emergency medicine for medical students. The national attention that had been focused on emergency medical services starting with the NAS/NRC report in 1966 (see Chapter 3), and then through ACEP, UAEM, and the American College of Surgeons, spilled over into medical education. A required, 52-hour course in emergency care was instituted by the George Washington University School of Medicine and Health Sciences in 1976. The course was given to first-year medical students and was derived from an emergency medical technician training program. By 1976, ten medical schools offered courses in emergency care or first aid for first-year medical students. Seven medical schools offered emergency medicine experiences in the third or fourth year. A required clerkship in emergency medicine was developed at the New Jersey Medical School of the College of Medicine and Dentistry of New Jersey.[84] Notably absent in the list of schools that offered emergency medicine training for medical students were the traditional, top-ranked medical schools.

At the same time that emergency medicine was developing as a new entity, some educators were bemoaning the lack of practical knowledge possessed by graduating medical students. For some, the ED came to be viewed as a training site for medical students where they could help care for undifferentiated patients and learn "bread and butter" aspects of many clinical problems as well as critical care. In the 1980s, more medical schools began offering training in emergency care as part of the curriculum. A 1984 survey found that one fourth of U.S. medical schools had a required emergency medicine experience in the first year, but less than 15% had a required experience in the third or fourth year of medical school. Over 90% of schools offered an emergency medicine elective in the fourth year.[85] Even with these advances, emergency medicine remained a minor player in the overall picture of medical education. Medical students were discouraged from considering emergency medicine as a career option even a decade after the field became a recognized specialty. A familiar refrain from internists, surgeons, and others who advised medical students in the 1980s was that emergency medicine was a risky career move, that burn out was high, and that emergency physicians functioned mainly as triage officers in the medical system. Despite these negative influences, the allure of emergency medicine for medical students increased, and emergency medicine residency programs saw their numbers of applicants rise, along with the quality of those applicants.

THE 25-YEAR WAR: EMERGENCY MEDICINE IN NEW YORK CITY

New York City is usually an epicenter for new movements and cultural change. But in the field of emergency medicine, particularly in terms of academic development,

New York was like a ponderous, creaking metal door, slowly pushed open over three decades. New York State was not necessarily hostile to emergency medicine. In fact, one of the earliest Alexandria Plan–type groups was started upstate in Binghamton by five full-time emergency physicians in 1965.[86] But emergency medicine elsewhere in the state had little influence on what happened in the city. The size and complexity of the New York hospital system, the huge burden of indigent, uninsured patients, and stubbornness of a few key opponents created a battlefield unlike any other for emergency medicine. In most other cities, the emergency medicine struggle was played out within the halls and meeting rooms of academic medical centers. In New York City, the battle for improved emergency care and training was in city and state governments and played out on the front page and editorial pages of newspapers and the television evening news.

When Lewis Goldfrank came to the Bronx to complete his residency training in internal medicine from 1971 to 1973, he was focused on helping the underserved in the community. He gravitated to the emergency departments of his training sites—Montefiore Hospital and Morrisania Hospital in the South Bronx—because this was where the patients with greatest need presented for help. Unlike many of the early leaders of emergency medicine, Goldfrank's migration to emergency medicine was totally from a public health perspective. He says, "I wasn't sure that emergency was the solution for what I saw as this ambulatory care problem."[65] He initially focused on trying to improve ambulatory care clinics, and if he had thought he could do the most good in this area, he probably would have stayed in internal medicine. But, in the EDs of New York City, Goldfrank saw a public health crisis around which he could build a career. When he completed his residency, Golfrank became the director of the ED at Morrisania Hospital. He remembers,

> We began to institute systems, to triage patients using volunteers and nurses, establishing critical care and trauma rooms and a separate place for children. When we required that all patients' vital signs be taken, we found severe hypertension in large numbers of people. We saw ten people a day who appeared asymptomatic yet had diastolic blood pressures greater than 130 mm Hg, 15 to 20 patients a day with critical asthma, five to ten patients with heroin overdoses, multiple patients with gun shot wounds and stabbings, child abuse and neglect, and a gonorrhea and syphilis epidemic. All of these patients had problems that led us to innovative solutions. This was a unique era in medicine.[87]

The hospital EDs were totally staffed by interns and residents, and Goldfrank was not provided the resources to hire many attending physicians or faculty. He remembers,

> I think my wife and kids would have said it was very difficult. I'd go to work, get to work early and leave late. I would have to be reminded sometimes, there was no one else, so every time I left I felt someone was just dying. There wasn't any support.[87]

A high percentage of patients who presented to Morrisania Hospital ED had nonurgent problems or were seeking primary care. Goldfrank used a public health approach by creating a referral system to get patients into ambulatory and primary care sites. He had internal medicine residents work in the ED and then provide follow-up clinic care to the ED patients they saw. He was able to show a decrease in hospitalizations for asthma, diabetes, and other chronic diseases.[88] Goldfrank also found the time to conduct research in this busy setting. He had a long-standing interest in toxicology and trialed the use of naloxone for opiate overdoses. Goldfrank as a researcher did not approach specific research questions or try to focus on one area. He saw the whole picture and research as just one component. In emergency medicine, he felt that it was "obvious that we could define a medical problem, investigate, develop a solution, and confront great political issues."[87] In the realm of emergency medicine, Goldfrank remained a loner, focused almost entirely on serving the needs of his community. He did not become involved in emergency medicine organizations at this time. He notes,

> I'd gone to an ACEP meeting once and I didn't like the people at all, I just never felt at home. They talked about money and about a shared practice and I said I don't know

there is any money in the job at all. I can't imagine how you would make any money doing emergency medicine, I'm more a public servant than I'm anything else, so it wasn't the talk I could share....[65]

Elsewhere in New York, others were approaching the care of emergency patients with as much vigor as Lewis Goldfrank. The Albert Einstein College of Medicine was formed in the 1950s with a commitment to educate and care for people without regard for race, gender, or social standing, and the physician educators of this medical school had a history of being socially active. At one of its clinical affiliates, Jacobi Hospital, the ED was bustling, and in 1974 Sheldon Jacobson, M.D., started an emergency medicine residency. As the only emergency medicine residency in a huge metropolitan area, the Einstein/Jacobi program was able to recruit talented residents. One of the early graduates, Mark Henry, M.D., became, in 1979, the first emergency medicine residency–trained physician to become director of a department of emergency medicine in New York City at Booth Memorial Medical Center in Queens. One problem for those physicians who were considering careers in emergency medicine in New York City in the 1970s and 1980s was the poor rate of pay. While New York City internists in the 1980s might make $100,000 per year, the average emergency physician salary was $30,000 to $40,000 less than this. One of the reasons for low salaries was that the great majority of New York City hospitals had internships and residencies, and could staff their EDs with these low-cost employees. Also, there was an ample supply of foreign physicians who had completed internships in New York City hospitals but could not get into residency programs. With no standards for training or quality in the EDs, these physicians could be hired cheaply. This ED staffing model had sufficed for New York City hospitals from the 1950s to the late 1970s, but a number of pressures would mandate change. As it became clear that other large U.S. cities had multiple emergency medicine residencies, with hospitals mostly staffed by career emergency physicians, some questioned why New York lagged behind. The EMS system of New York was developing rapidly in the 1970s, and as Goldfrank notes, this "created a gap between the newly organized prehospital care and the persistent chaos of most hospital EDs."[87] The EMS Act of 1973 and the update in 1976 required potential grant recipients to develop regional, organized systems, and hospital and physician leadership in these efforts could not come from interns assigned to the ED.

All New York City public hospitals were controlled and owned by the Health and Hospitals Corporation (HHC). The HHC was established in 1970 in response to the continuing deterioration of medical care and facilities in New York municipal hospitals and was housed under the city's Health Services Agency.[89] Goldfrank remembers the HHC at that time as "a relatively impoverished, socialized system." Once the HHC was in existence, it was clear that any major changes in emergency care in New York City municipal hospitals would need to be brokered through the HHC. Since the mayor appointed the HHC board, the entire process was political. While most would have viewed working with the HHC as an undesirable situation, Lewis Goldfrank was in his element, quoting Virchow, who said, "Medicine is a social science, and politics is nothing more than medicine on a grand scale."[87]

In 1979 Goldfrank moved to Bellevue, the oldest public hospital in the United States, where he was appointed as a tenured associate professor of medicine and director of emergency medical services. This was a challenge he actively sought. He remembers,

I think the political part of me would say that we are doing great things in the South Bronx, but no one cared. It was too far for CBS or New York Times to go and look, and who cared what you did, the people were so poor in the South Bronx it didn't affect the affluent people on 5th Avenue so that by the end of the [19]70s, I thought the way to show how important emergency medicine is and to change the perspective of society was to go to a place like Bellevue.[65]

Bellevue Hospital was in a sorry state and had just been rebuked by the Joint Commission on the Accreditation of Hospitals for numerous areas of substandard care, including the ED. Goldfrank would need to once again institute changes, programs, and systems to help the underserved patients who came to the Bellevue ED. He would also need to deal with Saul Farber, M.D., the powerful chairman of internal medicine at NYU and Bellevue. Farber, as an internist, would prove to be every bit the foil to emergency medicine as Oscar Hampton had been as a surgeon. Goldfrank sensed from their first meeting, when he was interviewing, that Farber would be a major opponent. Farber was not welcoming to Goldfrank, saying that he felt his job "was not necessary."[65] Goldfrank negotiated with the dean and hospital director to be an independent entity in the hospital and medical school—he did not push for departmental status as he felt that his public health mission was based on service and he did not need academic status. This approach later came back to hurt Goldfrank and the faculty members he hired when they found they had no avenue for promotion, and no one would sign off on research grants they might write. Just before starting his new position, Goldfrank learned that the dean had left to take a government position in Washington D.C., and Saul Farber was named the new dean.

Within a few months, Farber tried to fire his new emergency director, but Goldfrank was tenured and had enough support to make this untenable for Farber. Goldfrank was then instructed that he should refrain from talking to the media. He argued with Farber over this and then ignored his request. The media was an essential tool in the quest of Goldfrank and other New York City emergency physicians to enact change. As noted above, increased media exposure was one of the primary reasons Goldfrank came to Bellevue. Goldfrank wrote:

> We were observing and making history. Everything that happened in New York City's physical and political environment altered patient needs and disorders: the weather, the closing of hospitals and psychiatric facilities, new reimbursement strategies. We knew first which societal experiments were succeeding or failing. We were the six o'clock news and tomorrow's headlines in the Daily News. I translated medicine for the media and assisted reporters on their projects—I had long ago learned of their importance—and assumed that ultimately I would need their support.[87]

For emergency medicine in New York City, change seemed only to come following tragedy. Mark Henry remembers that publicity from two cases of missed ectopic pregnancy with bad outcomes in hospital EDs prompted the formation of a 911 Receiving Hospital Committee. This committee included ED directors, HHC officials, health department representatives, and community leaders. It proposed minimum standards for staffing and supervision for first New York City, and then the entire state. Hospitals with "911 Certified" EDs had documented capabilities to care for ill patients and some level of supervision of house staff. But in the early 1980s as New York hospitals were managed to run at extremely high occupancy and ED visits increased, the problems were not solved. Mark Henry recalls,

> An old lady came to this hospital, Flushing Hospital, from a nursing home, and they diverted the ambulance. The nurse went out and said we are too busy, go next door. That was our hospital, Booth. Then she died. She probably would have died wherever she went, it was her time. It became a celebrated case because they turned the ambulance away…a heart attack patient gets turned away and dies. So the politician, he decided he was going to do a law so you could never do this again, that's why the 1-year jail term. But, when he actually sat down with parties from the state and the city from the hospitals it was a bigger problem.[90]

Mark Henry and other emergency physicians worked with the city and state to develop the Emergency Medical Services Reform Act. The Act required some minimum standards for EDs and outlawed the inappropriate diversion or transfer of emergency patients.[90,91] Emergency medicine leaders then pursued, with the support of the state, the development of new standards for emergency departments and staffing of EDs.

One case, however, had a greater impact on emergency care and graduate medical education in New York City, and eventually the entire United States, than any other. The death of 18-year-old Libby Zion in March of 1984 did not occur at one of New York City's overburdened municipal hospitals. Ms. Zion presented to the ED of

New York Hospital, the nearby, private hospital antonym of Bellevue. Zion presented with fever and altered mental status and, after an ED evaluation by an unsupervised junior medical resident, was admitted to the internal medicine ward team, also run by an unsupervised intern and resident. Zion was prescribed meperidine, with the house staff apparently unaware that she had been taking phenelzine. The combination of these two agents, and possibly other drugs the patient was taking, was later felt to be responsible for causing extreme hyperthermia and delirium. When Ms. Zion became agitated and more delirious she was restrained and given a sedating agent. She suffered a cardiac arrest and died several hours after she was admitted.[87,92,93]

It is possible, even likely, that many other cases of missed diagnosis and inappropriate treatment occurred in New York City hospitals. In most cases, events like this went unrecognized or unreported. Ms. Zion's case was different—she came from a well-connected family. Her father, who was an attorney and writer for the *New York Times*, aggressively sought answers. He convinced the New York County district attorney, Robert Morgenthau, to initiate a grand jury investigation into the death. Lewis Goldfrank learned of the case and saw that this sad outcome might be a vehicle for change in emergency care in New York City. Goldfrank rides the train from his home in Ossining to Manhattan each day and had come to know John Freed, the assistant district attorney of New York County, who rode the same train. He remembers,

> John Freed came to see me after Libby Zion died when Sidney Zion and Elsa Zion went to Morgenthau and the mayor and said this was criminal—he came to see me that night, a week after the event. I said I knew about the case, it had been discussed with me and we went over it and we plotted out…back and forth, 4 to 6 months, morning and night, to go over this case. I said I didn't have time to do more than that. I went to work but we organized things and met with Morgenthau many times and designed a strategy that this was a systemic failure and this was a societal failure….[65]

One of the grand jury recommendations was that all level I emergency departments be staffed by a physician who had 3 years of training. In response to the grand jury investigation, David Axelrod, M.D., the state health commissioner, formed the New York State Department of Health Ad Hoc Advisory Committee on Emergency Services, Supervision, and Resident's Working Conditions. The Committee was chaired by Bertrand Bell, M.D., a prominent New York physician from the Albert Einstein School of Medicine, who had a hand in the formation of the first emergency medicine residency in New York City. Goldfrank, who was a friend of Bell, sat on this "Bell Commission" as it developed its recommendations, which then were codified into New York State law.

Goldfrank was at this time pushing for an emergency medicine residency at Bellevue. His clinical volume was over 100,000 patients per year, and he had a few residents and some moonlighting physicians to handle this load. Several of the young faculty physicians he hired left because of the poor working conditions and limited opportunities to advance at Bellevue and NYU. Saul Farber's reflexive reply to the proposal of an emergency medicine residency was "over my dead body." In the Bell Commission activities, Goldfrank saw a way to bring this issue to the forefront. He remembers providing input at meetings:

> They'd say how will you ever get to an attending physician around the clock? It's obvious—you have to have an emergency medicine residency in every state school in New York State and you have to get all the others to have emergency medicine residencies that is the only way you are going to save the people.[65]

The Bell Commission recommendations were published in 1987, and adopted in 1989. New York State became the first governmental body in the United States to limit resident work hours and require a certain level of supervision in teaching hospitals. The regulations did not directly target emergency care, but did affect ED staffing by requiring 24-hour supervision of residents by attending physicians, which meant that interns and residents could not longer work alone in EDs. The regulations also limited moonlighting by residents by including these hours in an 80-hour work week limit.[94] However enforcement was lacking, and many programs and physicians openly violated the regulations.[93] As Goldfrank and others tried to implement the supervisory regulations, they knew that they would create "a necessary deficit of formally trained emergency physicians, which, in turn, would affirm the need for emergency medicine residencies."[87] Goldfrank also knew that the fight would be toughest in his own backyard. A committee that reviewed the proposal for an emergency medicine residency at Bellevue, in a refusal note signed by the associate dean in February 1988, said that it was "aware that its recommendations are at variance with the current practice of the American Board of Emergency Medicine," but stated that emergency medicine "draws on knowledge of other specialties," that these specialties were "extremely well represented" in the ED at Bellevue, and that they provide "the highest level of specialty care" that was "hard to match in any hospital."[95] A year later, the Bellevue Hospital Center Medical Board overwhelmingly passed a resolution that an emergency medicine residency program was "premature and could be detrimental to patient care." The resolution noted that a program must have qualified faculty to teach residents, and that Bellevue did not have enough emergency medicine faculty to support a residency.[96] This was an evil conundrum. The resistant actions of Saul Farber, and Goldfrank's own failure to push for academic standing for his faculty when he took the job, prevented the development of a "qualified faculty" in emergency medicine, and this was now being used as a reason to withhold a residency program. Farber and others knew that without approval for a residency, Goldfrank would not be able to find willing academicians to join him. They seemed to have him in an effective stalemate.

Farber and the other opponents may have underestimated the power of the connections Goldfrank had cultivated in medicine and the media over many years in the trenches in New York City. When Goldfrank made this situation public, articles appeared in the *Daily News* and *New York Times* and pieces were aired on local television news programs. Goldfrank even cooperated in writing a book with New York author Edward Zeigler, titled *Emergency Doctor*, and published in 1987.[97] The book provided an in-depth look at the Bellevue emergency department and chronicled the challenges that Goldfrank and others faced, both in terms of patient care and medical politics. The media attention on the question of an emergency medicine residency was not one-sided—supporters of Farber wrote letters to the editor and opinion pieces in the *New York Times* and other papers, explaining why emergency training for physicians was not needed at Bellevue. After some spirited discourse, the Community Board of Bellevue Hospital, which was very supportive of Goldfrank, played its own power game. The board declared that NYU medical students would not be allowed to train in the Bellevue ED unless an emergency medicine residency was established. The board also called for the resignation of Saul Farber. At least one member of the Health and Hospitals Corporation also called for Farber to resign. In the end, Farber and the Bellevue Hospital Center administration were forced to concede, and an emergency medicine residency was started at Bellevue/NYU in 1992. The residency was successful from its inception and attracts quality resident physicians.

Goldfrank's next fight was to gain academic departmental status at NYU School of Medicine. Robert Glickman, M.D, a new dean replaced Saul Farber. Glickman was not as strident in his opposition to emergency medicine as Farber had been, but he opposed an academic department for emergency medicine at NYU, and set up roadblocks and diversions, which would take another decade for Goldfrank and his colleagues to navigate.

Elsewhere in New York City, emergency medicine, after being slow to take off in terms of residency training programs, received a significant boost from state reimbursement procedures for graduate medical education. In an effort to increase the number of primary care resident physicians, New York State began paying for these residents at a higher rate and specialist resident physicians at a lower rate. Emergency medicine, thanks to lobbying from emergency medicine leaders, was considered like a primary care field and hospitals found it lucrative to start emergency medicine residency programs. The result was a 1990s boom in the number of emergency medicine residencies in New York City. The war to establish emergency medicine in the Big Apple was over, and after thousands of little skirmishes and a few big battles, emergency patients were the clear winners.

BECOMING A HARDY PERENNIAL

The flower analogy to describe the field was used, and overused, by some of the early leaders of emergency medicine, but in many ways it fit. Emergency medicine did sink roots and bloom in the 1980s. By the end of the decade, 75 healthy emergency medicine residency programs dotted the landscape in every region of the country, and by 1991, 22 academic departments of emergency medicine had formed at U.S. medical schools. The newness and inexperience of the field was detrimental in many ways, but in some ways it was an advantage. Unencumbered by long-standing traditions or practices, emergency medicine could be innovative. Another aspect of being new was that many emergency medicine leaders carried a chip on their shoulders. They were so accustomed to being criticized and treated like second-class citizens that when they embarked on projects, they felt like they had to do a better job than physicians in other fields. They set standards that in some cases exceeded those in other specialties or defied the norm. In this way, emergency medicine became a model for supervision and on-site teaching of residents and medical students. ABEM used cutting-edge educational methodology in creating and administering its examination. Emergency medicine textbooks were as good as others in medicine and the journals eventually became that way. Emergency medicine became an increasingly popular career choice among medical students, and the competitiveness of the field approached or exceeded that of many of the traditional medical specialties. Quality research was beginning to be done by a small cadre of dedicated investigators. Excellent scientific meetings and continuing medical education were adequately serving the needs of emergency medicine academicians and practitioners.

Despite this success, some in medicine continued to view emergency medicine as an invasive species. For every emergency medicine program that had relative harmony in its environment, two or three had to justify their right to exist on a daily basis. The numbers for emergency medicine, if viewed with a glass-half-empty perspective, were not that impressive. Many residency programs were at large teaching hospitals, centered in the Midwest, and as of 1990, emergency medicine had not infiltrated many of the academic institutions that set the tone for academic medicine in United States. Research funding in emergency medicine was lower than in any other medical field. Only 18% of medical schools had academic departments in emergency medicine, and emergency medicine was a minor player in medical education. One encouraging fact was that not many emergency medicine programs had folded, and the growth rate of new residencies and academic departments was steady and during some periods exponential. Therefore the harsh climate was being met, tolerated, and adapted to in most institutions. By 1990, emergency medicine had become a wizened, hardy perennial and would move forward as part of the landscape during a period of time when the climate for all of medicine would become harsher.

8 Experiencing and Exploiting Success

Rapid rises to success often become cautionary tales. Although it seemed for many early emergency physicians like it took forever to gain specialty status, the process was quite quick by the standards of American medicine. Thousands of emergency physicians were in full-time practice by the middle of the 1980s, where 20 years earlier there had been less than 100. Of the other medical specialties, only family practice had experienced such enormous growth in practitioners, residency programs, and boarded physicians in such a short time span. In the case of family practice, it was an upgrade in training for general practitioners, but with the same type of practice. In emergency medicine a new type of practice and training was created, and became a unique entity in medicine. The emergency physicians of the 1980s were a diverse lot, and their demographics provide some insights into the field.

The Demographics of Emergency Medicine

Exact data on the population and characteristics of emergency physicians before 1980 are difficult to obtain. The primary reason for this is that emergency care was provided by a mixed bag of full-time, nonresidency-trained physicians, a small cohort of residency-trained emergency physicians, and a large number of part-time physicians, many of whom would not self-identify as emergency physicians. Most full-time emergency physicians in the late 1970s were members of the American College of Emergency Physicians (ACEP); therefore ACEP member counts are representative of the relative growth of the field. ACEP membership increased from around 1,000 members in 1970 to 10,203 in 1980. Growth was much more modest in the next decade—by 1990 there were 13,681 ACEP members.[1] As would be expected for a new specialty, the growth rate of emergency physicians greatly outpaced that of U.S. physicians in general. Between 1970 and 1986, the total active physician population increased by 66%. The emergency physician population increased 1000% between 1970 and 1980 and 98% between 1980 and 1986. Still, by 1986 emergency physicians accounted for just 2.4% of all U.S. physicians.[2] According to American Medical Association (AMA) data from 1986, 51% of U.S. emergency physicians were not board-certified in any medical specialty. This low number of board-certified physicians was not unique to emergency medicine—at the same time 46% of practicing anesthesiologists and 42% of general internists were not board certified.[2]

The founders of emergency medicine were white men. Although a few women became emergency physicians in the 1970s, the field remained much less gender-integrated than many other medical specialties.[3] The percentage of women enrolled in U.S. medical schools increased from only 9.2% in 1970 to almost 30% by 1980. Emergency medicine attracted some women physicians in the 1980s, but lagged behind other fields. As the percentage of women medical students exceeded 40% in the 1990s, the percentage of women emergency medicine residents increased, but only to around 20% and is currently static at 27% to 28%. Compared with other medical specialties, emergency medicine is similar in its percentage of women to surgery, the surgical subspecialties, and ophthalmology. In fields like internal medicine (40%), pediatrics (65%), and family medicine, the percentage of women physicians is much higher.[4]

Going back to 1971 when the AMA approved the Medical College of Pennsylvania (MCP) emergency medicine internship with its statement that it would be good for women so they "could have scheduled hours," the perception was that emergency medicine would be a good choice for women physicians who wanted to raise families.[5] But, it was not that simple. The ability to schedule shifts and work part time provided some flexibility. However the fact that two thirds of emergency department (ED) shifts were evening or night shifts, and the challenge of working late into the night and then having to tend to children or other family duties during the day made it difficult for some women to function long term in emergency medicine. Pamela Bensen, the first woman emergency medicine resident at MCP, was fortunate in that her husband was available and supportive in child rearing and helped to tend to home and family issues. Bensen remembers "at the 1972 scientific assembly sitting outside the lecture room with the door ajar, nursing my son while listening to the lecture."[5] For Judith Tintinalli, who divorced and became a single mother when she was an emergency medicine faculty member at Wayne State/Detroit Receiving, raising her children was "a wonderful life achievement." She notes:

> I have three kids…I managed to juggle raising the kids, living in downtown Detroit, which was great. We lived like urban pioneers and had just a wonderful, wonderful time…I told the kids, I remember they were…little and I put them together and I'm like really busy and I have to do all this work, so you guys are going to have to take care of a lot of these things yourself. So I taught them how to wash their clothes and everything, they were always pretty self-sufficient.[6]

According to Bensen, discrimination against women physicians in ACEP in the 1970s and 1980s was not openly apparent. However on a more subliminal level, it was difficult for women to crack the "old boys' club." In the 1970s, ACEP nominated one woman for the board of directors each year. The nominees were selected by the ACEP Nominating Committee and voted on by the council. For male nominees, according to Bensen, no person who had been put forward as a nominee for 3 years had ever failed to be elected to the ACEP board of directors. Pam Bensen, Ellen Taliaferro, or Vera Morkovin was alternately nominated each year, but after 9 years of women nominees, none had been elected. Bensen remembers when the Nominating Committee "called me for the fourth time, I said no."[7] They called back twice more, asking her to reconsider, but she still refused. She was no longer interested in being the "token woman" on the ballot, but was eventually persuaded to once again run.

ACEP held a "Meet the Candidates" session at the scientific assembly. Bensen was asked what she brought to the board. Her answer included a double entendre: "I bring more estrogen and a broad perspective."[7] During this session she told the story about how she previously ran for the board and lost. She was at a reception for the ACEP Council when an ACEP member came up to her and said, "I don't know why you lost, but you know us Southern gentlemen couldn't vote for a woman!" Bensen noted that she almost hit him. She concluded her remarks by saying, "Don't vote for me because I'm a woman, but I ask you to not vote against me because I am a woman."[7]

Bensen won the election and in 1982 became the first woman to serve on the ACEP board of directors. When she was to attend her first meeting she received a memo telling her to wear a dark suit, white shirt and tie for the Board of Directors annual photo. She took it in good humor. At the board meeting when the time for the photo came, she yelled out, "Wait, wait!" Holding up two gaudy ties, she said, "Which tie should I wear?" This broke the ice with the board. Bensen made another observation at one of the early board meetings. After having an intense discussion, the board broke for lunch. The discussion continued as the board members left the room and the male members filed into the men's room. Bensen, cut off from the conversation, briefly considered following them. When the meeting reconvened after lunch Bensen raised her hand and said, "I make a motion that when we are having a substantive discussion, all discussion stops at the door to the men's room." The other board members laughed, but Bensen remembers, "They didn't realize what they were doing."[7]

In her practice in Maine, Bensen encountered some gender discrimination, usually from older surgeons, but she became the first woman to direct a multihospital emergency medicine group. Those who opposed her because she was a woman found that she was a formidable presence. Bensen notes, "I have a very strong personality and I tend to bulldoze and pit bull people around. I stick with things and fight through it."[7]

For Judith Tintinalli, at Detroit Receiving Hospital it was not gender discrimination that led to her eventual departure to Beaumont Hospital in nearby Royal Oak, Michigan, in 1984. Tintinalli remembers,

> It was a very sad time because I loved Receiving, but I sort of had my fill with city/county medicine. To be honest, if somebody calls me a motherfucker one more time on the floor, that's it. They did it one day, and I had had it. It was a sad time because of course I recruited the residency program that began there....[6]

Like Bensen, Tintinalli's strong personality may have served as a shield against discrimination. She notes,

> I think I have my nose to the grindstone and never, I've never had a mindset that because I'm a woman somehow I'm being treated differently. I don't think of myself as a woman. I think of myself as an academic emergency physician first. I suppose if I had issues, maybe I haven't noticed them.[6]

She offered similar sentiments when she was interviewed by the *Detroit News* in 1987 after she became ABEM President:

> For me, being elected president of the board is the highest honor in my field. But being a woman has nothing to do with it. I'm not a token. I do my job and when I have a problem, it never enters my head that the problem exists because I am a woman.[8]

Tintinalli, who was often the only woman in the room as she rose to higher levels in emergency medicine organizations, was asked to type documents because she was a fast typist, and perhaps because this was a role that the men expected. But Tintinalli did not feel lonely or left out. She remembers being part of the social scene at the University Association of Emergency Medicine (UAEM) and ABEM meetings, "I remember Dave Wagner is a good dancer. We used to dance a lot. No, we had a lot of fun. I could drink better than most of them."[6]

Tintinalli was the first female president of ABEM, and in 1991 the first woman to rise to the level of chair of a U.S. academic department of emergency medicine at the University of North Carolina.[6] She contributed to the increase in women in emergency medicine in a very direct way—her daughter went to medical school, trained in emergency medicine, and is now a practicing emergency physician.

An organization called Women in Emergency Medicine was formed in 1983, with Trish Blair, M.D., as its first president. The group eventually became the Section of American Association of Women Emergency Physicians within ACEP. As more women joined the ranks of emergency medicine they began to meet at ACEP to discuss advancement and promotion, gender equality in work and pay, and balancing professional and child-rearing commitments. It is difficult to tell, given the smaller number of women in emergency medicine and the relative youth of the field, if a glass ceiling exists in academic emergency medicine for women. However a study of academic emergency physicians done by the Society for Academic Emergency Medicine (SAEM) in the late 1990s found that 10% of male respondents were chairs of their departments, compared with only 1% of women.[3]

Women in emergency medicine have contributed in special ways to women's health issues in the ED and in society at large. Ellen Taliaferro, M.D., an ACEP charter member became a national leader in the study of domestic violence, and in advocacy for reducing violence in society. She and another long-time emergency physician leader, Patricia Salber, M.D., co-founded an organization called Physicians for a Violence Free Society.

At the time that emergency medicine residencies were first developing, a national movement to increase underrepresented minority medical students was under way. This was modestly successful in increasing the percentage of minority medical student from only 2.2% in 1970 to 6.8% in 1981.[2] The race and ethnicity of emergency medicine have paralleled that in medicine in general. Despite the fact that emergency patients were much more likely to be underrepresented minorities, the proportion of minority physicians who chose to practice emergency medicine was not higher than in other medical fields. The percentage of black physicians in emergency medicine is 5% to 6%, and the percentage of Latinos is less than 4%. Both numbers remained constant through the 1980s and 1990s, although some data suggest that the number of Hispanic emergency medicine residents may be declining. In the 1980s and 1990s the number of U.S. physicians of Asian descent increased dramatically, but the percentage of Asian physicians who chose careers in emergency medicine (around 10%) was much lower than for most other medical fields (up to 25%).[4]

Although the early leaders of ACEP, UAEM, and ABEM were almost exclusively white men, many emergency physicians became known for their egalitarian and nondiscriminatory views. Most emergency medicine practice settings engender in the emergency physician a strong empathy for the plight of underserved patients who are often underrepresented minorities. Caring for such patients often creates a sense of frustration with the inability of government and society to provide a proper system for attention to the poor and underserved. James Mills, Jr., set the tone for involvement beyond the workplace in his efforts to provide better health care for poor and minority patients in the greater Washington, D.C., area. Lewis Goldfrank has dedicated his career to caring and advocating for underserved patients.

Despite the general sense that emergency medicine was a good base from which to serve and advocate for minority patients, a compelling move to emergency medicine by minority physicians never materialized. A handful of black and Hispanic emergency physicians could be identified in the early years of the specialty. Harry Tunnel III, M.D., was a black emergency physician who became president of the Indiana Chapter of ACEP in the middle 1970s. Jack Mitchell, M.D., a black ex-surgeon, founded the emergency medicine program in Bakersfield, California, and was an early associate editor for the *Journal of Emergency Medicine*. After retiring, he helped to develop an emergency medical services (EMS) system in the Bahamas.[9] But for the most part, emergency medicine was white and male. The lack of diversity was even worse in academic emergency medicine. A study done in the late 1990s by an SAEM task force found so few underrepresented minorities in academic emergency medicine that it was unable to do a meaningful analysis.[3]

The small number of minority physicians who trained in emergency medicine often gravitated to jobs where they could serve minority populations. The pressure on minority emergency physicians to serve minority patients, but also to become role models, mentors, and advisors for other medical professionals, was immense. Two notable black emergency physicians, Marcus Martin, M.D., and Emanuel Rivers, M.D., have been successful in their own careers and have played key roles as mentors for others. Martin's life has been a series of firsts—first black football player at North Carolina State University, first black medical student at Eastern Virginia Medical School, first black emergency medicine resident at the University of Cincinnati, and eventually the first black chairman of emergency medicine in the United States at the University of Virginia.[10] Emanuel Rivers is from Detroit and went to medical school at the University of Michigan where he developed a strong interest in critical care and resuscitation. He did his residency training in the combined emergency medicine/internal medicine program at the Henry Ford Hospital in Detroit and did fellowship training in critical care. He then joined the faculty at Henry Ford and developed a highly productive and innovative resuscitation research program. Working with an urban population with a high percentage of black patients, Rivers has become a prime example of an academic emergency physician giving back to his community.

The ethnic backgrounds of emergency physicians are diverse, but not as international as some other fields. Although many of the early emergency medicine leaders were white, Anglo-Saxon, and Protestant, the field was welcoming to all ethnicities and religious persuasions. Leaders like Rosen, Krome, and Levy who were Jewish did not in general feel discriminated against by their emergency medicine peers, although they sometimes detected anti-Semitism from those they battled in their efforts to advance emergency medicine. Emergency medicine had fewer foreign medical graduates in its ranks than most other medical fields. Since the inception of residency training in emergency medicine, the proportion of international medical graduates (IMGs) in the field has been dramatically lower than in internal medicine, surgery, family medicine, pediatrics, and most other medical specialties. Where IMGs account for nearly 40% of residents in internal medicine, and more than that in family medicine residencies, they account for less than 5% of emergency medicine residents.[4] This is a reflection of the popularity of emergency medicine as a residency choice for graduating U.S. medical students. U.S. senior medical students grab all but a handful of the available emergency medicine residency positions in the annual matching program. IMGs often resort to finding unfilled positions that are left over after the regular match, and these positions are more plentiful in the less competitive specialties. The percentage of IMGs in emergency medicine is therefore more similar to orthopedic surgery (2%) and other competitive specialties than to the primary care fields.[4,11]

Osteopathic medicine experienced a growth surge at the same time that emergency medicine was rapidly developing. Between 1970 and 1981, the number of osteopathic medical schools doubled from seven to 14, and the number of graduates tripled to about 1,200 per year.[12] The field was born in Kirksville, Missouri, and like emergency medicine, was strongest in the Midwest. The development of an organizational infrastructure for emergency medicine within osteopathic medicine paralleled that in allopathic medicine. In 1973, a group of osteopathic emergency physicians founded the American College of Osteopathic Emergency Physicians (ACOEP) in Toledo, Ohio. The ACOEP developed similar membership criteria, requirements for continuing medical education, and national meetings as ACEP. The AMA-equivalent for osteopathy, the American Osteopathic Association approved emergency medicine as an osteopathic medical specialty in 1978, and a board was established in 1980. Osteopathic emergency medicine residency programs developed more slowly than in allopathic medicine—by 1979, there were five approved programs.[13]

In 1980, there were 18,820 U.S. osteopathic physicians (DOs). There were 25 times as many allopathic U.S. physicians.[2] The percentage of DOs in emergency medicine has been small. Only 3% of the original 3,200 "charter" members of ACEP were DOs.[1] From the start, most allopathic emergency medicine residencies were open to accepting qualified DO graduates. Osteopathic medical school graduates have consistently accounted for 5% to 7% of entering residents in allopathic emergency medicine residency training programs.[4] Once in emergency medicine residency, DO graduates are generally considered and treated as equals with medical doctor (MD) graduates, and several osteopathic-trained emergency physicians have become notable educators and researchers in emergency medicine. For example, the most successful faculty researcher in emergency medicine at the University of Michigan in the late 1980s and 1990s was Ronald Maio, a DO who did an allopathic emergency medicine residency at Michigan State University. As would be expected with their small numbers and some inherent negative biases from MDs osteopathic physicians have had less of an impact in organized emergency medicine. However in 2004 Robert Suter, D.O., became the first osteopathic physician to become president of ACEP.

The practice demographics of emergency physicians changed as the specialty matured. The single-hospital contract, Alexandria Plan–type group emergency practice was the early model. A 1975 survey of community hospitals found that 30% had a physician group on contract to provide emergency department staffing. By 1985 almost all larger community hospitals had a contract with an emergency medicine group. Multihospital emergency department management groups began to proliferate by the end of the 1970s, and became the major employers of emergency physicians in many regions of the country. The reach of emergency management companies also began to extend into a new realm—freestanding emergency centers, usually referred to as urgent care centers, or the more pejorative "doc in a box." Urgent care centers were sometimes staffed by emergency physicians, but more commonly by part-time physicians with a variety of backgrounds.

The board examination in emergency medicine was quickly ramped up in 1980, and by 1991 more than 10,000 physicians were ABEM certified. About two thirds of these physicians were eligible for the ABEM examination through the practice track mechanism, and one third were emergency medicine residency graduates.[14] The practice track candidates were required to have no less than 60 months and 7,000 hours of ED practice time to sit for the ABEM examination. The pass rates for both the written (part I) and oral (part II) components of the ABEM examination were much higher for emergency medicine residency graduates than for practice track–eligible physicians. ABEM data from 1981 showed that practice track–eligible physicians had a first-time pass rate of 65% for part I and 52% for part II compared with respective rates of 89% and 76% for emergency medicine residency trained candidates. Five years later, in 1986, the pass rate for practice track physicians on part I had fallen to 45%.[14,15] Thousands of people were ineligible for or unable to pass the ABEM examination, and this created a group of physicians who felt competent and committed to emergency practice but were not able to become board-certified. The disenfranchised feelings of these physicians would create significant controversy in the organizations of emergency medicine.

The early emergency medicine residency graduates, as would be expected, had no trouble finding desirable jobs. A 1978 survey of about 300 residency graduates found that 56% had taken a job in a medical school or medical school–affiliated hospital. Most graduates, appropriately or not, were put into supervisory or leadership positions right out of residency. A third became ED directors or assistant directors, and 5% became residency directors. The most common work environment was an urban community hospital with a moderate volume ED, and salaries were reported to be in the $41,000 to $60,000 range for most respondents. Seventy-nine percent of respondents worked in only one hospital, and most worked 40 to 59 hours per week. One fourth of residency graduates worked for emergency medicine corporations, but 32% reported they were not part of an emergency physician group and were presumably paid by the hospital.[16] The survey results indicate that early emergency medicine residency graduates were more likely to choose academic positions, were less likely to work for "corporate" emergency groups, and were more often put in leadership positions than nontrained emergency physicians. The 1984 to 1985 Physicians Costs and Income Survey found that practicing emergency physicians had similar work hours (50 hours per week) but saw more patients per hour than physicians in other specialties. About one third of emergency physicians were employed by a hospital and one third by a physician or corporation. While half of other physicians worked in a solo practice, only 6% of emergency physicians did so. Emergency physicians had an average net income of $93,150 (1983 dollars), and those employed by corporations had the highest net income. Emergency physician salaries were higher than family practice physicians and medical specialists, but lower than surgeons.[17]

Demographics and statistics do not provide a true picture of emergency physicians of the late 1970s and 1980s. Although high-achieving, more "normal" medical students were choosing emergency medicine as a career, the cowboy element persisted in practicing emergency physicians. Bruce Janiak, who was the director of the emergency department at Toledo Hospital, remembers some of the physicians he hired to staff his ED in the late 1970s:

> I could tell you that I had six doctors in my department, amongst those six doctors there had been 14 wives and four of them were dead by violent means. Okay, that's the cowboy image. One guy who ran into cows twice and killed two wives in his Corvette. I mean, give me a break. It was just, that's the kind of image that we don't need![18]

The issue of high attrition or "burn out" has always followed emergency medicine. Since for many years, those who worked in emergency departments did so transiently, the impression was that no one could do emergency medicine long term. Many medical students in the 1970s and 1980s who considered careers in emergency medicine were cautioned they had a high likelihood of burning out. Some data existed to support this idea. A survey done in 1990 of a random sample of 1350 emergency physicians with a mean age of 41 years found high rates of depression and occupational stress, and 12% of respondents said they were very likely to abandon emergency practice within 1 year. However this study had a low proportion of residency-trained emergency physicians and only 26% were fellows in ACEP.[19] It is likely that many of those who reported stress and dissatisfaction and were planning to leave the field were older emergency physicians who were not trained in emergency medicine, could not become ABEM certified, and were losing the choice jobs to residency-trained physicians. Data began emerging in the late 1980s that for those physicians who were fully trained and board certified in emergency medicine, the attrition rate was no greater than it was for other medical specialties. A study published by Hall and colleagues from Cincinnati in 1992 found that emergency medicine residency graduates had an attrition rate of about 1.5% per year, and a 10-year retention rate in the field of 84%.[20,21] Nonetheless, it has been difficult to extinguish the burn out myth—the decades-old image of a migrant, poorly trained physician still persists in the minds of many in medicine when they think of emergency medicine.[17]

Throughout the 1980s, a patient presenting to a community hospital ED might be cared for, in decreasing order of likelihood, by a nonresidency trained, non–board-certified career emergency physician; a board-certified, non–residency-trained physician; a physician trained and possibly certified in another specialty; a non–residency-trained, non–board-certified, part-time or moonlighting physician; or, lastly, an emergency medicine residency–trained, ABEM-certified physician. Despite the proliferation of emergency medicine residencies, a shortage of emergency physicians existed, and continues to this day. Since the late 1980s, it has been estimated that around 25,000 emergency physicians are needed to staff all U.S. hospital emergency departments. Even into the 1990s, for every ED position occupied by an ABEM-certified emergency physician, there was at least one position filled by a noncertified emergency physician. Estimates are that it will take until at least 2012 to train and certify enough emergency physicians to staff all U.S. EDs.[20] The chronic shortfall, like most physician work force inequities, is as much a problem of distribution as it is numbers. It is difficult to entice residency-trained, board-certified emergency physicians to staff small, low-volume EDs, where the caseload may not be robust or exciting enough for professional satisfaction and salaries are usually lower. In other medical fields there is no practical mechanism to make up for a specialist shortage—other physicians cannot, for example, assume the role of an orthopedist or neurosurgeon. However in emergency medicine, nontrained physicians were commonly hired to function as emergency physicians. In some cases, independent study, innate talent, and practice experience allowed this large group of non–emergency trained physicians to adequately man the positions in U.S. emergency departments. In other cases, poor training and a lack of professional development caused these physicians to be pushed down the ladder to staff emergency departments in the least desirable, backwater, or urban hospitals. Large, multihospital management groups were very effective at shifting the least competent emergency physicians to practice sites where they would be the least noticed and hopefully do the least harm. Another common method for meeting the emergency physician shortfall was for local family practitioners to form a small group to provide ED coverage in low-volume hospitals in their communities.

AMERICAN COLLEGE OF EMERGENCY PHYSICIANS MOVES SOUTH AND FEELS SOME HEAT

The American College of Emergency Physicians was, in the late 1970s, experiencing growing pains. The organizational structure and facilities in Lansing had been expanded in response to growing membership and increasing national involvement in organized medicine. The executive director, Art Auer, capably managed the headquarters but ACEP had continual financial struggles. In the 1975 fiscal year, ACEP had a deficit of $190,000. ACEP was surprisingly candid about its financial misadventures in its 10-year anniversary publication, stating, "the College has occasionally been more aggressive in its fiscal practices than its budget would allow."[22] Some ACEP leaders and members were becoming upset with the lack of financial stability, and the matter came to a head in 1977 and early 1978. Karl Mangold was ACEP president,

Leonard Riggs, Jr., was on the board of directors, and J. D. McKean, M.D., was chairman of the Finance Committee. The three men were very business-oriented and realized that the ACEP budget process and finances needed a major overhaul. Riggs recalls,

> ...we just didn't think that the physicians were looking at the finances of the Association in a business like way and part of the problem was incomplete information. I won't say it was inaccurate, but it might have been that. I don't mean to imply that Art Auer and his staff purposely were trying to hide something, I don't think that was the case, I think they just didn't have a very clever, sophisticated accounting system for the budgeting that we were trying to do. As I remember this was a budget crunch problem. So, Art got a little lost in it all too and lead to some of the guys just having some doubts about the credibility of the numbers...but it was the first bit of sort of agronomy we had as a group, really a problem that we had that didn't involve our primary goal which was to get specialty status. It was something more mundane, which was the administration of the association.[23]

A special ACEP Board of Directors and Council meeting was called in April 1978 in Tarpon Springs, Florida, to address two crises—the budget, which according to John Wiegenstein "was in chaos at the time," and the ABEM-modified conjoint board issue.[24] During the day, John Rupke, Ron Krome, Mangold, and others participated in the rancorous meeting where the "young Turks" on the ACEP Council battled against the modified conjoint board proposal. Then the board of directors met in the evening and allowed McKean to propose major changes in the way ACEP handled its finances. Dues were increased, expenses were slashed, many budgeted items were reduced or dropped, and free benefits for members and staff were eliminated. The discussion was intense, and the marathon meeting did not end until after 2 AM. The end result was a leaner, more fiscally accountable ACEP. Many ACEP leaders cite the work of McKean when they speak of ACEP's financial turn around. The term "J.D. factor" was coined to refer to the extra fees and revenue generating techniques ACEP used to become profitable. The organization also adopted Mangold's maxim—never do anything for free. By 1981, ACEP was showing revenues over expenses of $6,000, with another $450,000 of capital in land acquisition in Dallas.[25]

As ACEP grew, the Lansing, Michigan, location for a headquarters became more and more undesirable. Lansing lacked a major airport and was difficult to travel to in the winter months. The board found that much of its business was with government activities in Washington, D.C., or with the many other medical organizations based in Chicago, Illinois. Complaints grew until in 1978 the board decided to relocate the ACEP headquarters. Four cities were initially considered: Washington, D.C., Chicago, Atlanta, Georgia, and Dallas, Texas. The two Southern "Sun Belt" cities were chosen because they had booming regional economies, and land and building costs were cheaper than in Washington and Chicago. Washington made sense from a political lobbying point of view, but some ACEP members were leery of getting "Potomac fever"—an overemphasis on federal government affairs—if ACEP moved to Washington.[23] Other national medical organizations had found Dallas a welcoming relocation site. For example, the American Heart Association moved its headquarters in 1975 from New York City to Dallas. Leonard Riggs, Jr., M.D., ran a multihospital emergency medicine group in Dallas at this time and was a member of the ACEP board of directors. But, Riggs was not on the Relocation Committee, and was surprised when Dallas was considered. He remembers,

> I kind of almost laughed when they said Dallas. I had no idea they would consider that. So, somebody said, well we are going to be gathering information from these cities, Leonard, might you have any idea who we might get information from? I called some business friend of mine and...he sent me to...Texas Power and Light. The electric utility had great interest in more people coming here...There was a guy whose job it was to promote Dallas. When the committee sent him the questionnaire he sent back this notebook back. I couldn't believe it. The thing was 6-inches thick, weighed about 4 pounds and...he compared everything there was to compare between the four cities. He did their work for them, almost. It was unbelievable. He had all the stuff in the

computer, which people could barely spell computer then, he had it all organized. He was quite a character. It ended of course with the records of the four football teams. The Dallas Cowboys were starting to do pretty well about then.[23]

Riggs says he never lobbied for Dallas to be the headquarters location, but he remembers,

Then the board came here for a meeting or two......and I showed them around and all that. Dallas was, we had the joke about the state bird of Texas was the construction crane, everywhere you looked there was buildings being built. All happened before the great bust of [19]83–[19]85.[23]

After a year's deliberation, the ACEP board selected Dallas as the site for the new headquarters and decided to set up a separate, small office in Washington, D.C. Land was purchased and a new building was designed. Art Auer had mentioned to the ACEP staff that a move was planned, but according to staff members said it "wouldn't happen for 20 years."[26] When it was announced that ACEP was moving to Dallas a few months later, it was a shock to many of the long-time staff at ACEP. Still, over half of the staff (around 30 employees) elected to move to Dallas with the organization. They arrived in Dallas in the middle of one of the worst heat waves in years.

One thing that ACEP did not bring to Dallas was the UAEM. UAEM had shared space in the ACEP headquarters in Lansing since 1973 and was under a management contract with ACEP. When UAEM found out that ACEP was moving, it had to decide whether to tag along or try to function on its own. The organization had almost no resources, and ACEP had assigned as its executive manager Mary Ann Schropp, a diligent, smart, efficient woman, who was only 21 years old. Schropp remembers cringing when she had to tell Ron Krome that he had fewer UAEM members than he thought, and she prodded the UAEM leaders to compile the "quarterly newsletter that they sent faithfully once a year."[26] The UAEM executive council decided not to move to Dallas, and asked Schropp to serve as its executive director. Schropp remembers that the ACEP move came quicker than she expected. After organizing and running the 1980 UAEM annual meeting in May, she returned to Lansing to find that ACEP had begun the moving process. Schropp was in a panic—she had not secured new office space, and finances were another issue. ACEP handed her a tardy final bill for their management services, and there "wasn't enough money in the account to cover it." Schropp remembers,

I think I just looked in the yellow pages and looked at some commercial property and found this basement of a dentist's office. Really dinky, really bad. It smelled like those dentist's offices...But, it was cheap. So I rented this place...I rented a truck, like one of these panel truck things and I got some guy who was working for ACEP loading these things up. I said, "I need you."[26]

Schropp went to Art Auer and asked what items she could take from ACEP to the new UAEM office. She remembers him saying, "Well you've been working within ACEP you get nothing. You're done." Schropp took what she thought she was entitled to— two desks, two chairs, a typewriter, some pencils, and memo pads.[26] She remembers,

I just went through this thing and I boxed up these...supplies and loaded them in the truck myself. I got the guys to do the furniture and I said, practically in tears, could you please drive it to my new office? I rode with him in the truck...we just threw everything, we just threw it in, because I had to go back to ACEP. About 11 o'clock that night I got a call from the cops. When I finally had gotten home I was just exhausted, mentally exhausted and physically exhausted—I'd left the door open on my brand new office! I not only left it open, I had tied it open to carry the desks in. So, the police are driving by, they see this door and they think I'm getting robbed....[26]

Just before Auer left for Dallas, he showed Schropp "a big floor plan of the new office in Dallas, and he pointed out the office that was going to be the UAEM office when I failed."[26] As it started life out from under the skirts of ACEP, UAEM was as humbly resourced as ACEP had been a decade earlier, but Schropp's determination and the emergence of some new leaders in the organization quite rapidly moved it to a position of credibility in academic medicine.

Art Auer did a good job orchestrating the move to Dallas, but as the ACEP leadership changed, an undercurrent of dissatisfaction with Auer persisted. The "cocktail chatter" among ACEP leaders was that Auer had botched ACEP finances, lacked vision, and that the organization had outgrown him. Some ACEP leaders had witnessed better management leadership in their involvement in other national organizations. In addition, some felt that Auer's persona was not what the new ACEP wanted to project. John McDade, the Alexandria pioneer who served as ACEP president in 1979 to 1980 recalls that some ACEP leaders "didn't like Art because he had a crew cut, he wore funny green sport coats, and he had earth shoes. They said we can't deal with that."[27] The ACEP board directed Auer to hire a consulting group to examine the ACEP executive office. Although the official report of the consultants did not indict Auer for ACEP's troubles, the message behind closed doors was that he should be replaced. Leonard Riggs, Jr., who was president-elect of ACEP at the time and B. Ken Gray, M.D., who would follow Riggs as president, decided to "take the bull by the horns."[23] At a meeting in the Virgin Islands, as ACEP board members walked on the beach they decided to put it to a "quiet little vote," and the majority favored replacing Auer.[23] The person who as a young man had designed the ACEP logo and had literally grown up with ACEP was fired after serving the organization for a decade.

The ACEP board of directors then used the same consulting group to recruit Auer's replacement, and the obvious choice among three candidates was Colin Rorrie. Rorrie's background was in government. Educated, with a doctorate degree, bespectacled, serious-appearing, and with Washington-style attire, he was a marked contrast to Auer. Rorrie had taught hospital administration and health planning at Washington University School of Medicine and then worked for 11 years in the Department of Health Education and Welfare (HEW) in the Comprehensive Health Planning Program. He was in Washington during the Watergate scandal, and experienced the ups and downs of changing federal executive branches. Rorrie remembers that John McDade and George Podgorny, representing ACEP, visited him at the HEW Bureau of Health Planning to learn more about how his initiatives might affect emergency medicine. He notes that ACEP was one of the few medical organizations to do so and that the AMA regarded his bureau as "the evil empire."[28] After working on the plan to rationalize health care and use federal regulations to control costs, the "free market" Reagan administration came into power and Rorrie was given the unpleasant task of dismantling the program he had helped to create. It seemed to be a good time to move on, and Rorrie found out about the ACEP executive director job. He flew to Dallas, interviewed with Riggs, McDade, Brooks Bock, and the rest of the search committee, and was offered and accepted the job on the spot. He remembers he went back to Washington,

> …submitted my resignation and on the 18th of January 1982, showed up…walked into this office…looked around, I said, "Well, it's 8:30 here, it's 9:30 in Washington. On Monday morning I'd be having a senior staff meeting right now. What the heck do I do here now?"[28]

Leonard Riggs remembers thinking that Rorrie may have been overqualified for what they wanted him to do, but Rorrie quickly changed the ACEP staff structure, hired, fired, and greatly improved the management structure and finances of the organization. Rorrie created a strategic plan for ACEP and encouraged the board of directors to take ownership. He felt that more ACEP members needed to become involved in their hospitals and other organizations, and felt,

> …we had too many of these high flying guys who came in with their sandals and their long hair and they came in and pulled a shift and they left. I said we are not going to survive if we don't start getting a group of people who are integrated within the medical structure of the organization.[28]

Rorrie inherited two ACEP programs, which were "political dynamite," but seemed to him to be of questionable value and took up a large amount of the board's time. The first was an endorsed malpractice insurance program administered by I. David Gordon in New York City. The program was a service to some ACEP members, but Rorrie questioned whether it was central to ACEP's core mission, and it was gradually phased out. The second area was ACEP activities in Washington. Since the 1970s, ACEP had employed a Washington contract lobbyist named Terry Schmidt. ACEP leaders like John McDade and Richard Stennes, who were very involved in lobbying efforts for ACEP, were very fond of Schmidt, and he had become almost like one of the ACEP staff. Schmidt was heavily involved in the lobbying efforts around the EMS Act of 1973, and the revision in 1976. Rorrie, as a former Washington insider, believed that Schmidt was more of a "hired gun slinger" representing multiple, and sometimes competing interests.[28] Incoming ACEP president Brooks Bock heeded Rorrie's advice, and the relationship with Schmidt was ended in favor of a single person who worked only for ACEP in a small Washington office that was established in 1985. This upset McDade and some of the early ACEP leaders, who had a long, productive relationship with Schmidt, but ACEP used its Washington presence very strategically in influencing federal health policy and regulations. By the 1990s, ACEP was one of the most influential medical specialty organizations in the nation's capital.

Colin Rorrie helped to make ACEP a more functional and professional organization, but the mission and purposes of the organization seemed unclear to many in emergency medicine. Part of the reason for this was that ACEP was responsible for representing an extremely diverse constituency with different needs and expectations. It was the professional organization for career emergency physicians who lacked residency training, many of whom would never become board certified. For these individuals ACEP was most valuable in providing continuing medical education programs and protecting them from restrictions on their practice due to their lack of training. ACEP was also the primary "trade" organization for board-certified emergency physicians, both residency-trained and those who had grandfathered in via the practice track. These individuals also benefited from good educational programs each year at the scientific assembly, but were most interested in ACEP advancing emergency medicine at the national level—in the AMA, at the big academic medical centers, and in government. ACEP was also the organization for those emergency physicians who were the business leaders of the specialty. For these entrepreneurs, ACEP was used as a venue for recruiting physicians and as a political vehicle to help protect the market place for multihospital emergency management groups. On a higher, ideological level, ACEP wanted to serve and represent the interests of all practicing emergency physicians, regardless of their training or certification.[29] On a more practical level ACEP, like most medical specialty organizations, is financially dependent on its members, with member dues accounting for almost all revenues. Policies that alienate or exclude any significant contingent of the membership are a form of financial suicide. The large corporate groups often required their members to join ACEP, and this provided a steady increase in members for ACEP.

ACEP found itself in a dilemma, watching emergency medicine advance as a boarded specialty, but with its member ranks swollen with many untrained, noncertified emergency physicians. The maneuvering of ACEP to try to please everyone resulted in two major errors of omission that diminished ACEP's reputation and created discord in the ranks of emergency medicine. The first was ACEP's failure to take a stand against the exploitation of emergency physicians by the large emergency management corporations. The second was the failure of ACEP to take a strong stand in supporting emergency medicine residency training and board certification as the superior standard for emergency practice in the United States.

During the 1980s some emergency physicians, particularly those in the academic realm, came to perceive ACEP as being dominated by the interests of "corporate" emergency practice. A common refrain was that the board of directors and ACEP presidents were all businessmen, and were looking out for their interests, rather than those of the common emergency physician. A review of the board of directors' members and ACEP presidents shows that this claim was partially true, but probably overstated. Some of the early leaders, after starting out with single-hospital ED contracts, managed contracts at multiple hospitals. This included James Mills, Jr., in the Washington, D.C., area, William Haeck in the Jacksonville, Florida, area, and John Rupke in Western Michigan. Phillip Buttaravoli graduated from the University of Cincinnati emergency medicine residency and moved to the Washington, D.C., area in the middle 1970s. Buttaravoli, ever the idealist, envisioned setting up a "democratic" emergency practice group where all employees became partners and emergency medicine–residency-trained physicians would provide top quality care. He experienced first hand the cold-blooded game of emergency contract acquisition when he competed against Mills's group for the ED contract at the newly built Mount Vernon Hospital. He remembers,

> I was energetic. I was one of the first residents trained in emergency medicine and I had all these great ideas that I wanted to do. In fact, they selected me; they chose me to be the head of their department. I got a lesson in politics because Mount Vernon Hospital was being built by Alexandria Hospital. I mean it was the same corporation or whatever. There was an enormous political network that Jim Mills and his group and John McDade were all a part of…Well, when the search committee selected me, I thought I had it, it was in the bag…Well, they ended up getting it overturned.[30]

Buttaravoli lost the contract at Mount Vernon and then tried to set up a group practice in Maryland. This venture also failed as he was out maneuvered and eventually eliminated from the group by his partner who wanted to form a large corporate group practice, with a limited number of partners and a profit-minded approach.

The first large-scale emergency management businessman to become ACEP president was Karl Mangold in 1977, who had been managing multiple ED contracts in California since 1966. Although Mangold was a businessman, he was a champion of specialty recognition and residency training in emergency medicine and was one of the most outspoken and influential emergency medicine leaders of his day. Between 1980 and 1993, more than half of the ACEP presidents and about one third of members of the board of directors could be viewed as coming from the "big business" realm of emergency medicine. The most notable of these entrepreneurs were Leonard Riggs, Jr., who founded EmCare, Robert Williams who co-founded Emergency Consultants, Inc., and Richard Stennes, who founded Associated Emergency Physicians Medical Group in Southern California. One of the reasons that the big business leaders rose to the top of ACEP leadership was that they could afford to, both in terms of time and money. Pam Bensen, who after graduating from the MCP emergency medicine residency initially ran a single hospital group, notes that when she served on the ACEP board of directors from 1982 to 1985,

> …it cost me $10,000 a year to be on the ACEP board out of my pocket. A lot of emergency physicians didn't want to put in the additional cost to be involved… [I]t got to be easier for me as our group got larger because I didn't have trouble covering shifts…I paid to have my shifts covered. But when you don't have anyone to cover you it is hard to go to an ACEP board for 3 days.[5]

Within the ACEP office, Art Auer, the executive director who was terminated in 1981, expressed his concern to John Wiegenstein, who had founded ACEP but was no longer on the board of directors. Wiegenstein remembered,

> …Art let me know that he felt that the original mission was being diverted and that the people who were more interested in making lots of money are getting in charge and he was worried that the mission was going to be changed and so forth.[24]

When asked if the entrepreneurial side of emergency medicine became too influential in ACEP in the 1980s, John McDade, who was one of the original Alexandria four, and ACEP president in 1979 to 1980, says:

> I had a sense that some of them had too much influence, but I don't think it got to be way too much, because there were enough people around that weren't going to let

that happen. I wouldn't let it happen. Haeck wouldn't let it happen. Wiegenstein wouldn't let it happen.[27]

George Podgorny notes that before ABEM approval,

The practicing guys, the multigroup guys, the academic guys, the in between guys…were very much together and had very little real friction. Everybody's effort had a single channel and that was specialty recognition. After that, things came apart because there wasn't anymore single unified overriding goal.[31]

ACEP was very conscious of the issues surrounding contract management and multihospital emergency physician group practices from its early years. John Rupke was the first chairman of the ACEP Socioeconomic Committee, and he wrote ACEP's "Principles of Ethical Practice" in 1971. These principles were then codified in the 1972 revision of the ACEP constitution and by-laws. The second principle spoke to the issue of groups stealing contracts from one another:

The emergency physician shall not negotiate for a position as emergency physician in a hospital without first notifying the incumbent emergency physician concerning the proferred [sic] position and his interest in it.[32]

This simple principle was honored by most for several years, and the principles were updated in 1977 to even more explicitly advise emergency physicians to avoid exploitation, fee splitting, and stealing hospital contracts. But, in 1979, ACEP, reportedly acting on legal advice that such principles might violate antitrust and other economic laws, abandoned its official stance and removed those principles from its ethical guidelines.[33] In the early 1980s, as large emergency medicine contract management groups increasingly swooped in and out-competed smaller, single-hospital emergency groups for contracts, ACEP was largely mute on an organizational level. With some corporate emergency groups profiting by hiring poorly trained, itinerant physicians to staff some of their EDs and limiting emergency physician practice through exclusivity clauses in their contracts, a contingent of emergency physicians became rankled. Editorials and speeches decried ACEP's lack of backbone in this matter. One author noted in 1979, "if these trends are allowed to continue without any intervention by the College on behalf of its membership, it seems likely that we are destined to end up right where it all began…".[34] The mega-group leaders were assailed as "buckmasters" and "menaces" who employed "hired guns" or "transient physicians" who "will work cheap" to staff their EDs. ACEP was accused of being "dominated by these so-called entrepreneurial physicians who in concert with a business manager and a lawyer present…one of the greatest threats to the specialty of emergency medicine."[34–36] Finally, as the written debate became more vitriolic, Ron Krome, as editor of *Annals of Emergency Medicine* wrote in 1982, "we do not intend to continue this debate within the pages of the journal." Krome encouraged members and readers to "express their sentiments directly to ACEP officers, chapter presidents, and councilors."[36] Even lay periodicals were calling attention to the corporate controversy. A 1978 article in *New West* magazine was titled: "Fast-Buck Medicine." It declared, "…the franchising of ER's offers the physician an opportunity to combine the roles of American medicine man and business tycoon…".[37]

ACEP's standard response to the barrage of criticism was that "restraint of trade legislation precludes ACEP's intervention on behalf of either party."[38] Resolutions introduced in the ACEP Council to limit the avarice and inappropriate practices of corporate emergency medicine died on the vine, or failed to gain support at the level of the ACEP board of directors.[36,39,40] On the other hand, ACEP did not initiate any actions in the 1970s or 1980s that specifically helped corporate management groups. Brooks Bock, M.D., who was an ACEP board member and president in 1983 to 1984 notes,

I never, ever, during my time from [19]78 until I left in [19]85 saw anything on the ACEP board that I could have related to supporting mega groups, never, not even one time. I don't even remember a discussion along that line.[41]

Peter Rosen, who was critical of the practices of corporate mega-groups in emergency medicine, thought that the answer lay in emergency physicians banding together and successfully competing against the corporate entities for hospital contracts. He thought that ACEP had little role to play in this area and advised, "it is not wise to expect the College to legislate this affair."[42] Still, many academic emergency physicians and community-practice emergency physicians who were threatened or hurt by the presence of large emergency management groups came to view ACEP's silence as complicity in eroding the quality of emergency care and limiting the opportunities of practicing emergency physicians.

The second major error of omission by ACEP in the 1980s and early 1990s was the failure to provide strong support for the concept that emergency medicine is best practiced by residency-trained, ABEM-certified emergency physicians. The practice track for ABEM certification closed in 1988, leaving many practicing emergency physicians who started practicing in the early to mid-1980s without a mechanism for gaining certification other than going back to complete an emergency medicine residency. This contingent became vocal in ACEP and pushed ACEP to come up with alternatives for certification. There were definitely some sympathetic ears in ACEP, as many early leaders had used the practice track to become certified or were practicing without certification. William Haeck, M.D., a key early ACEP leader who never became board certified in emergency medicine, notes, "I grieve a little bit…," referring to the plight of nonboarded emergency physicians who were unable to sit for the ABEM exam, and became ostracized by some in emergency medicine.[43] An ACEP Manpower Task Force in the early 1990s advocated for the establishment of an "alternative" residency program for the "have nots" in emergency medicine. The program called for 12 weeks of mentored training in established emergency medicine residency programs for practicing emergency physicians over a 2-year period and then allowing the physician to take the ABEM examination.[29] Those who had worked to make emergency medicine credible and legitimate by establishing ABEM and developing emergency medicine residencies were strongly opposed to this proposal, which withered without ever gaining widespread support. Despite ACEP's support for nonboarded emergency physicians, it was not able to do enough to satisfy them. Some of those who were disenfranchised by the closure of the practice track and who felt like ACEP was failing them created a new organization. The group, formed in 1993, was initially called the Association of Disenfranchised Emergency Physicians and then became the Association of Emergency Physicians (AEP). The singular goal of AEP was to find a way for all qualified emergency physicians to become board certified.[44] The organization has a few hundred members and has not gained any measure of political power or influence in organized medicine. The competing demands of a diverse constituency would become very difficult for ACEP to manage in the 1980s and 1990s. ACEP became like a parent with squabbling siblings. At the same time one child was accusing the organization of not representing the needs of nonboarded emergency physicians, another was whining about the lack of support for residency training in emergency medicine.

One area where ACEP steered a safer course was in the representation of "free-standing" emergency centers, and those who worked in the centers. From its inception, ACEP labored to be involved in all aspects of emergency medicine. When it was based in Lansing, the organization had management contracts with UAEM and other organizations and was dabbling in malpractice insurance, EMS agencies, the Emergency Nurse Association, and research funding through the Emergency Medicine Foundation (EMF), in addition to trying to represent emergency physicians in the AMA, the American Board of Medical Specialties (ABMS), and the academic world. When Colin Rorrie took over, he tried to focus ACEP, but the predilection to have an iron in every fire of emergency medicine continued. The free-standing emergency center movement came about when hospitals became less generous and more demanding in their emergency department contracts. Hospitals began to advocate at a national level for control over emergency physician fee schedules and threatened the status of the emergency physician as an independent contractor. Some advocated that a portion of the emergency physician's professional fee be used to purchase ED equipment and supplies. Karl Mangold in a 1978 article accused the American Hospital Association of "price fixing," and potential "restraint of trade."[45]

The difficulties experienced by some emergency physicians with hospitals were coupled with a changed American cultural mentality. As Mangold noted, "We have a 'McDonald's society' that wants what it wants, when it wants it; and wants it 24 hours a day."[46] The first privately owned nonhospital emergency care center was started in New England in 1975 by Robert L. Gordon, M.D., who said that such centers "provide a means for emergency physicians to practice their specialty in the private sector."[33] While many entrepreneurial emergency physicians were part of the free-standing emergency center or urgent care expansion, those who actually practiced in urgent care centers were often family practice–trained physicians or physicians with only internship training. Moonlighters constituted a major part of the workforce of early urgent care centers. Some of the businessmen in emergency medicine advocated for ACEP to take a role in setting standards and representing urgent care physicians. An interesting debate ensued. It was clear that practice in a free-standing emergency center would be more like other ambulatory medicine practices and posed a threat to family practice physicians and other generalists. Was this emergency medicine? Ron Krome argued that early emergency medicine leaders had to fight off the stigma of being doctors whose practice was defined only by their location—the emergency *room* doctor—and that emergency physicians should be able to practice wherever they can use their special skills. Although he did not advocate that emergency medicine organizations should set standards for free-standing emergency centers, Krome opposed a philosophy that would restrict the definition of emergency medicine practice to the ED.[47] Others opposed the idea that free-standing centers be called "emergency" care centers, and believed that extension of emergency medicine into outpatient urgent care would diffuse the specialty and create uncertainty about what was the key role of the emergency physician.[33] H. Arnold Muller, M.D., an early emergency medicine leader in Pennsylvania was on the ACEP board of directors from 1976 to 1984, and served as ACEP president in 1982 to 1983. Muller opposed the migration of ACEP and emergency medicine into setting standards and becoming politically involved in urgent care realm and was eventually successful in squelching initiatives by others on the board and in the ACEP membership to increase ACEP's involvement in free-standing emergency centers.

The Business of Emergency Medicine: Profit at a Price

Emergency medicine grew up at a time when all of American medicine was becoming more "corporate." The rise of hospitals, medical insurers, and medical specialists along with the sheer magnitude of the money that was changing hands as medicine worked its wonders meant that health care would become a major industry. Corporations were seen as the solution, even for the care of indigent, or "charity" patients in urban, municipal hospitals, as seen with the New York City Health and Hospitals Corporation. The national solutions to health care funding involved what Colin Gordon refers to as an elaborate "corporate compromise."[48] The number-one concern of health leaders in the 1970s was spiraling costs. The federal health maintenance organization (HMO) act of 1973 promoted corporate means of containing costs, but the lobbying strength of the AMA and American Hospital Association, prevented any significant reforms that would make medicine in America anything but a free-market free-for-all. As the small emergency contract groups of the 1960s began to show they could be profitable, and Medicare and Medicaid allowed reimbursement of services in patients who had previously been charity care, it became widely appreciated that "there was gold in them there hills" of emergency services. In a gold rush, the lure of huge profits for those who can capitalize first causes some measure of chaos and at times the erosion of ethics and professionalism. This was certainly the case in emergency medicine in the 1980s.

The first significant business issue to be addressed by emergency physicians in the first decade and a half of practice was contracts for service. When James Mills, Jr., and then others established contracts with hospitals for their emergency groups, some in medicine decried this new professional relationship between physician and hospital.

Surgeons, internists, and obstetricians of the 1960s and 1970s did not contract with hospitals for their services. John Rupke, who ran an emergency medicine group in Grand Rapids, Michigan, and collaborated with John Wiegenstein in the formation of ACEP, was very pro-business for emergency medicine, but he wrote about the dangers and lack of necessity of establishing formal contracts with hospitals. He preferred a hands-off approach for hospitals and insurers and advised emergency physicians to "stay out of the bright lines of contract."[49] Rupke's sentiments were not widely shared, and most community emergency physicians who were establishing group practices followed the lead of the great guru of emergency department contract management, Karl Mangold.

As was noted previously, Karl Mangold was a master at learning "how things work," and devising methods for the efficient distribution and management of emergency department staffing. He established contracts with two hospitals and tapped into a "pipeline" of resident physicians and fellows from military bases and teaching hospitals in the San Francisco and Oakland areas. Mangold notes that in the late 1960s, "I could have gotten ten hospitals' a year contracts, just by answering their phone calls. I couldn't find good enough doctors...."[50] Mangold eventually managed to find more doctors and began to expand his business in the 1970s. He then thought about what kind of company he would form with his partner, Herschel Fischer. He remembers,

> ...my first idea was to form a big group of doctors, what they now call a democratic group. I went around to a CPA [certified public accountant] and an attorney and I went around to a couple of other doctors and the message kept saying, "don't form a group, you don't want a lot of guys that have ownership and voting rights, and will not be very involved and this and that" ... [A]nd the advice I got was, you keep the ownership with Fischer and then you structure something that you can substantially keep good doctors with you for 30 years. I said well how can you do that if there's no partnership track. So I sat down and I started making a list of what would it take to keep me with this group. Autonomy, no influence on my medical decision making, it was incentive based reimbursement that if I build a big department I would want to share in that revenue immediately not wait for something. It would have to reward my seniority, it would give me as much time off, if I wanted to take six months off to go to Harvard or go to Nepal I could do that. It would give me a total kind of freedom...The only way I figured I do this is I have to be real smart in collecting the money so I could offer more money to get the best quality doctors I could. That was the basis of the group...You've got to align the incentives with the employees or the subcontractors or your vendors otherwise it is not sustainable. So, I started this group.[50]

Fischer Mangold became the largest provider of emergency department staffing in the country and the first to hold contracts in multiple states. Mangold would eventually have 300 doctors subcontracting for him, and his company had 200 employees to manage the recruitment, scheduling, billing, and contract management with hospitals. When he started in the 1960s, he never dreamed it would become so large.

> At the time I envisioned maybe having ten hospitals. When I was at one, I never thought of two until I got the concept that this was going to work. The thought of having large multihospital groups of 40, 50, 100, 300 was never in my mind. And yet, they developed because there were 500 doctors that could get ten hospitals and do it right.[50]

The problem was that some in the emergency medicine contract management industry would do it wrong. Karl Mangold was a wheeler-dealer, and could persuade almost any hospital administrator into signing an emergency department contract, but he relied on his wife to handle the organizational details of his company. He borrowed money, without his partner's help, to form a billing company and his wife, Jan, who had a nursing background, attended to the details of physician scheduling, billing for services, and information management. Mangold notes that Jan was "a real organizational genius and it sort of complemented my personality, who seems to have big picture sort, but, with the details I'm a little bit lacking."[50] Jan Mangold went back to school and got a degree in information systems management and rose to the level of vice president of administration and finance in their company.

Mangold's approach was to hire the best-qualified physicians he could find at a time when almost no residency-trained emergency physicians existed and those who graduated frequently started their own emergency groups. He was viewed by most as a fair-handed employer, and many of the physicians he hired for the choice jobs in desirable emergency departments worked for him for decades. Mangold was almost giddy with the possibilities, in terms of business opportunity and because he believed he was improving the quality of emergency care in the United States by staffing emergency departments for hospitals.

> It was fulfilling my sense of—I see this sweeping the country and I don't want be one doc with one hospital when I see this group thing that can't miss. You see, hospitals wanted groups. They didn't want individuals. They wanted people with experience. Hospital administrators thought doctors as unmanageable. It is not true. People buy in; doctors are the easiest people to manage. All you have to do is buy into the values and get the hell out of their way, they are going to do the right thing, they're doctors, they are good people, they care about patient care. They care about resources and space and curriculum and cash flow. I mean, you just got to get out of their way. You can't treat doctors like they are not knowledge workers.[50]

As Fischer Mangold grew, it became more difficult to find qualified physicians to staff EDs at some of the smaller and less desirable hospitals. An expected trickle-down occurred, where the best emergency physicians got the best ED positions and in some cases marginal-quality physicians were scheduled in marginal-quality institutions. Residency-trained emergency physicians were hot commodities in the 1970s and 1980s, and Fischer Mangold and other large emergency management companies had to pay a premium to attract them. Peter Rosen remembers speaking with Mangold about this, "He once berated me...for not producing more resident graduates because he couldn't hire resident trained emergency physicians cheaply."[9]

Mangold also stuck to his principles in terms of billing and making sure that his company did nothing for free. Michael Callaham, M.D., remembers a story related to him by Tom Evans, M.D., an emergency physician who is now deceased. Evans was a product of the sixties—a true "hippie" and "eccentric with a ponytail and full beard." Callaham relates,

> ...he did a locum tenens as I recall for Karl Mangold in Louisiana somewhere down in the bayou for a month or two and Tom had a huge empathy for the poor and the unfortunate...down there where the people were all poor, and so he charged his professional fees out accordingly. There were no coders so you did your own billing. He charged people $5 to $10 pretty much regardless of what he did because it was all they could really afford. So he finishes his locum tenens, of course he's getting paid by the hour or the shift, and a month or so later gets summoned down to Mangold's office by Mangold who is in a rage and asks him, "Are these your bills, what's this, pneumonia, admit to the hospital, ten bucks, extensive lacerations, five bucks, what is this crap?" "These people are poor they can't afford anything," and Mangold says to him, "What are you the god-damned Robin Hood of emergency medicine?" If you knew Tom, that is exactly what he was, he was the Robin Hood of emergency medicine.[51]

The label of emergency medicine robber baron was affixed to Mangold almost from the start. John McDade thinks that part of this criticism of Mangold and other early entrepreneurs from other physicians came from "insane jealousies—they wanted to be as rich as the other guys."[27] Mangold's response to critics was always the same:

> ...the best I can answer is that it's a free country. This is America. We are a competitive based, capitalistic, free enterprise society. If you want to beat me at what I'm doing you have to get out there and do the same thing and do it better and take my business away. That's the way it works for soap, or for cars, or everything else.

You are not going to change the American economic system. I thought this was the most inane, stupid kind of argument.[50]

In many ways, Mangold had fulfilled the American dream. He came from a relatively humble background, saw a great opportunity, worked hard, and capitalized on being the first person to form a business to manage multiple EDs. In the beginning he undoubtedly improved the care in the EDs he staffed. As his business grew, and competition increased, he encountered problems with staffing and ensuring quality at some of his hospital EDs.

While Karl Mangold was the first to become a true entrepreneur in emergency medicine, he was followed by a contingent of men who had similar paths and experiences. They were in the right place at the right time, had the ability to recognize a great business opportunity, and became more interested in management and systems than in seeing patients themselves. Two of these men, Leonard Riggs, Jr., M.D., and Robert Williams, M.D., were both native Texans. Williams came north to the University of Michigan for medical school and then returned to Parkland Hospital in Dallas for his internship. Riggs did his internship in Memphis and then worked for 6 months as an emergency physician at Baylor University Medical Center. He earned enough money to buy a new Corvette. Williams did a similar thing—moonlighting as an emergency doctor at a small hospital in Grayling, Michigan for 3 months. Williams remembers, "I worked 12 days straight in August, never left the hospital."[52] In this Vietnam War era, military service was required, and from 1970 to 1972, Riggs and Williams had very similar experiences as flight surgeons in the U.S. Navy—Williams was based at Jacksonville, Florida, and Riggs was in Pensacola. Williams returned to Michigan and partnered with James Johnson, M.D., another University of Michigan Medical School graduate who also had a doctorate in pharmacology. Johnson had started a surgery residency, but took a year off to work in the small hospital emergency department in Grayling, Michigan. Grayling is a small northern town whose population and emergency visits swell in the summer with the annual influx of tourists. Williams and Johnson were both excited and satisfied with ED work and liked the relaxed, outdoor environment of northern Michigan. They incorporated in 1972 as Emergency Medicine Consultants, Inc. (ECI). Much like the early American College of Emergency Physicians, they had a grand name for such a fledgling enterprise. Williams explains how it came about,

I remember reading a book by Walt Disney about that time, it was Walt Disney's philosophy that to be truly successful you had to take something that nobody wanted and make it something that everybody wanted. His model, of course, was Disney World, because before then Coney Island and circuses were seedy. He took something that nobody wanted and made it a good thing and people wanted it. When we first started, again it was our notion that we would work as much as we wanted to, which was a fair amount, and then we would have a lot of free time and we'd work some recruiting people like ourselves, who were primarily part time or might do one on an occasional basis. Once we realized what the potential was—where hospitals literally would call us. Remember in the early 70s, there was no organized emergency medicine in northern Michigan. People…staffed on a rotational basis, by the on-call physician, who lived up there all year to have the summers off, and then they get inundated with people. It was really a godsend to them to have anybody that would work in the department. Where ever we went there was a tremendous opportunity. If you could provide the service, which at that time meant a warm body, there was a huge demand for it. It didn't take us long, probably 6 or 7 years before we realized for this to work, we had to work at it full time, not try to be clinicians and learn how to be better business people. That was the major turning point for us. We quit practice and said let's run a business instead of a clinical practice.[52]

Johnson and Williams set up what John Rupke called "their trap line" of ED contracts in the small hospitals of northern Michigan, charging the hospitals a start-up fee of $100,000 for their services. This provided the capital for them to enlarge and expand. They initially employed primarily moonlighting residents from the University of Michigan and Grand Rapids residency programs, and then hired family practice physicians. In the early years, Williams and Johnson had to run around the state, filling in vacancies in the schedule and "putting out brush fires." In the middle 1970s, they were able to hire some emergency medicine residency graduates, and Williams notes,

> …we kind of expanded everywhere. We took contracts in Colorado and Texas and Florida and Georgia and Louisiana. That was a big mistake because we were too spread out to make it work properly. Then our group went through kind of a period of consolidation where we primarily dealt with small hospitals.[52]

Leonard Riggs had intended to do a plastic surgery residency when he finished his military commitment, but did not want to commit to that many years of residency. He then signed on for an ophthalmology residency, but had a year to wait to start the residency. He had very much enjoyed working in the Baylor ED, and he returned to Texas and resumed his job. The ED was run by B. Lewayne Lambert, M.D., who had formed a group called Emergency Health Services Associates. Lambert knew something of ACEP and the national move toward specialty status, and was trying to make his staff appear credible. Riggs says,

> I remember after I had been there 4 or 5 months one day he said, "You know you really ought to go sign up to be a member of the medical staff." I said, "What does that mean?" He said, "Well you go up there and fill out some papers and stuff and that way you can be on the medical staff." So I worked at Baylor in [19]69, all of [19]72 and finally the first record they have of me working at the hospital is in 1973 when it dawned on us that I probably ought to go down there and get medical staff membership and privileges. That is how these things were in those days.[23]

Riggs recognized a great opportunity in emergency care and says, "I liked it so much that I called the ophthalmology residency and turned them down and said, I'm going to stick this out for a while—I kind of like what I am doing over here." The Baylor University Medical Center was a well-respected teaching hospital, and Riggs took over the contract there when Lambert left. He remembers, "we were getting called, it seemed like daily…by all these little hospitals in the area around here begging us to come and provide a similar service." He expanded to five northern Texas hospitals and eventually formed a new entity, EmCare, Inc., which would become one of the largest emergency medicine management groups in the country. In the early years Riggs, like Williams and Johnson, "could barely find enough qualified, good guys to work with us at Baylor much less to try to staff some other places," and he found it difficult to both work clinically and manage his new business.[23] Riggs notes,

> I was running around, you know you can imagine, with a shoebox in the back seat to collect money to cover the bills, pay the doctors—one thing I always did was make sure that the doctors got paid correctly and on time. I was trying to get the other members of the group to become involved in the running of it, I just could not get them interested. They didn't want the responsibility, they didn't want to do the extra administrative work, some of them didn't want the liabilities, financial or otherwise. Malpractice was almost unheard of in those days. I remember the first time I bought a good policy it was $0.25 per patient. When it went up to $1 a patient I was outraged…So I had a hard time finding others who wanted to be partners, that is why sometimes I'm amused about this democratic group stuff, I couldn't get anybody who wanted to be part of the group. It is really the reason that I formed a management company on the side—I couldn't get the guys to participate. Maybe we were just attracting guys who wanted to work their shift and go home. We all know that is still an issue. A lot of people do that. I continued working, pretty much a full clinical load, while running around to these other hospitals.[23]

Riggs became familiar with ACEP and attended the scientific assembly when it was held in Dallas in 1973. He met the leaders of the field and entertained them in Dallas. Some remarked that there was not much to do in Dallas, and it was therefore ironic that 7 years later Riggs would help orchestrate the relocation of ACEP to the city. Riggs came into the good graces of the ACEP leadership, and he notes, they "took an interest in marshalling me forward." He believes that this was partly due to the fact that his group held contracts in larger, respected teaching and community hospitals. He remembers meeting Karl Mangold, and says, "in many ways Karl was a bit of a mentor for me." They met at an ACEP Winter Symposium in Palm Springs, California, and while walking to dinner found that the biggest challenge for both "was trying to attract and retain high-quality doctors."[23]

Riggs even became involved in the ABEM test development process, preparing the questions on facial injuries. He helped start the Texas Chapter of ACEP, and remembers the early meetings had six or eight people in attendance. As his group became larger and more stable, he had more time to devote to national organizational activities. By 1976, Riggs was elected to the ACEP board of directors, and in 1980–1981, just 7 years after beginning work as an emergency physician he was the president of ACEP. His rapid rise to success had its personal costs. Riggs says, "I was totally consumed by my career. I had a failed marriage. I got married in [19]77 and it was ended in [19]79."[23]

One of the things that Mangold and Riggs discussed, and Williams and Johnson came to appreciate, was the concept of incentive-based compensation for their emergency physicians. The standard model, initially, for large group practices was to bill for their physicians services, pay their malpractice insurance, take out a management fee (for ECI this was 13% or 14% of revenues), and provide the remainder as salary to physicians. Riggs came to recognize that "people do what you pay them to do." He remembers how he went beyond that approach,

> A brainstorm came to me from one of my business advisors. He said, "One of the things that you are complaining about is, they won't fill in their fee sheets," which we had to do to get the charges done properly and transform it into codes, and he and I came up with this idea, why don't we put them on a percentage of what they produce versus an hourly guarantee. In one month after it started they started using all the fee sheets and their pay jumped from $16 an hour to $25 an hour. They were nervous wrecks about it, but I guaranteed them that it wouldn't go any lower than it was. Putting everybody to work for us on the same deal, I didn't differentiate between, they were doing the same work, it didn't make sense to me to pay a resident less than a moonlighting resident less than a staff man. What we were trying to do was encourage full-time career oriented people, anyway…If you incentivize them the right way you get the right behavior.[23]

Williams also adopted an incentive-based method of compensation and this allowed ECI to become more profitable and to pay physicians more, which was a big factor in the retention of physicians. He notes,

> …once we reach budget 85% of any additional revenues are distributed as an incentive plan for the doctors. That is how you get a 92% retention rate, and you show people the numbers. I think that is fair. I don't think it is unfair to do the things we do for a 13% or 14% management fee to arrange malpractice, to do the billing, to take care of the scheduling, recruiting. But if people are making 50% margins, which, it has never happened in our organization, and the physicians were earning $200 an hour and they were being paid $50, then that would be exploitation. That is a very rare situation in my experience.[52]

Those who formed emergency medicine "mega groups" often had one or two hospitals that served as their showpieces for quality and employee satisfaction. At these flagship hospitals many of the emergency physicians were well trained, ABEM-certified, were well paid, and had long tenures of employment at that hospital. Riggs was proud to have the first collection of all ABEM-certified emergency physicians at Baylor University Medical Center. These physicians often became prominent members of hospital committees and active in the community. At these places, the annual retention rate might be as high as the 92% quoted by Williams. This was the best face of what became to be known as emergency medicine contract management groups, or CMGs.

(The industry, which also developed in other medical fields became known as physician practice management, or PPM.) The profitability was far different away from the flagship hospitals. As Williams notes, at smaller hospitals in less desirable locations and where the patient payer mix might not be as good, ED contracts would operate at a loss if not for the subsidy paid by hospitals.

> ...most emergency physicians in my experience work in situations where they do not earn their own salary. In our organization with 66 clients we probably have ten where we survive strictly on fee-for-service revenue, the other 50 there is not enough money there to hire residency-trained people, for example.[52]

The fact that hospitals were often eager to pay a large sum of money to ECI or other emergency medicine management groups to run their emergency department attests to the difficulty of finding qualified emergency physicians. A mega group through the ED contract would provide the hospital with reliable staffing of the ED, assume the malpractice risk for the physicians, and address physician problems or complaints. For beleaguered hospitals and medical staffs, especially the smaller hospitals that had always struggled to staff their EDs with anything other than a rotation of the medical staff or poor-quality itinerant physicians, contracting with a mega group was usually a winning proposition.

As the first emergency-medicine–residency-trained physicians became available for hire, hospitals began to inquire about these qualifications in the physicians supplied by the emergency medicine management groups. This was a tough request to meet. First, many early emergency medicine graduates formed their own small groups or went to work in academic centers. The trickle of residency-trained physicians was going into a desert of need. Karl Mangold remembers the situation in the late 1970s,

> There must have been 100 emergency residency–trained in the country, and all these medical staffs are saying we want...residency trained emergency physicians. I said we want them too. That's what I've been working for all my life![50]

The residency graduates expected to command higher salaries than non–residency-trained emergency physicians, but contract groups did not necessarily see it that way. In some cases, emergency medicine residency trained physicians did not outperform those who were already in practice. Given the meager residency education of most early graduates, this would not have been surprising. Leonard Riggs found that those emergency medicine residency graduates who performed the best were those who had practiced in an ED and then done residency training.[23] He found that many of his long-time practice-trained emergency physicians functioned as well as, if not better than, the new residency graduates. If the large contract groups were able to attract residency-trained emergency physicians, they placed them at their premier hospitals, where reimbursement and physician's pay and practice environment were usually better.

Few emergency-medicine–residency-trained physicians worked in the backwater hospitals, and these locations became the sore spots and breeding grounds for exploitation in corporate emergency medicine. The PPMs often secured the ED contracts at these places and resorted to staffing with physicians who were not much better qualified than the legendary itinerant emergency room doctors of the 1950s. Although Mangold, Riggs, and Williams strongly state that they attempted to find the best available physicians to staff their EDs at a time when not many qualified physicians were available, they struggled with this quality chasm. Many of their peers who were not in the business side of emergency medicine understood this dilemma, and have "a hard time painting with a uniformly black brush" when critiquing the early PPM leaders.[53] These men profited greatly from emergency medicine, but also made valuable contributions to specialty recognition and to the organizational and clinical advancement of the field.

The 1980s are remembered as a time when prosperity was sometimes accompanied by selfishness and greed. The dour mood and financial malaise of the 1970s was replaced by a freewheeling, "get it while you can" attitude as the economy heated up.

The Reagan administration was as pro-business as any in U.S. history. Taxes were cut and regulations diminished. In the medical world, two factors dominated the outlook for the future. The first was that health care costs were skyrocketing and that some type of control would be needed. Health maintenance organizations (HMOs), with their new, rationed, business-model approach, were thought to be the answer to controlling costs. The rise of HMOs brought new approaches to outpatient and hospital care, but few restrictions were placed on emergency care. However at the federal level, Medicare cuts were an annual refrain, and it became clear that the golden days of physicians submitting a bill for services and being handed a full payment check in return were rapidly fading. These economic factors made the entrepreneurs of medicine feel that it was imperative to make lots of money fast, because the window of time for major profits was shrinking. The second dominant factor in shaping the mood of medicine in the 1980s was the feeling that an oversupply of physicians existed and that it would be difficult for physicians to find jobs in the coming decades.[54,55] In emergency medicine, this was coupled with the idea that hospitals would be closing as HMO care became more prevalent and that with primary care increasingly handled in HMO clinics, the number of emergency visits would decrease.[42] Although none of these forecasts turned out to be true, by the middle of the 1980s a sense of urgent competition was fostered for both individual emergency physicians and the PPMs. They had serious concerns that their earning potential would be reduced in the coming years.

The PPMs found a niche in the competition for hospital emergency care that was not being adequately filled by others in medicine. Many emergency medicine–residency graduates were staying in academics or forming their own groups at desirable hospitals. Other ABEM-certified physicians were in stable, smaller groups and some in regional PPMs. But thousands of emergency physicians, many of whom were incompletely trained and not board-certified, were working in less favored EDs. The mentality of many of these physicians was to work their shifts, much like laborers in other industries and then to enjoy their lives outside of medicine. But, as Mangold, Riggs, and other early physician management groups found, this shift-worker attitude was also present in many career and residency-trained emergency physicians. It became apparent that emergency physicians often chose the field so they could have a satisfying, challenging medical job, without any of the worries of upkeep, overhead, or management. Emergency physicians, when compared with their colleagues in the traditional medical fields, were more likely to be mobile and to have other hobbies, activities, or side careers. It was not uncommon to find an emergency physician who was an international adventurer, airline pilot, or small business owner in his or her "spare time." By offering flexibility and the ability to pursue outside opportunities, emergency medicine also fostered a lack of commitment and reduced involvement in the management of hospital EDs by a significant cadre of its members. Into this vacuum stepped the PPMs.

Although they may not have intended for it to happen, men like Mangold, Williams, and Riggs created the formula from which a monster would grow in emergency practice. The corporate expansion of emergency medicine took off in the 1980s, far beyond what the early entrepreneurs had ever imagined. The scale of some PPMs went up another order of magnitude. Job opportunities listed in the *Annals of Emergency Medicine* in 1988 included prominent advertisements from California-based companies. Fischer Mangold offered positions in nine different states. Emergency Physicians Medical Group and California Emergency Services competed for contracts across the state. Coastal Emergency Care boasted in bold letters of its "quality assurance," and EmCare listed opportunities in Texas, New Mexico, Louisiana, Florida, and New York. And a relative newcomer to the field had become the biggest PPM of all—Spectrum Emergency Care had an ad proclaiming that it was "serving over 400 hospitals coast to coast." Spectrum was apparently appealing to a certain type of emergency physician. Its advertisement included a photograph of a black doctor's bag, with a European travel book sticking out the top, and a set of keys to a BMW lying in front of the bag.[56]

In some cases, the incentive-based compensation model favored by Mangold, Riggs, and Williams was eschewed. PPMs hired part-time or moonlighting physicians, paid them a low hourly rate, and skimmed profits off the top at a rate exceeding 30%. The PPMs also limited competition by locking their full-time physicians into contracts with exclusivity features. These contract clauses were also known as restrictive covenants. In the event that the PPM lost an ED contract with a hospital, the restrictive covenant prevented the emergency physician from working in that ED for the new contract group. The restrictive covenant clause was usually in effect for 2 or 3 years. Exclusivity clauses also kept physician employees from banding together as a new entity and outbidding the parent PPM for the hospital ED contract. In its most extreme iteration, the restrictive covenant also prevented the emergency physician from working for any hospital within a certain distance from the original hospital.[57]

The net result of the PPM movement was the perpetuation of an underclass of emergency physicians who were sometimes ABEM-certified, but usually had limited training—often only an internship. These low-level staff physicians could be shuttled from hospital to hospital and had no prospects of long-term career advancement. Whereas the standard practice in a democratic group was for a member to rise to full partnership after a trial period of a few years, the large PPMs offered almost no chance for becoming a partner. In one PPM, there were four levels to advance through before the physician would receive a full profit share, and 10 years of service were required to become a senior partner.[58] Graduating emergency medicine residents would sometimes jump at the chance to become the ED director at a PPM-run hospital, only to find that they were not able to rise to become a partner in the organization. Data from the late 1980s and early 1990s demonstrate how the PPMs focused on physicians who were lesser trained. A survey of emergency medicine groups found that those groups allowing "equity participation" or the ability to become a partner in the group within a few years were far more likely to have a majority of board-certified emergency physicians as members.[59]

As the PPMs began competing with each other for contracts, the connection between quality emergency care at individual hospitals and the corporate mission was harder to make. The extent of the business motive in emergency medicine, which had been viewed by some in the early years as inappropriate, now became almost obscene. The huge resources of the large PPMs allowed them to rip contracts out of the hands of smaller, local "democratic" emergency groups. In the tried and true practice of big-business franchises, the PPMs could outbid a smaller group for a less lucrative hospital ED contract, even if it meant operating at a loss, to lock up more desirable contracts in an area or within a particular health system.[34]

Hospital administrators and medical staff leaders were the disbursers of hospital ED contracts, and they became essential for the rise of PPMs in emergency medicine. PPMs employed recruiters and managers who sold their product to hospitals. These individuals became very adept at wooing hospital administrators with glossy brochures, fancy meals, and inducements like sports tickets or free hotel lodging. They talked about the things that were appealing to hospital administrators like quality assurance, risk management, and efficiency of care. They pledged to staff the ED with high-quality physicians. In some cases, the PPMs would initially supply their best emergency physicians to give the appearance of a quality staffing model. Gregory West, M.D., an emergency physician who worked for Sterling, EmCare, and National Emergency Services, said in a recent interview,

> CMGs are notorious for using "startup doctors" who are board-certified, residency-trained and experienced when they first take over a contract. The startup doctors are then moved to the newest hospital and replaced with physicians without board certification. I was the only board-certified ED doctor of more than 15 doctors at two of the hospitals where I worked for one CMG. They would showcase me when competing for new contracts.[60]

It appears that in many cases, hospitals were willing to overlook the complaints of patients and their medical staff about weaker emergency physicians due to the money saved in a contract with a large PPM.[57]

The ability of smaller emergency medicine groups, even those with all residency-trained and ABEM-certified physicians, to compete with large PPMs had been greatly reduced by the late 1980s. During this time of increasing corporate presence in medicine, hospitals and health systems were financially strapped and some were going bankrupt. They became increasingly concerned about cost savings. The argument that residency-trained emergency physicians could provide higher quality, more stable emergency care became less convincing when placed against the financial concerns. The large PPMs, which could pay lesser trained, part-time, or moonlighting physicians a low hourly rate, could bid lower on contracts because their payout in emergency physicians salaries was far less. They were also able to move much more rapidly to acquire contracts for larger hospitals or for health systems where smaller hospital contracts might be packaged with a large hospital ED contract. As Leonard Riggs notes,

> The small democratic group can't recruit fast enough to do that kind of stuff and pay the build up of accounts receivable which is significant, at least 8 months worth before the pipe line gets filled up.[23]

Although often well intentioned and egalitarian, the smaller group had much less experience with negotiations and could not offer the glitz or inducements of the PPM managers. When it came to big-time ED contract acquisition, they were like high school athletes trying to compete with the pros.

The next phase of corporate growth of emergency medicine occurred when competition between PPMs escalated. In the never-ending move to get bigger and raise capital, some of the PPMs went to Wall Street and became publicly traded companies on the stock exchange. Leonard Riggs remembers that his company, EmCare, was trying "to be in the better quality places," but that it was hard to remain "pure" in the very competitive PPM business:

> The other large groups kept trying to buy us or merge with us...The problem was that when we'd go try to compete for an important, busy place that could command a residency even for example, these bigger competitors could under cut us because they had more financial resources than we did. We had 50 or 60 contracts, they had 200 or 300. Even thought some of those were smaller, they still had a lot bigger company, and I came to this conclusion that we were going to have to continue to grow or you will fail to survive if you stop growing. I didn't want to just grow willy-nilly so I decided we had to have some sort of financing in place to help us weather the storm against these bigger guys and that's how we eventually wound up with some investors from New York....[23]

Then, like other large companies whose shareholders demanded high performance, the pressure was on to expand into other areas of medical and even nonmedical services. The big PPMs established contracts with hospitals to provide physician staffing for ambulatory primary care clinics. At least one PPM bought hospital vending machine contracts—profits could then be realized from care of the emergency patient and from the soda pop or candy bars that the patient's relatives purchased in the hospital vending areas. The contrast between the simple ED staffing contract signed by James Mills, Jr., and his three colleagues with Alexandria Hospital in 1961 and the status of the business of emergency medicine 30 years later could not be more striking. By the early 1990s, some publicly traded PPMs had 300 or more hospital ED contracts and were run by physician businessmen who had not cared for an emergency patient in years, or even worse, executive officers who had little concept of the state of emergency care. The business of emergency medicine had become like nothing ever seen in American medicine, and seemed to some like an animal eating its young. The incomes of emergency medicine PPM leaders surpassed the most exorbitant salaries of the other high earners in medicine. Corporate reports in the 1990s show base salaries for the chief executive officers of PPMs of $400,000 to $500,000, with stock options ranging from $2 to over $20 million.[58]

Other medical fields in the 1980s found that forming group practices facilitated work schedules and could be more profitable than solo practice. Radiology, anesthesiology, and pathology, which like emergency medicine were hospital-based specialties, sometimes formed incorporated physician groups and secured contracts at multiple hospitals. These small, regional groups were much like the early group practices in emergency medicine, but other medical specialties did not mushroom to the next level of national, multistate, corporate mega groups. One of the reasons for this was the presence of internal controls in other fields. While ACEP, the primary national organization of emergency medicine, neglected to take a position against the excesses of corporate management in emergency medicine, other specialty societies advanced codes of ethics, or guiding principles that attempted to restrain exploitation and business improprieties. For example, in 1991 the American Society of Anesthesiologists issued a policy statement about how professional income should be derived. The statement noted that exploitation of anesthesiologists by other anesthesiologists is improper and that members of a group practice should receive appropriate, proportionate income.[61] These codes or guidelines were not backed up with any significant enforcement methods, but did give the sense that someone was monitoring the business side of these fields. The best that ACEP could offer at this time was a weak "value statement" in 1990 advocating for the "fair and equitable" relationships between emergency physicians and business entities.[59]

At a time when all of medicine was becoming more business-oriented, emergency medicine evolved into the most fertile field for corporate growth, profits, and exploitation. The entrepreneurs were clever about keeping a step ahead of government regulations and the health care marketplace in building their empires. Although PPMs gained a reputation for exploiting physicians, not all PPMs were exploitative, and it was clear that smaller business arrangements in emergency medicine could also result in exploitation. Karl Mangold notes,

> The biggest exploitation I've ever seen, it was where one doctor had one hospital; it was well connected to the medical staff, the board of trustees, the administration, and not infrequently the mayor and board of supervisors. They never wanted to have another full-time career emergency physician with them. They just wanted to rotate residents and military, and fellows through forever because they could make a big amount of money.[50]

Exploitation could also occur in the academic setting if the emergency medicine director chose to skim profits from the billings of junior faculty members and unfairly reward him- or herself or senior faculty members. In fact, it may have been easier to financially exploit faculty in emergency medicine than in other academic fields, because in many cases there was little oversight from medical school administration or the hospital, and emergency medicine was allowed to tend to its own business. Even by the early 1980s, the problem of corporate practice and exploitation of emergency physicians was concerning to emergency medicine leaders. Robert Simon, M.D., who was then assistant residency director at the UCLA emergency medicine program, wrote in 1983,

> The entrepreneurism of large corporations and some multihospital groups and even many single hospital groups with one or two individuals receiving a large portion of the "pie" has resulted in very few being able to maintain the same group of physicians in the same hospital for more than a few years…I believe this practice is truly destructive to the future of emergency medicine in that highly capable physicians…are finding it increasingly difficult to find a stable and fair group.[62]

The early emergency medicine entrepreneurs were minimally trained, often not board-certified, but academic emergency medicine eventually began to produce the next generation of emergency medicine businessmen. Perhaps the most prominent of these is Stephen Dresnick, M.D., who graduated from the UCLA emergency medicine residency program, and became chairman of emergency medicine and founding director of the emergency medicine residency program at Orlando Regional Medical Center. In 1987, Dresnick co-founded Sterling Healthcare Group, Inc., which became a leading PPM. From its inception, according to Dresnick, Sterling contracts with emergency physicians did not have exclusivity clauses or restrictive covenants.[63] By 1994 Sterling had gone public, and was sold to San Diego–based FPA Medical Management, Inc., in 1996.

If ever a book was written for a waiting, receptive audience, it was *The Rape of Emergency Medicine: A Novel by the Phoenix*.[57] The book was published anonymously in 1991, and the author later identified himself to be James K. Keaney, M.D. The book was "a fictionalized recounting of his many years working for multihospital emergency department contract management groups."[64] Keaney wrote the book in the style of Samuel Shem's 1978 novel, *House of God*, with an irreverent, humorous tirade directed at what he called "the largest covert health care swindle in the history of American medicine." The villains in Keaney's book, some of whom seem to be amalgamations of various early PPM entrepreneurs, engage in corporate skimming, stealing of contracts, and the exploitation of their physician workforce through restrictive covenants and unfair firings. The heroes expose the corporate greed of the "suits" and Keaney provides disturbing descriptions of poor-quality emergency physicians and their mishaps in emergency care. *The Rape of Emergency Medicine* was widely read by emergency physicians and created head-shaking discussions by practitioners in community and academic settings. Most knew that Keaney's account, although fictional and in some cases exaggerated and unsubstantiated, was a fairly accurate description of the excesses of PPMs. Keaney touched a nerve for many emergency physicians on what had gone bad in emergency medicine.[57]

For a number of years, editorials in emergency medicine journals and barroom talk at national meetings had murmured that if something did not change with the marauding PPMs and ACEP's failure to do anything substantial to oppose them, a new organization would have to arise in emergency medicine to address the issues. After Keaney was revealed as the author of his book, he received many calls from emergency physicians who wanted to do something about PPMs in emergency medicine. With the encouragement of a like-minded fellow emergency physician named Scott Plantz, Keaney decided in 1992 to form the American Academy of Emergency Physicians (AAEM). Ironically, this was the "fictional" name Keaney chose in his book to lampoon ACEP. In 1993 Keaney appeared on the television show "60 Minutes" as part of an expose on emergency care and PPMs. After this, AAEM membership grew to hundreds of physicians. Robert McNamara, M.D., who trained in emergency medicine under David Wagner at MCP and had seen his own graduating emergency medicine residents hurt and exploited, became a crusader for AAEM against PPMs, and was a strident critic of ACEP's reluctance to take a strong stand against the improprieties of PPMs.[58] The resulting political battle, which is still playing out, caused ACEP to rethink its positions and become more supportive of its board-certified, practicing emergency physicians and less visibly involved with PPMs.

The solution to the mega group dilemma and exploitation of emergency physicians, as Peter Rosen noted, would have been for well-trained emergency physicians to form small, democratic emergency medicine groups to compete favorably against the PPMs for hospital ED contracts at all U.S. hospitals. In the 1980s and even to the present, this has turned out to be a pipedream. The reason that PPMs were able to secure contracts in the smaller, more rural and even some larger urban hospitals was because smaller emergency physician groups did not want to work in those environments. Pamela Bensen, who ran a regional emergency medicine group in Maine says, "To the day I left practice in 2001, I could not hire board-certified emergency physicians—they wouldn't come."[7] Even if they did look to work in the less desirable hospitals, the higher salary expectations of trained emergency physicians made it difficult for financially strapped hospitals to come up with a reasonable contract offer. Adding to this problem was the fact that some hospital administrators remained unconvinced that board certification or training in emergency medicine was really necessary. The administrator of a small hospital in Texas, in discussing the merits of ABEM certification for emergency physicians said, "But hands-on experience is better than any test you can take." He also noted,

If you have a board-certified emergency medicine physician you will advertise it. The public thinks it's great. They perceive it having greater quality. I don't think there is any difference.[65]

The end result is that even with the extensive development of emergency medicine as a medical specialty, thousands of ED positions are left unfilled by residency-trained or board-certified emergency physicians in the small and less appealing hospitals of America. In 1994, there were an estimated 3,200 ACEP members who were not eligible for board certification in emergency medicine, and probably an equal or greater number of non–board-eligible emergency practitioners who were not affiliated with ACEP or organized emergency medicine. PPMs became the default job brokers for this underclass in emergency medicine—matching physicians to hospitals where the tentacles of interest for more qualified emergency physicians did not reach. It can be rationalized that if this gap exists, and PPMs are allowing needy hospitals to have rudimentary ED staffing, this is better than what might otherwise be managed. But as in any situation where need is great, supply is limited, and workers are vulnerable, the specter of exploitation lingers. Some PPMs did a fairly honorable job of providing low-end emergency physician services to low-end hospitals, but the few that used unethical and abusive practices created a bad odor that permeated the entire atmosphere of contract emergency medicine. Some smaller hospitals never bought into the PPM movement, or after being burned, stopped contracting with PPMs. For these hospitals, ED coverage is provided by a local contingent of physicians (often family medicine doctors) who are paid directly by the hospital. Other small hospitals use physician's assistants or nurse practitioners to staff their EDs, with physician back up and liberal transfer policies for sicker patients. The problem of emergency physician staffing in rural hospitals and in some "undesirable" municipal hospitals remains unsolved by the growth and advancement of the field.

As the economics of health care became more profit-driven, cost conscious, and cutthroat in the 1990s, some unraveling occurred in the PPM world. Spectrum Healthcare came under intense legal scrutiny and was successfully sued by two North Dakota emergency physicians who had been under restrictive covenants in their contracts. The North Dakota Supreme Court found that the contracts were void because they "restrain the physicians from negotiating for and securing future employment."[66] Spectrum was also sued unsuccessfully for violating laws against the corporate practice of medicine in Texas. Spectrum and EmCare, Inc., also ran into legal problems in the 1990s when they were charged by the federal government with Medicare fraud for up-coding emergency patients' bills. The actual fraudulent billing charge was leveled against Emergency Physicians Billing Services (EPBS), which was run by J. D. McKean, M.D., whose financial expertise had helped bail ACEP out of its financial difficulties in the late 1970s. EPBS was also sued. In the settlement with the federal government, EmCare paid $7.75 million in 1997, and Spectrum paid $3.1 million in 1998.[67,68]

Emergency medicine contract groups suffered the same fates as many new service industries in the 1990s as mergers, buy-outs, and bankruptcies changed the entire landscape of the business. As noted before, Dresnick's Sterling Healthcare, Inc., was bought out by FPA Medical Management, Inc., which went bankrupt in 1998, and Sterling was sold to Coastal Physician Group, which changed its name to PhyAmerica Physician Group, which also filed for bankruptcy in 2002. Leonard Riggs and his partners sold EmCare, Inc., to a Canadian company, Laidlaw, Inc., which specialized in school bus transportation services, ambulance companies, and waste management, and was looking to expand into the emergency medicine PPM business. Within 2 years, Laidlaw was looking to dump its EmCare acquisition. Karl Mangold and his partner sold Fischer Mangold to MedPartners in 1997, which was then sold to venture capitalists and became Team Health. By the end of the 1990s, the PPMs of emergency medicine had become true corporate giants like telecommunications businesses or the auto industry, with five or so large companies controlling most nonacademic ED contracts in the country. As Robert McNamara wrote in the late 1990s,

> Certain geographic markets are so dominated by the PPM industry that they essentially control the only jobs available to graduating EM residents. Such areas include Florida, Texas, Michigan, New Jersey, and Washington, D.C.[58]

Emergency medicine always carried a chip on its shoulder, struggling to be recognized for excellence by the traditional medical specialties and trying to be innovative and better at delivering care than other fields. By the 1990s emergency medicine could claim a dubious dominance in one area—it was champion of the PPM industry. The big businesses of emergency medicine had evolved to be as different from the small physician staffing groups of the 1970s, as ACEP, now a large specialty organization in the 1990s, was from the small, 30-member group that had formed the organization in 1968. Emergency medicine became a ripe orchard for the PPMs to pick partly because it was a new field, without the limiting burdens of tradition or a professional code that resisted corporate overtures. It was emergency medicine's mindset to be different, so new types of practice arrangements were more welcomed than shunned. Emergency physicians were consenting adult shift workers who provided a distinct, portable service that could be nicely packaged and sold. And for a few years, when PPMs remained smaller and more accountable, the PPM system often did work, without a great degree of exploitation. However the massive enlargement and degree of corporate impropriety of the late 1980s and 1990s erased the credibility of the emergency medicine PPMs.

Emergency medicine could lay claim to being the leader in the PPM movement and the expansion of corporate medicine, but other medical fields were soon discovered by corporate interests, including primary care, pediatrics, oncology, and pathology. PPMs in these fields rapidly developed into publicly traded companies in the 1980s and 1990s. The number of PPMs in other fields may be less than in emergency medicine, but profits were comparable. U.S. Oncology, Inc., employed 900 physicians in 32 states, and had revenues of $2 billion and a net profit of $71 million in 2003.[69]

The debate still rages about whether PPMs have destroyed emergency medicine. For the most part, the academic emergency medicine world has stayed out of this practice issue, but has occasionally directly benefited from the largesse of PPM leaders who made it big. In 1996, Stephen Dresnick, who had done his undergraduate schooling at the University of North Carolina, gave a $1 million gift to establish the Stephen J. Dresnick, M.D., Distinguished Chair of Emergency Medicine, and Judith Tintinalli became the first endowed chair. Cynics would say that Dresnick was just trying to buy influence with graduating emergency medicine residents and North Carolina hospitals. The more charitable view of this charitable contribution was that PPMs, which had profited so greatly in the business of emergency medicine, were now giving something back to help develop the specialty.

Becoming a Primary Board

The relationships between emergency medicine leaders who were elected to the board of directors of the American Board of Emergency Medicine (ABEM) and the physicians from the other medical specialties who were appointed to the modified conjoint board by their respective boards evolved in a most interesting way. As the emergency physicians in ABEM demonstrated that they could administer a top-notch, innovative certifying examination and contribute in a meaningful way to discussion and policy decisions in the ABMS, the nonemergency medicine directors of ABEM were transformed from skepticism and sometimes opposition to the field. As noted in Chapter 6, the representatives of other specialties became true believers in emergency medicine and coached the emergency physicians on how to best move toward primary board approval. ABEM fully funded the participation of these representatives from other boards, and many became friendly with the emergency medicine ABEM leaders and their spouses. Unfortunately, this level of collegiality did not necessarily extend back to the parent boards of these ABEM representatives. Internal medicine, in particular, seemed to be waiting for a chance to undermine emergency medicine.

Despite the conjoint board label, ABEM functioned as an independent board from the start. Benson Munger, the executive director, was a bright, fair, extremely organized, and efficient administrator and was responsible for much of the respect that came ABEM's way. Munger initially was concerned because most of the other boards were run by physician presidents or executive directors, and he thought he might be treated differently because he was not a physician. However Munger's talent was appreciated by the other board directors, and he was quickly viewed as a peer within ABMS. By 1987, ABEM had certified 5,371 diplomates in emergency medicine, and the board was running smoothly. The makeup of the ABEM board of directors changed in 1986, when for the first time new directors were required to be diplomates (board-certified) of ABEM. Munger and the ABEM leaders decided that it was time to push for primary board status. The other nonemergency medicine representatives on ABEM agreed. In fact, family medicine had dropped out in 1986 as a sponsor on the conjoint board because it believed that ABEM should be a primary board. Even as it moved forward in pursuit of primary board status, ABEM intended to keep representatives from other boards on it board of directors, because these individuals had provided valuable counsel for the new specialty. The main difference between an ABMS primary board and conjoint boards was that primary boards could offer subspecialty certifications. The obvious subspecialties in emergency medicine were critical care, pediatric emergency medicine, and toxicology. The latter two did not turn out to be much of a problem, but the critical care issue became a thorn in the side of ABEM.

Emergency medicine had a logical interface with critical care going back to the early 1970s when the Federation for Emergency and Critical Care Medicine was formed to aid in specialty recognition for emergency medicine. Although the Federation did not last, a small subset of emergency physicians continued to think that subspecialty certification in critical care was valuable and desirable. In the middle 1980s four boards, internal medicine, pediatrics, surgery and anesthesiology, tried to create a common subspecialty certificate in critical care. When this fell through, each of the four applied separately and was approved by ABMS in 1985 to offer subspecialty certification in critical care. ABEM, still in its modified conjoint board status, in 1986 also proposed to issue certificates of added qualification in critical care. The American Board of Internal Medicine (ABIM) sent an official letter of opposition. Pediatrics also objected, and Benson Munger remembers that they "were paranoid about the idea of emergency physicians working outside of the emergency department."[70] John Benson, Jr., M.D., a staunch opponent of ABEM in the 1970s who grudgingly gave approval to the modified conjoint board, was still president of ABIM, and still was up for a rousing battle over the critical care issue. In the ABIM objection, Benson wrote a fairly condescending opinion that emergency medicine training only dealt with the short-term critical care and that emergency medicine residents needed at least 2 years of internal medicine training to have a broad enough background to pursue additional critical care training.[71] This flap over critical care was part of what pushed ABEM toward applying for primary board status.

ABEM prepared a reasonable, well-substantiated argument in its 1987 application for primary board status. But, in a similar manner to what had happened with the 1977 application to ABMS, the ABEM leaders were reassured by individuals from other boards that ABMS would be supportive, but underestimated the political maneuverings and opposition of some of the other boards. With a two-thirds vote needed for passage, 48 ABMS representatives voted for ABEM approval as an ABMS primary board and 52 were opposed. All the representatives from internal medicine, pediatrics, obstetrics and gynecology, and surgery voted against. ABEM was highly disappointed, but the response from practicing emergency physicians was not nearly as dramatic as the 1977 negative ABMS vote. Emergency physicians seemed secure that they had a certifying board and were not too concerned with the details at the upper level of the organizations. But, for men like James Mills, Jr., Gail Anderson, Harris Graves, R. R. Hannas, Ronald Krome, David Wagner, and George Podgorny, who had fought the initial battles for specialty recognition and were still on the ABEM board of directors, this final challenge was of great importance. They teamed with Ben Munger to develop a plan that would lead to primary board approval.

Internal medicine and pediatrics, as they had been from the time ABEM was first proposed, were very concerned about the migration of emergency physicians into areas they traditionally controlled. Emergency medicine had become one of the top-three most competitive fields for the residency match, and internal medicine feared that it would lose more potential internists if emergency medicine also offered a path to subspecialty certification in critical care. Some leaders in internal medicine challenged the sanctity of emergency medicine training by proposing the development of a fellowship year in emergency medicine following an internal medicine residency. This would have done great damage to emergency medicine's credibility and improved internal medicine's ability to attract medical students. Another hot-button topic for internal medicine was the ability of internists who worked in the medicine/surgery-segregated EDs of academic centers to become board-certified in emergency medicine after the ABEM practice track closed in 1988. These internists complained to ABIM, seeking a path for ABEM certification, and ABIM advocated for this in the negotiations.

Judith Tintinalli was on the ABEM board of directors at the time, and served as president in 1989. She remembers how the debate evolved.

> So, internal medicine started agitating, they are like, we are going to finally kill emergency medicine…We are going to kill it by developing a subspecialty certificate in emergency/internal medicine. Ped[iatric]s decided they would do that at the same time. It took, first thing I had to do, we actually had special retreats of the board that year. We had about three of them because I needed all of the directors of ABEM to have a single vision on what we were going to do, how we were going to fight this attack and it was out of that that everybody finally agreed okay, let's go to them with another proposal. Let's have a combined program, with an offer they can't refuse. So we came out with the idea of the combined EM [emergency medicine]/IM [internal medicine] programs, combined Ped[iatric]s/EM programs. We had grandfather clauses for boarded internists who worked in academic centers. It made the academic people feel like they were getting something out of the deal and they were able to buy into emergency medicine. There was a lot of dissension within emergency medicine at that time…the real hard liners versus the flexible people. The real hard liners said no straight ER [emergency room], nothing else. This is actually how we came to the 5-year [combined] programs, is because emergency medicine would not back down from a 5-year training program."[6]

Most emergency physicians were not aware of the continued pecking of the traditional medical specialties at the kernels of the new specialty. The average board-certified emergency physician was thinking about his or her ABEM recertification examination. ABEM field-tested a recertification examination in 1985 to 1986, and first offered both oral and written recertification examinations in 1989.

After intense discussions, ABEM decided to give up the critical care issue to gain ABIM approval for a primary board in emergency medicine. It proposed 5-year combined-training programs in internal medicine/emergency medicine and pediatrics/emergency medicine that would lead to dual-board certification. ABEM also acquiesced by creating a mechanism for academic internists to sit for the ABEM examination after meeting practice and teaching experience requirements. Harvey Meislin, who trained under Peter Rosen in Chicago, and eventually became chairman of emergency medicine at the University of Arizona, and the president of ABMS in 2004, notes,

> There was a letter…, which is still flashed now and then, which says we will not be a specialty that works outside this geographic environment. This was brought up at the critical care negotiations…We agreed not to have a practice outside the emergency department and nobody wanted the emergency department. So, we fulfilled the need that everybody had. In the argument with critical care, that paper was still flashed. There was a concern of taking the domain of somebody. There is a lot of politics at the ABMS level—there is a lot of politics.[72]

With these concessions in place, ABIM gave its full support in 1989 to emergency medicine as a primary board in ABMS. In the letter of support, Benson wrote about the "constructive, congenial dialogue it has enjoyed" in dealing with ABEM over the primary board issues.[73] The ABEM leaders bit their tongues and accepted the compromises to finally gain the highest level of recognition available for a medical field in American medicine. The ABEM primary board approval voice vote in ABMS was unanimous, and Joseph Clinton, M.D., who had taken over from Tintinalli as ABEM president, sent out a mailgram, saying "September 21, 1989—a great day for emergency medicine."[74]

ABEM and the specialty celebrated the new primary board status, but some active issues with the disenfranchised emergency physicians who were unable to take the ABEM examination remained. Then a bizarre set of events caused ABEM to have to cancel its written examination in November 1989, just a few months after ABEM's primary board approval. One of the physicians scheduled to take the November 6th ABEM written examination was being stalked and harassed by a former acquaintance. The stalker apparently did not want the physician to become board certified and extended the threats to ABEM by throwing a brick through a window at the ABEM offices and mailing a threatening package. Munger hired an ex-CIA (Central Intelligence Agency) worker to do a threat analysis. When the analysis suggested that the stalker might try to disrupt the examination, ABEM was forced to send out urgent letters canceling the examination in all eight of the cities in which it was to be given. Hundreds of examinees were affected. One said, "When I opened the letter I thought it was a hoax. Had I been studying for the test? That's probably the understatement of the year."[75] The matter was eventually resolved with the involvement of the Federal Bureau of Investigation (FBI), but ABEM became the first ABMS-member board to have to cancel one of its examinations due to threats of violence. As Munger notes, "This was a first ABEM could have done without."[70]

A problem that would not easily go away was the dissatisfaction of many practicing emergency physicians with the closure of the ABEM practice track in 1988. Hundreds of physicians were close to having the ABEM-required 60 months and 7,000 hours of ED practice time to sit for the board, but did not quite make it by 1988. This group believed that another mechanism for board certification should be available. ABEM had given prominent and frequent notices to emergency physicians at least 8 years in advance that the practice track would eventually closed. The board's position was that the emergency physicians had enough notice to plan to acquire the requisite hours, or to do an emergency medicine residency to become board eligible. Legal action was bound to come, and in 1990 Gregory Daniels filed a suit against ABEM. The suit was transferred to Federal Court in Buffalo, New York, and an additional 176 plaintiffs joined. After a decade of legal squabbling and distractions, the judge dismissed the case in 2003. Throughout the legal action, and in all of its discussions with those who challenged the legitimacy of the certification process in emergency medicine, ABEM repeated the mantra: "It's not just the test, it's the training." This message conveyed the important point that even though ineligible physicians were focusing on the ABEM examinations, it was residency training that had become the accepted path to eligibility. Residency training was the backbone of all U.S. medical specialties, and if emergency medicine left open other paths to certification, it would jeopardize the quality and credibility of the field.

ABEM moved forward as a primary board and began offering subspecialty certifications in pediatric emergency medicine, sports medicine, and medical toxicology. Each of these subspecialty areas has multiple sponsoring boards. For example, sports medicine fellowships and subspecialty certification are offered by the boards in emergency medicine, pediatrics, internal medicine, and family practice. When ABEM was initially approved in 1979, ABMS by-laws did not permit multiple sponsoring boards for subspecialty areas. However this was changed in the 1980s, and no new primary boards have been approved since this path for subspecialty certification was allowed. Benson Munger, who is in the best position to understand the workings of the ABMS, says,

> I am convinced that if the ABMS had allowed multiple boards to sponsor subspecialty certification in the 1970s, emergency medicine would have been a subspecialty under multiple other boards. The modified conjoint board for emergency medicine was what got the other boards thinking of this type of arrangement. But, if it happened today, I believe that emergency medicine would be a subspecialty in ABMS.[70]

Pediatric Emergency Medicine

Despite the fact that, on average children represent one fifth of ED patients, the organizations of emergency medicine did not pay much attention to pediatrics in the 1970s. At the specialty board level, significant animosity existed between ABEM and the American Board of Pediatrics during the fight for ABEM approval. Pediatrics was extremely concerned that emergency medicine would draw patients away from pediatrician's offices, and very few pediatricians had declared themselves as pediatric emergency physicians by working solely in EDs. The climate changed somewhat in 1981 when Robert Schafermeyer, M.D., and some like-minded colleagues gave a presentation on pediatric emergency care at the American Academy of Pediatrics (AAP) meeting in New Orleans, and then formed the Section of Pediatric Emergency Medicine within the AAP. Schafermeyer and others developed the extremely valuable advanced pediatric life support (APLS) course, which became a staple for emergency medicine residency training. In 1985, Gary Strange, M.D., brought emergency physicians into the mix, and ACEP began to collaborate with the APLS course. Other key figures in the early development of pediatric emergency medicine were Stephen Ludwig, M.D., from the Children's Hospital of Philadelphia and Gary Fleisher, M.D., from Boston Children's Hospital. Ludwig and Fleisher co-edited the first U.S. textbook of pediatric emergency medicine, published in 1983.[76] Practicing emergency physicians, many of whom believed their pediatric training was limited, welcomed both the APLS course and the new textbook. In 1987 ACEP reestablished its Pediatric Emergency Medicine Committee and Gary Fleischer became the chair. Two years later, ACEP created a formal Section of Pediatric Emergency Medicine.

One of the first activities within ABEM after primary board approval in 1989 was to develop a subspecialty examination in pediatric emergency medicine. Robert Schafermeyer was instrumental in this process and became the chairman of the subboard in pediatric emergency medicine. By the mid-1990s, a few emergency physicians with pediatric emergency medicine fellowship training and more pediatricians with pediatric emergency medicine fellowships were passing the subboard examination and becoming certified pediatric emergency medicine specialists. This small contingent of experts began to populate the EDs of children's hospitals and large academic medical centers and is now heavily relied upon to educate both pediatric and emergency medicine residents.[77]

Pediatric emergency physicians sometimes live in a Neverland between the two disciplines. Although they are better understood by and more in synchrony with emergency physicians, they are more likely to be housed under departments of pediatrics. Some emergency physicians have distanced themselves from pediatric emergency medicine due to the activities of the AAP and the media in recent years. In an apparent attempt to discredit emergency physicians and their care of pediatric emergency patients, the AAP and pediatricians made a number of disparaging statements about emergency physicians in children's health magazines. The old stance of pediatrics against emergency medicine seemed to be reemerging, although pediatric emergency physicians were not part of the negative campaign, and spoke out against it.

Academic Emergency Medicine Organizations Come of Age

When Mary Ann Schropp moved UAEM to the dentist's basement in Lansing in 1980, she was a very young person to be the executive director of a national academic medical society. Two years before, when at the age of 19 she had attended the UAEM meeting in San Francisco, she remembers,

> ...it was my very first time on a plane, my very first time I stayed in a hotel, I took a towel and wash cloth with me because...I didn't want to ask anybody whether they were provided. I had probably eaten in a restaurant five times in my entire life. You know we were like major hicks.[26]

Now Schropp had a small office in Lansing with a single typewriter and a newly purchased photocopier. She hired a temporary secretary but let her go within a year because there was not enough work. Schropp was directing a poor organization that had an annual meeting, but little activity throughout the year. Committees existed, but Schropp remembers,

> *I was thrilled if the committee chair knew he was the committee chair…They were not particularly productive. But, on the other hand, I don't know what they were going to produce. In the beginning years maybe having ten people sitting around a table just shootin' the breeze and trying to work something out was as valuable as anything that they could have done.*[26]

The major event for UAEM was its annual meeting, which was the only real forum for emergency physicians to present their research in the 1980s. The meetings drew around 300 to 400 people and the research was sometimes primitive, but the feedback provided at meetings stimulated emergency researchers to explore new methods and areas of research. Because most emergency medicine researchers worked in academic isolation, the opportunity to interact with and learn from other researchers and develop collaborative or mentor relationships was greatly appreciated. In the early years, attendance at oral scientific abstract presentations was sometimes sparse. Schropp remembers,

> *We had these big halls, and you'd have seating for 400 even though you only had 150 people there, and on the last day the poor schmuck who has to present his paper, it would be me and his wife and the moderator.*[26]

As the last of the surgeons finished their leadership roles in UAEM and went back to their original academic roles, a group of new, emergency medicine–residency-trained physicians became active in the organization and quickly rose to leadership positions. The first was Joseph Waeckerle, who had finished his emergency medicine residency under the guidance of W. Kendall McNabney in Kansas City and was one of the founders of the Emergency Medicine Residents Association (EMRA) in 1974. McNabney was the UAEM president in 1980 to 1981, and then handed over the reins to Waeckerle, who was president in 1981 to 1982. Richard Levy, from the Cincinnati program took his turn at president in 1984 to 1985. Stephen Davidson who was heavily influenced toward service by David Wagner when he did his residency at the MCP was UAEM president in 1985 to 1986.

Even though the association had humble beginnings and a small-time feel, the early academicians in emergency medicine were very enthusiastic about UAEM. The meetings were annual pilgrimages that invigorated faculty, through the new research and educational advances they saw but also as a commiseration forum for those who were still struggling back at their home institutions. UAEM came to embody academic emergency physicians as a lean, no-frills organization with a clear mission and purpose. When compared with ACEP it had a more defined constituency, and seemed less polit-ical, more efficient, and was not struggling with the corporate practice issues. UAEM members came to be proud of their "little engine that could" organization, even if it did not have much standing in the world of academic medicine.

ACEP was used to being the dominant organization in emergency medicine, and had tolerated UAEM, even serving as its landlord in Lansing. Now that the two organ-izations were separate and true emergency physicians had replaced the academic surgeons in the organization, UAEM was seen as somewhat of a threat. On paper, the strengths of the two organizations were not even close. ACEP had thousands of members, and UAEM only reached the 1,000-member mark in 1988. ACEP had a huge staff and its own Washington lobbying office, where UAEM had a staff of three people. But, ACEP still wanted influence in the academic world, and in 1988 it started its own Academic Section. According to Mary Ann Schropp, the two organizations were holding an officers' meeting when the ACEP president said, "So we just started an academic section of ACEP. Why does your organization even exist?" Schropp notes, "…that meeting was pretty short…They discussed dismantling our organiza-tion. It wasn't going to happen."[26]

Within the world of academic emergency medicine, the other organization, the Society for Teachers of Emergency Medicine (STEM), had developed out of ACEP, initially as a paper organization and then took on a life of its own. It was a key element in the development of emergency medicine faculty as teachers. As noted in Chapter 5, STEM was viewed as the home of the educators and teachers in emergency medicine, where UAEM was considered more of a research organization, although it also had a major education component. However the two organizations had major cross-pollination in terms of membership, including the elected leadership, and held joint annual meetings. As UAEM became a larger and more credible organization and began to have some financial resources and stability, STEM remained a poorly resourced subsidiary of ACEP. Given all the common ground, it was not surprising that talk of a merger began in the 1980s. The discussions became formalized in 1987 and 1988 when Dr. Ernest Ruiz, who founded the emergency medicine program at Hennepin County Medical Center in Minneapolis, was UAEM president and led an Amalgamation Committee to explore the merger of UAEM and STEM. As Mary Ann Schropp notes,

> ...we called it an amalgamation, which is so silly, it's a dental thing...Nobody wanted to use any words that suggested either organization was discontinuing...that one organization was eating up the other organization, so we came up with this word that no one understood and that seemed to make people happy....[26]

Mary Ann Cooper, M.D., who was the STEM president in 1987 to 1988 and at the same time was a member of the UAEM Executive Council, coordinated the merger from the STEM side. The UAEM by-laws were changed, the transfer of leadership was arranged, and the 1989 STEM president, Gabor Kelen, was given a seat on the board of the new organization. Dues were made cheaper for the new organization than for the old organizations, and all STEM members were given a year of free membership. STEM felt strongly that a new name was needed to signify that they had not just been absorbed into UAEM. The negotiations produced the new name, the Society for Academic Emergency Medicine (SAEM), and the inaugural meeting of the new organization occurred without much fanfare in May 1988 at the annual meeting in Cincinnati, although meeting minutes do not indicate the new name until February 1989. Members of the organizations did not notice much difference—they still attended one academic meeting a year and had one less dues payment.

Perhaps it was the break with the past, or the excitement of starting anew, but SAEM began to succeed on a level that eclipsed what had occurred in UAEM or STEM. The society became much more involved in the national dialogue of academic medicine in research and education. Committees actually began to do work, develop products, and push the board of directors for more resources. SAEM grew to over 2,000 members in the 1990s and was financially on solid footing. It developed EMS and research training fellowships and partnered with the Hartford Foundation on an educational grant. The annual meeting became the showcase for the latest in research and education in emergency medicine. At the same time, the organization retained its small-town feel. It functioned with a staff of no more than five, frugally managed by Mary Ann Schropp. A "headquarters" was purchased in Lansing—an old gray house on a street corner.

Just as ACEP had spawned STEM, two new organizations arose out of SAEM and were supported by the parent organization. Both reflected the growth, maturation of emergency medicine, and the need for new, more focused entities. The Council of Residency Directors (CORD) was formed in 1989/1990 with Judith Tintinalli as its first president. CORD served as the clearinghouse for residency program directors— a function previously provided by STEM in a more informal way. One of the most important functions of CORD was to provide input to the Residency Review Commission (RRC) for emergency medicine. As Tintinalli remembers, "The RRC was trying to impose a lot of stupid rules and CORD was fighting it." The Association for Academic Chairs of Emergency Medicine (AACEM) was the other emergency medicine organization created in 1989. By that time there were enough chairpersons to make such an organization meaningful. This group functions mainly as a vehicle for information exchange, support, mentoring, and faculty development for chairs of emergency medicine.

Another part of the academic infrastructure for emergency medicine that developed primarily outside of academic institutions was continuing medical education. Although some academic departments of emergency medicine offered continuing medical education (CME) courses for local physicians, the focus of their educational efforts was understandably on resident physicians and medical students. ACEP offered a robust CME experience at its annual scientific assembly, and UAEM offered a more research-based CME experience, but for the average practicing emergency physician who was not residency trained, and perhaps not board certified, there was unmet need. Into this void stepped many proprietary CME providers. The most successful and famous of these was Richard Bukata, who was an early graduate of the emergency medicine residency at Los Angeles County/USC, who went into community ED practice in Southern California. Bukata had some experience with searching and condensing the medical literature in the 1960s when he worked for the McNeil pharmaceutical company during medical school. He and his friends pulled articles from medical journals and created a filing system for McNeil-produced drugs. After he finished residency, Bukata remembers,

> I basically got bored. I never had any kind of entrepreneur experience or desires…but…I kind of got to the point relatively quickly where I said is this the rest of my life, going in and doing these shifts? Is this emergency medicine for me?[78]

He started thinking about how he could advance the education of practicing emergency physicians.

> I was of the view that emergency medicine was knowing as much as you could of the first 2 hours of anybody walking in the door as possible, and that you really needed to look at the literature and the others areas to be up on that stuff and that there was no way to do that because there was so many of them, and so I figured well I'd start this abstract thing and I did and I just basically kind of stumbled along with it creating these 3×5 cards and listing every article that I thought was relevant to emergency medicine for physicians to kind of fast track that process for them if they were interested….[78]

Bukata started his abstract service in 1977 and called his product *Emergency Medical Abstracts* (EMA). He lacked the funds or business experience to make *EMA* much of a success, and within a few years, sold it to a businessman from New Jersey. But after a few years the company asked if Bukata wanted to buy it back. He agreed, and at this point, older and wiser, he devised a plan to make *EMA* work. Bukata had already started organizing literature-based CME courses in emergency medicine. He remembers starting this in 1980 with a conference in Hawaii. Two of his featured speakers were Ron Crowell and Jerome Hoffman. Hoffman, who had completed his emergency medicine residency at UCLA, was gaining a reputation as an educator. Bukata remembers, "People said you need to link up with this guy—he is really smart."[78]

Bukata then got the idea to put reviews of his abstracts and an essay commentary on audiotapes. At first he did this on his own, but recalls,

> It was a disaster…I remember being in Cancun one time and trying doing a tape down there myself and I was in the bathroom of my room because it was apparently the only place I could find a plug that would work…So I did it myself for a while. I guess maybe a year or so and then people said maybe you ought to consider bringing somebody else in. That was probably being very charitable. Why don't you ask that Hoffman guy? So, I did and Jerry was very talented. His ability to speak and be logical and compelling…basically were very apparent….[78]

Bukata and Hoffman created a spirited, often funny banter on the abstract tapes, with Bukata the practical emergency physician, and Hoffman the erudite academic. *Emergency Medical Abstracts* became a very popular and powerful source of CME for emergency physicians. Bukata and Hoffman played a big role in setting the national tone for emergency medicine in their reactions and analysis to new studies, drugs, and practice methods. Many other enterprises developed to provide CME to emergency physicians in the 1980s. Some were the typical vacation junkets of mostly play and a little learning offered in all medical specialties. Others were more intensive courses on trauma, cardiac care, or toxicology, or mixtures of emergency medicine topics. ACEP compiled these offerings in a monthly listing in *Annals of Emergency Medicine*.

Exporting Emergency Medicine: Canada, Europe, and Beyond

Emergency medicine was not an exclusively American endeavor. Canada closely followed, and sometimes created in parallel, its infrastructure for emergency medicine. As the first emergency medicine residencies were developing in the United States, residencies were also launched in emergency medicine at the Queens University in Kingston, Ontario, in 1971, and the Royal Victoria Hospital in Montreal in 1974. A Canadian Association of Emergency Physicians was started in 1978, and in 1980, just a year after ABEM approval in the United States, emergency medicine was approved as specialty by the Royal College of Physicians and Surgeons of Canada. The scope of emergency medicine was much smaller in Canada than the United States. For example, the residency program at Queens University admits only three residents per year. Part of the reason for this is the national health care system with tight control of the number of specialist physicians. Canada mandates that at least 50% of its graduates go into general practice.[79]

The mechanism for training emergency physicians is also different. In Canada, medical students who anticipate practicing emergency medicine in rural community hospital settings first complete family medicine postgraduate training (2 years) and then do an additional year of fellowship training in emergency medicine. Physicians who are selected directly out of medical school for an academic career path in emergency medicine complete a 5-year residency-training program. The academic centers for emergency medicine in Canada, particularly in Ottawa, Kingston, and Vancouver, became known for their contributions in research and education. The connection between Canada and the United States in terms of education and CME is strong. Given the limited number of positions in Canadian emergency medicine residencies, a fair number of physicians (like Ron Stewart and Gabor Kelen) came to the United States to get their training. In terms of faculty migration, more have wandered south than north, presumably because of the higher salaries in the United States. The national health care system in Canada did not prevent similar increases in ED patient volumes as were seen in the United States in the 1970s through the 1990s. However the absence of PPMs or major corporate influences prevented the controversies that plagued American emergency medicine. Some Canadian emergency physicians remark that they are exploited only by their government.

The other "Westernized," English-speaking countries such as the United Kingdom, Australia, and New Zealand, were also quick to engage in the development of emergency medicine as a specialty. Although medical education and residency training is different in these countries, the basic model of an extended period of postgraduate clinical training in emergency medicine is followed.[80] Australia had emergency practitioners as early as 1968, a society in 1981, and in 1984 the Australasian College for Emergency Medicine was incorporated. Formal specialty recognition came to Australia in 1993 and to New Zealand in 1995. Academic development for emergency medicine has been just as slow in these countries as in the United States.

Many early U.S. emergency medicine leaders were asked to provide consults for other nations, even before they had figured out how to run their own emergency medicine programs. Trips to Europe, Japan, China, and other countries were seen as part of the global development of the field. Many of the issues were similar to what been confronted in the early days of emergency medicine in the United States, but in "third-world" countries, the lack of infrastructure made it almost impossible to recreate what had been achieved in the United States. Two graduates of the emergency medicine residency at the University of Cincinnati did more than provide consults— they became founding fathers of emergency medicine in other countries. Jön Baldursson, who came from Iceland to train in emergency medicine in the late 1980s, returned to Iceland and played the leading role in developing emergency medical services systems and educational programs. John Fowler, M.D., had a strong missionary focus and moved with his family to Turkey around 1990 and from a base in a hospital ED in Izmir slowly built emergency medicine in that country. Fowler's early task was not to form an organization or specialty board in Turkey—it was to supply EDs with rudimentary equipment like cardiac monitors and defibrillators and teach emergency personnel how to use them. As emergency medicine started to have a more global feel, the first international conference on emergency medicine was held in London in 1986.

CREDIBILITY WITH A CRINGE

As residency-trained and board-certified emergency physicians began to populate more of the nation's EDs, the impression was that care for emergency patients was improved and this was supported by some data.[81] The American public appreciated and even applauded the development of quality emergency care, but government policy makers, HMOs, and many medical leaders of the 1980s were less embracing. The flip side of the success of emergency medicine was failure of the health care system to adequately care for patients and thus prevent some of growth in emergency visits. A big part of the concern was the perception that emergency care was expensive and that similar care for less sick patients could be provided at much lower costs in other health care settings.[82] Work in the 1990s would show that ED care was not such a bad bargain. However the thought leaders of medicine, just as they had in the 1960s, continued to wring their hands about getting nonemergency patients out of the ED. They never did come up with a solution as to where all those patients, many uninsured, were to go instead of the ED for their health problems.

By 1990, the profession of emergency medicine in the United States had achieved what many would never have thought was possible in 1970. A primary board was in place, emergency medicine training programs were thriving, and both prehospital and hospital emergency care systems had remarkably improved. The demographics of emergency medicine trainees came to resemble those of physicians in other competitive medical subspecialties. But even into the 1990s, emergency medicine was more like a side channel of the mainstream of medicine. Graduating emergency medicine residents were still asked by their relatives what specialty they were going to do after they finished working in the emergency room.

Emergency medicine, from its birth, has been inextricably linked with the needs and trends in American society. It is not surprising that in the municipal hospitals of New York City, emergency medicine became the social safety net, whereas in the suburban cities and smaller towns of Texas, California, and Michigan, the field emulated the no-holds-barred corporate aggressiveness of the 1980s. A collage of medicine in 1990 compared with one in 1960 would have many new, modernized features and one major new professional component—emergency medicine. Ron Krome, the man who as the president of ACEP, UAEM, and ABEM was in the center of it all, says in his delicate way, "We changed the face of fucking American Medicine."[83]

9 Epilogue: Back to the Future

Uncertainty was the constant companion of emergency medicine as it developed in America. From the first itinerant practitioners who were uncertain of their careers, or their roles in medicine, to the surgeons who advocated for good emergency care, but did not want to practice in emergency departments (EDs), to the great trepidation by the medical establishment for a specialty of emergency medicine, to the precarious position of emergency medicine residency programs and academic departments in medical schools, the subliminal fear was that it could all collapse or be taken away. This was voiced in the medical literature, in a 1981 article in the *New England Journal of Medicine* "Sounding Boards" section entitled "Emergency Medicine: Two Points of View." The first point of view was written by James Leitzell, M.D., who had worked full time in community hospital EDs for 6 years, but had negative, disparaging things to say about the nature of the work and claimed that emergency physicians "rarely last more than a few years." Although by this time the American Board of Emergency Medicine (ABEM) had been approved by American Board of Medical Specialties (ABMS) and had administered its first examination, Leitzell thought that the question of whether emergency medicine was a specialty, "has yet to be answered in the affirmative."[1] The second point of view solicited for this "Sounding Board" was from Leonard Riggs, Jr., M.D., who was ACEP president at the time. Riggs was given an advance notice of the general content of Leitzell's article, and he received advice and editing help from Peter Rosen in preparing the other point of view. Riggs's piece, placed after Leitzell's, was entitled "A Vigorous New Specialty," and he provided information on the history and recent development of emergency medicine.[2] He promoted the field with strong references to the American College of Emergency Physicians (ACEP) and ABEM and described why it was a legitimate medical specialty. Riggs's essay had a balanced, reasonable tone, and lacked the shrillness of Leitzell's essay. However the overall impression of emergency medicine gleaned by a 1981 reader of this "Sounding Board" in the *New England Journal of Medicine* would most likely not have been favorable.

The fear felt by those who practiced emergency medicine is analogous to the fears faced by most immigrants to the United States, and like many immigrants, the early emergency medicine leaders relied on their strong work ethic and a tenacious will to propel their descendants to positions beyond what they could achieve. Finally, by the new millennium, emergency medicine had gained enough staying power and importance in American medicine that its demise or absence would leave a gap that no other medical field could fill. Peter Rosen was in Wyoming in the late 1990s when he had an asthma attack and required emergency care. He remembers,

> *I was having a pretty bad attack and I was in trouble for two reasons. One was that I wasn't feeling well, but the other was I knew what the medical practice was like in St. John's Hospital from my days in Thermopolis, and that scared me more than the attack. In walked Rick McKay who was the chief of the (emergency medicine) group here, and he was a residency-trained graduate…The realization that in St. John's Hospital, in Jackson Hole, Wyoming, a resident graduate was going to take care of me, which was my dream that some day in this country you won't walk into any emergency department anywhere in the country without having a resident graduate there to take care of you. That's when I knew we had made it.[3]*

The evolution of emergency medicine in the past decade has been every bit as interesting and controversial as the previous four decades, but will not be covered in depth in this account. The analysis of history requires a certain amount of time for digestion and recent events have not had enough time to play out. Nonetheless, some important happenings occurred in the 1990s that merit at least a mention.

The Josiah Macy, Jr., Foundation has as one of its goals improved health care and medical education. In 1993 the Society for Academic Emergency Medicine (SAEM) board of directors came up with the idea of soliciting the Macy Foundation to host a conference on the state of emergency medicine in the United States and to make recommendations on its future. Given the amount of publicity emergency medicine was receiving at this time, it was not surprising that the Macy Foundation agreed to host a 3-day conference in April of 1994. This was another "we've made it" moment for the specialty, as the topics the Macy Foundation chooses for its analyses and recommendations are noticed, reviewed, and sometimes heeded by the federal government and organized medicine. The conference title was "The Role of Emergency Medicine in the Future of American Medical Care" and the 38 participants included some familiar faces from emergency medicine: Lewis Goldfrank, Louis Ling, who had just been SAEM President, Benson Munger from ABEM, Gabor Kelen, Peter Rosen, and others. But over half of the participants were not emergency physicians, representing other medical specialties, nursing, the federal government, hospitals, and industry. The representation was similar to the famous "Blue Book" conference convened by the American Medical Association (AMA) in 1973 to reach a consensus on the education of the emergency physician. Some of the debate and contentious issues had changed little in 20 years. Both surgeons and family practice physicians at the Macy conference expressed concern that emergency medicine was encroaching on their territory, both during training and in practice. Peter Rosen complained of the "enormous paranoia that we will spill out into areas that don't concern us, such as primary care."[4] But the spirit of this discussion was different from that in 1973. No one was questioning the right of emergency medicine to exist as a medical specialty or the important and valuable role emergency medicine was playing in improved emergency patient care and as the health care safety net.

The sessions in the conference were focused on defining clinical emergency medicine, the ED as the safety net for nonemergent care, education in emergency medicine, and research in emergency medicine. The six final recommendations from the group were not momentous. The first urged the U.S. Public Health Service to specify as a new goal "that access to high quality emergency medical care should be available to all persons who need such care." The second urged the Council on Graduate Medical Education to not reduce the number of emergency medicine residency positions. The third urged that SAEM, ACEP, and the Joint Commission on Accreditation of Healthcare Organizations (JCAHO) develop a system for classifying U.S. emergency departments according to levels of care that could be provided. The fourth called for improved education of medical students in emergency care. The fifth called for all U.S. medical schools to establish academic departments of emergency medicine. The final recommendation called on SAEM and ACEP to hold a conference to set a research agenda in emergency medicine.

The Macy Foundation conference was somewhat of a coming out party for emergency medicine on the national scene of health care. It made the participants feel important and was very much a validation that emergency medicine had arrived as a profession. The "Mom and apple pie" recommendations from the conference were on target with what emergency medicine needed to develop in the 1990s and were important in that they arose from a prestigious foundation and a multidisciplinary conference. However, other than allowing emergency medicine leaders to reference the Macy report when they advocated for the field, the recommendations did little to advance emergency medicine beyond what was already occurring. The recommendation to establish a classification or categorization of U.S. EDs was pursued with some trepidation by SAEM, never supported by ACEP, and after several years of work, was dropped with only one hospital ever becoming categorized.

Academic emergency medicine has clearly progressed in the past decade. After years of discussion about forming its own journal, SAEM started *Academic Emergency*

Medicine in 1994, with Jerris Hedges, M.D., as the founding editor. Although it has a much smaller circulation than *Annals of Emergency Medicine, Academic Emergency Medicine* became an important alternative for original scientific research and as a forum for publishing more in-depth consensus reports on key topics in emergency medicine. Residency programs continued to increase at a steady rate, so that in 2004 there were 132 emergency medicine residency programs in the United States generating about 1,100 new emergency physicians per year. Only internal medicine, pediatrics, and family medicine currently train more residents than emergency medicine. Slowly, steadily, and surprisingly to some, in the past decade emergency medicine has become one of the largest U.S. medical specialties. Acknowledgment of emergency medicine's rise to academic respectability came from prominent figures in medicine. Robert Petersdorf, M.D., the famed internist, educator, and former president of the American Association of Medical Colleges gave the Kennedy Lecture at the SAEM Annual Meeting in 1991, and noted,

> I have become a convert to emergency medicine because of your discipline's fundamental and unique contributions to prehospital care. This development has not only accrued to the benefit of patients but also has opened a new field of research, resulting in major advances in public education. The strong scholarship manifested by your specialty has catapulted it into academic prominence.[5]

Perhaps the most dramatic and important academic growth since 1990 has been the formation of 51 new academic departments of emergency medicine in U.S. medical schools. Many of the traditional academic medical schools have embraced, or some might say have succumbed to, emergency medicine in the past decade, including the University of Pennsylvania, the University of Rochester, Vanderbilt University, the University of Michigan, Emory University, the University of Pittsburgh, the University of Virginia, and in 2003, even New York University (NYU).

Lewis Goldfrank, who did not initially think that departmental status at NYU was that important for what he wanted to accomplish, found that his success in other areas could be used as leverage for becoming a department. He recalls how it came to be:

> Giuliani (New York City mayor) who had been pretty hostile with every thing we did would come by...when we were all working and hustling and he brought along with him his chief fund raiser who was the president of Home Depot, a guy named Langone, Ken, who came to Bellevue and was so excited and involved...he was supposed to stay 5 minutes and he stayed 2 hours. Thereafter, every time he saw the dean he'd say, if Goldfrank can cooperate with Giuliani and me, the capitalists and communists can work on these things for the devotion of the people and are committed to society, why doesn't this guy have a department? Every time he saw him at a public meeting, he'd start to rant and rave, tell them you got to have a department of emergency medicine, it's vital for this medical center, it's the most important thing people are doing. They are trying to help, these guys are the best. So, ironically because this guy is the head of the board of trustees and so devoted, the dean just said to hell with it, or he was about to when William Chang, one of my faculty, he happened to see on a Web site that there is a great teachers award for NYU, they give five each year for the entire University. He submitted my name...They have been doing it for many years, there had never been a clinical faculty member from NYU who had won the award. So I think they took great pride in deciding to select me as the awardee...and the week before I was to get this award the dean called me and said, okay, stop this, I agree to make you a department because at this award ceremony in front of the president of the university, and the chairman of the board of trustees...it was his job to say something good about me...Finally, I had the recognition, but really it was the recognition of our department—all the things we had hustled for all these years...the World Trade Center and that stuff. Ultimately it was people always. It was the people who we worked for who were the patients and the people who were outside of the academic environment.[6]

The organizations of emergency medicine have traveled an interesting path in recent years. The SAEM has developed in to a well-respected academic medical specialty organization. Its membership has grown slowly to around 2,400 academic faculty, with an equal number of resident, medical student, and other members. SAEM has moved to fund research-training fellowships in emergency medicine, and its annual meeting continues to showcase emergency medicine research. ACEP continued its strong influence in the 1990s, but its accomplishments in educating physicians and advocating for improved emergency practice were sometimes overshadowed by continuing criticism from others in emergency medicine. The formation of the American Academy of Emergency Medicine (AAEM) and the constant attack that ACEP was too much influenced by corporate megagroups led to some organizational soul searching. As Colin Rorrie, the ACEP executive director notes, "it became clear that we were going to have to start addressing those particular issues and concerns."[7] ACEP reviewed its stand on contracts and in 1999 came out with a new statement on contracts in emergency medicine. The statement did not go as far as AAEM would have hoped, but did take a strong stand for individual emergency physicians rights in a contract relationship with an emergency medicine business group.[8] Then ACEP took things one step further—it proposed revising its criteria for new members to include only emergency physicians who had completed residency training in emergency medicine. Colin Rorrie remembers how ACEP President Larry Bedard, M.D., first presented this issue in 1997 "at a leadership meeting where he stood up…saying time is now for the college to be focused on this, and boom he just dropped that sucker right in that meeting and the board of directors was looking around and holy cow!"[7] Many of the board of directors reeled with this suggestion, since it would clearly be seen as a slap in the face to those members who were not residency trained in emergency medicine. But, the fact was that the future of emergency medicine lay with those who had full training and board certification, and the ranks of practice-trained emergency physicians would eventually diminish. A more pressing concern was that a significant number of residency-trained emergency physicians had denounced their ACEP memberships in favor of the American Academy of Emergency Physicians, and ACEP needed to do something dramatic to keep more members from jumping ship. The new ACEP fellowship criteria went in to effect in January 2000.

The end result is that AAEM, and some academic emergency physicians who were not part of AAEM, pushed ACEP to adopt changes that many saw as far too late in coming. AAEM has grown and become a viable emergency medicine organization, with its own CME conferences, and journal—the *Journal of Emergency Medicine* became the official journal of AAEM. The presence of two practice organizations is viewed as undesirable by many in the field, particularly the early leaders. John Wiegenstein noted, "I regret that AAEM split off. I wish that hadn't happened, but I understand why it did."[9] Bruce Janiak phrases it a different way, saying, "I'm disappointed in the sort of schism right now in my view between the socialists and capitalists in emergency medicine."[10] The fact that emergency medicine no longer speaks with one voice is very troubling to many of the people who devoted so much effort to unifying the field and moving it forward to specialty status.

If there is one area where emergency medicine still lags when compared with most other medical fields, it is in research, and particularly the funding of emergency medicine investigators. It is interesting to hear from the early leaders, who were not researchers, how much research development meant to them. For example, Robert Dailey notes,

> I think that thing that has pleased me most about emergency medicine…is the kind of people who have gone into it and what has been accomplished as far as investigatory work. Whether you call it research, or whatever, but we have taken our practice and examined it. We have examined at the bench and we've examined it in the clinical work place. We've done it in a way that many other specialties much larger, more powerful have not, to whit surgery, to whit family practice, to whit many others. I think that probably more than anything makes me very proud that we have sought out our best practices and tried scientifically and objectively to determine what best practice is. It has benefited patient care immeasurably.[11]

William Haeck, the early ACEP leader has similar sentiments about research:

> I'm very proud of the specialty. I'm very proud of the things that it does today. It is like a kid you raised and you are happy to see the end product. I'm very content to have pushed it out on it's own at the point where I let go of it. I pick up the journal and read through it and go wow, wow. Lots of fascinating stuff going on. From the beginning the folks interested in academics always preached that research had to be a big part of it. I think we simply accepted it without knowing how much research could bring to the whole picture.[12]

Mickey Eisenberg, as someone who became a heralded researcher in cardiac resuscitation, a key area of emergency medicine, but who operated out of an internal medicine base, notes the poor track record for funding and sees emergency medicine at a critical juncture in terms of research,

> They (emergency medicine researchers) did get some chunk of federal dollars but really a very small chunk and I think what's happening, there is clearly a transition going on where the old guard is fading away in terms of those not trained in emergency medicine. The new guard, those who've come up trained in emergency medicine are now becoming associates and full professors and…I think the real challenge now is can emergency medicine grab its share of federal dollars, because if they don't I think they will always be at the periphery. I really think they will always be like family medicine.[13]

A few emergency medicine researchers have joined Blaine White in receiving the Holy Grail of federal research funding—the National Institutes of Health (NIH) R-01 multiyear grant. Several younger emergency medicine investigators have received career development ("K"-type) grants from the NIH. Others have received significant funding from the Centers for Disease Control and Prevention, the military, and foundations. Indeed, the NIH and other major research institutions have seemed quite supportive of emergency medicine investigators when they have submitted grants, and calls for a separate NIH institute for emergency medicine seem unjustified. The primary problem facing research in emergency medicine is that too few academic departments in emergency medicine have the mission, infrastructure, or personnel to support a young investigator to the level of becoming an established investigator. Fellowship opportunities in research are not highly sought after by emergency medicine graduates. The significant difference between salaries in community jobs and academic emergency medicine discourages young physicians, who often carry a high loan burden from medical school, from pursuing research training and academic careers. Emergency medicine has become a strong component of the clinical milieu at most academic medical centers. It remains to be seen if the field will develop a strong research component.

The development of most of emergency medicine in to corporate practices of varying sizes was something James Mills, Jr., never anticipated. In fact, according to John McDade, Mills never liked managing the business aspects of practice. He let the hospital do his emergency physician billing and collections. Mills told McDade that one of the reasons he left his general medical practice was to avoid the daily business hassles. The Mills group did secure other local hospital contracts, but never became a PPM. After Mills's death, John McDade took over the group and they took back the billing from the hospital by hiring their own billing person. In the first year the group made more than $1 million more than the previous year. McDade says, "I suddenly realized that this hospital had taken us to the cleaners."[14]

One of the nasty consequences of the "success" of PPMs in emergency medicine is that emergency medicine contracts have come to be viewed by some hospitals and administrators as portable, disposable, and easily replaceable units. Even the founders of the field were not immune from being replaced when contentious issues arose. McDade feuded with the board of directors and the chief financial officer of Alexandria Hospital over many issues, but unlike the days when Mills and his group were felt by other physicians to be "running the hospital," the power had shifted. The emergency physicians who had started it all with the Alexandria Plan were fired by the hospital after 30 years of service and replaced. McDade retired and moved to Florida. A few years later, he and his partners were summoned back to Alexandria by the mayor and city council to receive a special commendation and award for being the founders of emergency medicine.[14]

Other emergency medicine pioneers suffered similar fates later in their careers. Phillip Buttaravoli worked as the ED director in Palm Beach Gardens, Florida, for the large emergency medicine PPM, InPhyNet. After having squabbles with his hospital administrator, Buttaravoli was dismissed by the hospital he had worked with for 12 years.

> You have no protection. You might as well be housekeeping. In fact, the last hospital administrator that I had to deal with, and probably the last one I ever will be dealing with, said when discussing our department that we were going to be treated like the other hospital contracted services, housekeeping and food services. Not anesthesia and radiology, they were going to be treating us like the other contract services. That is how they treated us. It's got to be a very special individual to overcome those restraints. Basically you have no political power. You are at their mercy as to how, what direction to go, how high you jump, whether you jump at all, and so that puts a damper on everything, you can't really accomplish anything, I guess it sort of took the steam out of me over the years…There is very little downside to removing one group and replacing it with another. They are interchangeable parts. They have no sense for quality. Administrators just have no sense for quality.[15]

Likewise, Bruce Janiak, the first emergency medicine resident, after serving as chairman of emergency medicine for 18 years at Toledo Hospital, became disgusted at the lack of support by the hospital for the innovative measures he was trying to implement to improve efficiency and patient safety in the ED. Frustrated and worn out, he stepped down from his position.[10]

One of the continuing problems for emergency medicine, as well as medicine in general, is solving the workforce distribution problem. Even if there were enough emergency physicians to work in U.S. EDs, the smaller rural hospitals and urban hospitals where support is poor would be unlikely to attract board-certified emergency physicians. No clear solution has emerged for this problem, although recent discussions in ACEP have suggested that combined training programs in emergency medicine and family medicine might help. Since many family physicians currently provide ED coverage in smaller hospitals, the idea that combined training might allow a physician to have an office practice, and work in the ED seems reasonable. This type of training model has worked well in Canada.

In becoming a profession, emergency medicine has not outgrown or escaped the original problems that gave rise to the field. Despite the repeated predictions that changes in the U.S. health care system—Medicare, health maintenance organizations (HMOs), increased numbers of primary care physicians—would lead to reduced ED usage, the American population has defied the experts. Ironically, the annual rise in ED patient visits has become the most consistent aspect of health care in the past 30 years, and seems to be accelerating. Annual U.S. emergency department patient visits were 81 million in 1980, 96 million in 1992, and 114 million in 2002.[16] One of the factors thought to have accelerated the rate of ED utilization is the passage of the federal Emergency Medical Treatment and Labor Act (EMTALA) in 1986. This legislation was intended to outlaw the practice of patient dumping from one hospital to another. As the healthcare marketplace struggled in the 1980s, some hospitals refused to accept, or inappropriately transferred indigent or uninsured patients to other hospitals—usually to municipal or charity hospitals. A few highly publicized bad outcomes from this practice prompted Congress to act. EMTALA mandated that all hospitals participating in the Medicare program must provide an ED screening evaluation and stabilization or arrange an appropriate transfer without consideration for the patient's ability to pay. But as Robert Bitterman, M.D., an emergency physician and expert on EMTALA wrote, "Rather than address the real issue of uncompensated care, Congress simply decreed universal access for all, creating a federal right to emergency care for any person in the United States, citizen and noncitizen alike."[17] It was after EMTALA that ED visits began their latest surge, and the crowding of EDs was worsened by the closure of hundreds of mostly smaller U.S. hospitals and emergency departments in the 1990s.

Paralleling the increase in ED visits is an increase in the number of Americans who have no health insurance—estimated currently to be around 45 million people. A common assumption is that most of the increase in ED utilization is for nonacute or minor illness, and that it occurs mainly in urban metropolitan hospitals in uninsured populations. Data from the National Hospital Ambulatory Medical Care Survey have repeatedly shown that this is not the case. Insured patients have increased their rates of ED utilization as much or more than uninsured patients.[18] ED visits for sicker and critically ill cases (except perhaps for motor vehicle crash victims and penetrating trauma cases) have increased as the population ages and sicker people are managed outside of the hospital. Since the late 1950s, patients have figured out where they can and in some cases, must go when the health care system cannot provide timely care. People vote with their feet, and the steady march of patients to EDs in the United States and worldwide over recent decades suggests that emergency physicians are providing something that is lacking elsewhere in medicine.

Many have viewed this overreliance on emergency care as a significant problem, assuming that emergency care is more expensive and thus is a major factor in driving up health care costs.[19] This was disputed by Robert Williams, who after founding ECI, Inc., went back to school to get a doctorate in public health at the University of Michigan. Williams's work for his dissertation was on the marginal costs of medical care. His interest in this developed when he was ACEP president from 1992 to 1993, and was invited to meet with President Clinton when the Clinton administration was attempting to revamp the U.S. health care system. Williams remembers,

> When I met with him and told him who I was, his reaction was, "Oh you are the emergency guys. We really appreciate what you do." The second things he said to me was, "You know, we really got to work to get those people out of the emergency room who don't belong there." That was the genesis of me starting to think about it. So I left and got to thinking, he is the number-one policy maker in the world and that is what he believes and that is what a lot of people believe.[20]

Williams wrote a landmark article, published in the *New England Journal of Medicine* in 1996, describing a study of Michigan EDs. He says,

> The basic notion I tossed up when I was putting together my dissertation topic as a research topic that I believed then, kind of as a guess, that if you are going to make a commitment and have an emergency department, if the fixed cost is the driving factor, whether one person shows up or 70,000, once you make a decision as a community or as a nation...that you are going to have emergency services it was my premise that you are going to commit to that fixed cost. What you needed to know was what was the marginal cost to take care of that patient with the sore throat? If you read my article, basically what I found was that the marginal cost was incredibly low.[20]

The paper made health economists and policy makers pause and consider that emergency care was not a big factor in rising health care costs, and EDs might actually be good bargains.

The continual push by ACEP in the practice realm and SAEM in the academic world helped to contribute in the 1990s to a new, much more favorable and sympathetic view of emergency medicine in America. Media accounts of emergency care were no longer "shooting the messenger," but showed an understanding of why EDs were stressed and crowded. *Time* magazine had a cover article on emergency care in May 1990, with the title "Do You Want to Die?" Just as there had been major magazine feature articles on "the crisis" in emergency care ten and 20 years before, the *Time* article highlighted increasing patient volumes, uninsured patients, poorly resourced EDs and the effects of urban violence. In the early 1990s, the problems of emergency care were featured on almost every television news show and major magazine. The root problems described in the media remained the same, but the tone was different in 1990s. Now emergency physicians were in charge and had in some ways become the heroes with the broken health care system as the antagonist. EMTALA finally put into law the unwritten rule that most EDs lived by—that no one would be turned away regardless of the problem or ability to pay. This cemented the image of the emergency department as the social safety net in U.S. medicine. Gail Anderson speaks to the importance of this public health function:

> *I fully believe that the biggest impact on improving care in the past three decades for those who can't afford to pay for medical care has been the development of emergency medicine.*[21]

Health policy experts may cringe at this statement, but it is difficult to dispute.

A reinforcement of the new, positive image for emergency medicine came from network television. In 1994, NBC unveiled "ER," depicting the emergency department of a busy urban Chicago hospital and for the first time showing trained emergency physicians in action. The show used emergency physicians as consultants and produced authentic-appearing scenes of the hectic inner city ED, modeled after Cook County Hospital. More important, the show dealt with the major issues of emergency medicine—crowding, uninsured and destitute patients, hospital politics, insufficient resources, and the stress encountered by emergency physicians and nurses in providing care in this type of environment. Twenty years before, NBC had produced "Emergency!" and brought an awareness of EMS to the American public. Now, "ER" did the same for a new generation. Although the show, particularly in its first few years, did not clearly define its emergency physician characters and their careers, it did bring an air of legitimacy, and even honor, to those who practiced emergency medicine. Medical students gathered weekly to watch new episodes, and some claim to have learned aspects of clinical medicine from the show. Although a direct correlation is difficult to discern, a bump in emergency medicine residency applications was seen after "ER" debuted.

By the end of the 1990s, the new level of respect afforded emergency physicians was sometimes peculiar to those who had been so used to being scorned. But, the difference was also refreshing and invigorating. Stalwarts in emergency medicine who had spent decades fighting for their right to exist in medicine could now turn their attention and energy to their patients and those they were training. The abatement of opposition to emergency medicine also translated in to successes in the administrative realm as emergency physicians became deans of medical schools, and heads of government agencies. In the past decade, a number of emergency physician leaders including Peter Rosen, Jerris Hedges, Judith Tintinalli, William Barsan, William Baxt, Arthur Kellerman, Ian Stiell, E. John Gallagher, Blaine White, Lewis Goldfrank, and Stephen Ludwig have been elected to the prestigious Institute of Medicine of the National Academy of Sciences. Rosen describes it as "a singular honor," and Tintinalli says, "One day the letter came home and I just screamed and screamed and hollered, it was just so wonderful."[3,22]

WHAT ARE THEY DOING NOW?

The founders of emergency medicine are described, sometimes hyperbolically, as visionaries but it is interesting to note the difference between the risk-takers who created the field, and those who assumed control and had to manage it. From the formation of ACEP in 1968 to the approval of emergency medicine as a primary board in 1989, the band of leaders in the field was quite small. There was major cross-pollination and redundancy in leadership positions in the major organizations. For example, John Wiegenstein, R. R. Hannas, George Podgorny, Ron Krome, James Mills, Jr., Harris Graves, Bruce Janiak, and Brooks Bock served as presidents of both ACEP and ABEM. This small contingent of superleaders eventually was replaced by a somewhat broader group of leaders in the 1990s. For some of the founders, life after the genesis of the field did not involve positions as managerial leaders. These were restless souls who sometimes became bored or hopelessly irritated with the bureaucracy, compromises, politics, and routine of day-to-day emergency medicine management. As Ronald Stewart notes,

I believe there are phases of the development for anything and the first phase is a visionary phase. You have to have a charismatic, involved leader in the visionary phase. Then you have a phase of putting this vision into practical structure—it's called funding—and so on, and then you have the form phase…After the form you go into a reform phase. In any event I was the first phase. I was the visionary phase and…I always knew that around me there had to be practical people to keep my feet on the ground. If they were not there, then I was a disaster. So I always made sure that there were people there who shared my vision but who were practical, this is what we got to do, this is how we have to do it.[23]

Stewart has had one of the more unusual lives in his postemergency medicine founder phase. He returned to his native Nova Scotia and practiced emergency medicine at Dalhousie Medical School. With encouragement from his long-time friends, he ran for the provincial parliament and won. He soon rose to be the minister of health of Nova Scotia. A conservative turn in the mood of the electorate found him out of this office in the late 1990s, and he turned his attention to the medical humanities, particularly the interaction of music and medicine. Stewart now serves as the director of medical humanities at Dalhousie Medical School, and is restoring a lighthouse near his boyhood home. His new vision is to create and build a retreat and center for medical humanities on his native Boularderie Island.

William Haeck has been, like Ronald Stewart, a career wanderer. Haeck was a young man when he served as president of ACEP from 1974 to 1975, and the frenetic activity of those years, along with his busy emergency medicine group practice in Florida played a role in bringing out a chemical dependency problem which caused him significant personal and professional hardship. Haeck recalls,

I recall a trip with John (Wiegenstein) and John (Rupke) and Karl (Mangold) and some others a couple of days in Washington D.C. running full tilt, and getting on a 747, running to catch the plane with these guys and flying to San Francisco for God knows what next meeting, maybe the AMA or something and we got seats in that upstairs lounge and in those days at least up there, they just put out a bottle on the table. I don't know about anybody else, but I got shit faced. Fell asleep some where over the country and woke up in San Francisco.[12]

Haeck confronted these health issues like he had his professional challenges. After receiving chemical dependency treatment in 1979, he became interested in addiction medicine and began to work with patients and physicians who had chemical dependency. He learned a new specialty area, and became president of the Florida Society of Addiction Medicine. Then to cap off his career, Haeck became interested in medicine in correctional facilities. He became the medical director of the Broward County Jail and again rose to a leadership position by being appointed to a board seat on the National Commission on Correctional Health Care and in 2002 was chairman of the board.

R. R. Hannas was the oldest of the early leaders in emergency medicine. He had a long and successful practice as director of an emergency department in Kansas City and then retired at the age of 69. He then worked as a night watchman for a liquor store. Hannas moved to Tucson in the 1990s and came to like a local Irish pub so much that he eventually bought it. Hannas was managing the pub, there every morning to open the establishment, at the age of 84. Not surprisingly, Hannas was exploring the national organization of pub owners, wondering how things worked at the upper level of that organization.

James Mills, Jr., was active in ACEP and served as a leading voice of reason and a mentor to the rising leaders in the field until his death in 1989. David Wagner remembers what Mills brought to the field.

I'll never forget how he would be the one who would speak out at board meetings about what we need to really look for and find ways to develop compassion in our residents—residents who care about people. Jim was a very caring, compassionate person who cared about the feelings that people have. He was a hard worker who worked right up to the end…he was doing night shifts right until just before he died.[24]

Mills had traveled with his wife to London in February 1989 for one of their enriching, long vacations. Harris Graves wrote, "Jim loved Europe, perhaps because he had many of the Old World traits that are those of a gentleman." This time the vacation was cut short as Mills became seriously ill with an aggressive form of mye-logenous leukemia. He died in April of 1989, just 5 months before the final approval of emergency medicine as a primary board by ABMS. The reaction to Mills's death was intense. Stoic leaders were anguished and tearful at the sudden loss of a person who had served as a friend, strategist, consultant, and mentor for so many of them. John McDade, who was Mills's friend and partner for 30 years wrote, "His passing will leave some with the aching void a family feels when it loses a loved one." George Podgorny wrote a moving tribute with this closing: "The man of grace, the man of goodness, the man of quality is gone, but not his legacy. Let it be said that Jim Mills was the last man to bring forth a new specialty in American medicine."[25]

Key founders of the specialty of emergency medicine remained active in the field for many years after the field was secure. John Wiegenstein still stood tall and vigor-ous each year at the ACEP Scientific Assembly, and his opinions were solicited by the new leaders in emergency medicine. Wiegenstein remained the elder statesman of the field, and the man who many viewed as the founder of the specialty of emergency medicine. Wiegenstein had retired to Naples, Florida, in 2003 at the age of 73, but became somewhat bored with retirement and had applied and tested for his Florida medical license so he could practice medicine once again. He never got the chance. Wiegenstein was killed along with his grandson in a motor vehicle crash in late October 2004. The tragic news spread almost instantly around the emergency medi-cine community, and the shocking loss of this great leader remains difficult for many of his colleagues to fathom.

George Podgorny also remains active and involved in ACEP late in his career. He attends every ACEP Scientific Assembly, and keeps abreast of the issues facing organ-ized emergency medicine. After his incredible run of leadership as ACEP and ABEM president and head of the Residency Review Commission (RRC), Podgorny went back to practice emergency medicine at Moses Cone Memorial Hospital in Greensboro, North Carolina. He had medical school affiliations and helped others start emergency medicine programs, but he never became heavily involved in academic emergency medicine.

Another stalwart, Ron Krome, who had served as president of UAEM, ACEP and ABEM, as well as editor of the *Annals of Emergency Medicine*, moved from Wayne State/Detroit Receiving Hospital to William Beaumont Hospital, where he developed a new department and residency program and remained active in the further devel-opment of academic emergency medicine. In his "retirement," Krome spends time in Florida, but has returned to his old haunts, working part time in the ED at Detroit Receiving Hospital.

For Bruce Janiak, becoming the first emergency medicine resident may not be the most impressive accomplishment in his life. With his wife Michelle, who is a nurse, Janiak has foster parented or adopted scores of special needs children over the past 20 years. It started out when a pediatrician needed to move abandoned, infant twins out of the hospital, but they required special care. The Janiaks, who had three children of their own, volunteered to care for the infants and became foster parents. Many other foster children followed, but the Janiak's did not like the transient nature of being foster parents. They decided to start adopting special needs children, and ended up with 11 more members of their family. Janiak perhaps used some emergency medi-cine skills in managing such a large family. He notes,

> We want to give something back…you realize that the incremental workload for an extra kid is minimal because once you get so many they tend to take care of each other, they play with each other, and the issue becomes cleaning the house and doing the laundry and feeding them…We ended up buying a bus to travel.[10]

Staying power was a question for those who chose to go in to emergency medicine. The common conception was that longevity in emergency medicine was not possible. Many in emergency medicine have proven that to be wrong, but none more so than

David Wagner and Gail Anderson. When Anderson became the chairman of the first department of emergency medicine in a U.S. medical school in 1971, he did not know how the specialty would develop, or that he would serve as a chairman at Los Angeles County/USC for over 30 years. William Mallon, the current residency program director notes that Anderson,

> Lets people do their jobs, he doesn't micromanage. He hires good people and gives them pretty free reins. He is a grandfather figure—an elegant elder statesman. He never misses grand rounds, always there with his white coat on. He always supports residents when they are giving a presentation at SAEM or ACEP. He is always in the audience. He has unbelievable consistency.[26]

Anderson did not work clinical shifts in the ED, but he was a key figure as the advocate, diplomat, and politician for patients and his faculty and residents. He became, literally, a founding father, when his son chose to be an emergency physician. When Gail Anderson retired in June, 2002, well in to his seventies, the Los Angeles County/USC program had trained 463 residents, far more than any other emergency medicine residency, and Anderson was hailed by his Dean for his "illustrious career" and for being "a great leader."[27]

David Wagner was as much a fixture in on the East Coast in emergency medicine as Gail Anderson, Sr., was on the West Coast. Although he was not an official chairman for as long, Wagner has been at the Medical College of Pennsylvania Hospital for 40 years. The fealty and respect Wagner receives from his emergency medicine residency graduates is summed up by Steven Davidson's recollections of Wagner when he met him while interviewing for residency: "I was absolutely taken by the man. He was obviously a guy with vision, a guy who was a leader and a guy who was loyal to people and cared about them."[28] Wagner has always viewed residents as his main focus, saying, "You sort of serve at the pleasure of the residents. The residents are the I-beam of this clinically focused specialty."[24] It is no surprise, then that Wagner is held in high regard as a clinical teacher. He distills teaching down in to essential components,

> I think teaching is three things. Teaching is time, you've got to commit to some extra time, whether it is extra time on a one on one basis with a patient, or whether it is some extra time that you give each week. It isn't run by a time clock that you are punching. It's also interest. You have to be really interested in…the so-called the information transfer process. You've got to really feel, you've got to have passion about it…[A]nd then probably third on the list you've got to have some skills, ability and information that is worth transferring. But it's mainly time and interest. If you are willing to do that, and your people sense whether you are serious about things or not. It's a sense that comes through.[24]

Wagner worked night shifts in the MCP ED until he was 66 years old, and still works clinical shifts. He describes what has driven him to keep practicing and teaching emergency medicine in to his seventies,

> …the most important thing to me has been the anonymous rating that all of our faculty get…who are the people in their lives that are important to them as managers, as teachers? When I don't win that race, then I'm ready to hang it up. The residents mean a lot to me and so far I think that we mean something to them in terms of providing them useful information and a model, approach to emergency medicine that you don't get from the junior faculty. As I tell the residents often, I expect you to out knowledge me but I don't expect you to out doctor me. I think they understand that. As long as that holds I'm going to keep doing what I enjoy doing.[24]

WHAT GOES AROUND COMES AROUND

After the approval in 1989 as a primary board specialty, emergency medicine enjoyed a somewhat halcyon period from 1990 to 1997. New residencies were developing, academic departments were being formed, and the field was gaining respect for its clinical care and research. The bubble was burst by the Balanced Budget Act of 1997, and the burgeoning health care demands of the baby boom generation of Americans. The "BBA-97" legislation included provisions to try to control rising health care costs, and American EDs felt the brunt of reduced reimbursement, but even more so the shift of the burden of uncompensated and poorly compensated care to the ED. The belt tightening in hospitals, which included decreasing lengths of stay, increased the number of patients who were sick, but discharged, and who often bounced back to EDs for care. Primary care did not become the solution, as had been hoped for at the dawn of the managed care era. Primary care physicians were asked to see more patients, with fewer resources, in less time. Many patients who were now deemed too sick for an office visit, or who could not get appointments with their "regular doctor" were referred to EDs for care. Hospitals closed or beds were cut, increasing the stress on the remaining hospitals and EDs. Added to this was a nursing and health care worker shortage. Emergency patient visits climbed at an even higher rate, and crowding of EDs and gridlock in the system were the inevitable result. Gail Anderson describes his reaction to what has occurred in recent years,

> Well, the angst I have now is more national, regional, and local disappointment because when I walk out there, like tonight is Friday night, and I'll leave here 5 o'clock or whenever I leave, and I see this mass of people waiting on a hard stretcher for a bed the whole weekend. That's the angst and disappointment I feel. I feel we've done a lot and our best, but there's no reason in America why people have to lay on stretchers the whole weekend waiting for a bed. That's a disappointment…I certainly have screamed about it and pounded the table and still do, but it's not fair to the residents, it's not fair to the nurses because the nurses and doctors, residents in training, are wore out….[29]

The situation was remarkably similar to what had driven the development of emergency medicine in the 1960s. But now, trained, experienced, recognized emergency physicians were in place and were expected to do something about the problem. Only so much can be done to try to fix a systemic problem that is often miscast as being mainly a problem in emergency care. The leaders of emergency medicine have been creative in attempting to meet the new demand. They have hired physician's assistants and paramedics to work in the ED. They have created observation units to shift admitted patients out of the main ED. They have looked to other industries to develop streamlined approaches to improve efficiency and patient throughput. They have collaborated with other hospitals to set up ambulance diversion and reallocation of patients when EDs became hopelessly crowded. Some of this has helped, but it is far more difficult than trying to fix a static problem. The patients keep coming, millions more each year, so the improvements and changes have to anticipate even more demand. ED directors feel like they can never come up for air. The proverbial "do more with less" becomes trite and worn out as even emergency departments, the *de facto* safety nets of American medicine, begin to fray and unravel. Recently, some acknowledgment has been given to the fact that the "emergency department problem" is not an isolated issue, but merely the clanking noise signifying that the entire engine of health care needs to be overhauled.

WHAT WILL THE FUTURE HOLD?

The demand for emergency services has been a constant feature of modern health care in the United States and other nations. Even those countries with a national health care plan, like Canada, have experienced a steady increase in utilization of EDs. Since the 1950s, the cry that too many nonemergent patients are seen in EDs has been heard, but attempts to alter patient demand for the ED have usually been unsuccessful. The EMTALA legislation mandates that all patients who present for emergency care will be at least screened and evaluated, and attempts to change this have not been welcomed. Although health care policy makers are eager to reduce ED utilization, they need the ED as a place of last resort. Emergency medicine leaders have vacillated between trying to do something to reduce visits from less acutely ill or injured patients, and welcoming this group, especially those who could pay. Early in his career, Robert Williams realized that "these people who 'don't belong there' were paying the freight."[20] His work on marginal costs of emergency care has changed how people view the ED. Bruce Janiak notes,

> I think we've just scratched the surface in what we can offer to society. Instead, we sit there and worry about overcrowding and frequent flyers and all that stuff. We ought to be taking a more optimistic view. You don't hear General Motors saying, "There are too many people who want our cars, and we are really pissed. This is a crisis, we need Congress to intervene." What are you talking about? I mean, geez, look at it from that standpoint. We have too much business and are pissed about it?[10]

Other emergency medicine leaders suggest that the future will hold changes in the way emergency medicine is practiced and the environment of care. David Wagner notes, the population of the future is,

> ...going to get something and most of things that people get, particularly now that they live older, are chronic in nature and chronic conditions have acute exacerbations and we are going to have a plethora of acute exacerbations of chronic disease problems so much so that in our view it's going to be very difficult to encompass all these in emergency centers. We need to be thinking out of the box in terms of hand picking acute intervention or responding to acute needs elsewhere in other modalities and other locations. It is interesting to me when I hear people that are coming along now maybe starting to think about that.[24]

Richard Levy, who is regarded as one of the leading futurist thinkers in emergency medicine, takes this concept even farther.

> I think that emergency medicine is destined to become the diagnostician not just for a corner of the hospital but I think that we will become the diagnosticians of medicine and I think that will move us over time out of the emergency department out of the short-term diagnostic treatment centers to where we will eventually merge with [hospitalists]. But I think that will become a more serious kind of enterprise over time and it's more likely to shape up into a model where there are people who are clearly differentiated because of their time of association in the hospital, and those who are more likely to do outpatient medicine both diagnostic and nondiagnostic. I think that we are going to be the hospital types who do diagnostic medicine. But I think that we are more likely to move into the directions of intensive care and the direction of inpatient diagnostics as well and I think what you are going to see is an awful lot of, whether its radiologists, or cardiologists or surgeons, more and more of them are going to be consumed with outpatient medicine even the ones who you think of as inpatient types. I think that patients who are going to be left are the ones who truly have emergency needs and that come to the hospitals because they have highly complicated breakdowns of their systems and to a certain degree...undifferentiated and I think increasingly emergency medicine will take care of those patients all the way...Who assumes various roles is still up for debate and the idea that hospitals being increasingly places where very sick undifferentiated disease processes go and, because of technological advances, an awful lot of other patients will be taken care of outside the hospital. Those who are less differentiated, more complicated I think that emergency physicians will take on more and more roles in taking care of those people. Given enough time, given that same skill set that we keep sharpening and honing and at the same time, skill sets that in other people are atrophying and so that's why I project us moving into this.[30]

It will be interesting to see if Levy's predictions, coming from inside the field, will be more correct than the predictions of those over the years who have been outside the field, which have invariably been wrong.

The Constant: Caring for Emergency Patients

For all the work that went in to developing the organizations of emergency medicine, the training programs, the academic infrastructure and even the business of emergency medicine, the one constant and the aspect that provided the most joy for emergency physicians was the opportunity to care for emergency patients. The anticipation of not knowing what would come through the door next, the incredible variety, with no two shifts ever being the same—these were the compelling elements that made it worth the rest of the hassles associated with emergency care. As the originators of emergency medicine aged, some came back to their patients with even more passion than before. Phillip Buttaravoli despite his disappointment with the medical care system, notes,

> What I enjoy the most and still brings me satisfaction and what makes it worth while going to work for everyday, is that the practice of emergency medicine is interesting and full of excitement as it ever has been and now I'm a good emergency physician. I can do good. I feel like I am contributing to society, people recognize me. Working in a community where you live, people come up to me and say nice things about me. So, I like my craft. I can be frustrated by not having the equipment and supplies the way they ought to be and the inefficiencies of the department that could easily be corrected, if just anybody put a little energy into it. The fact is, people come in, they are in pain, they are frightened. I can come up a solution to their problem. I save lives. That is rewarding. It doesn't get any better than that. I guess if I didn't care, if I really detach myself from the political side of things, which is now that I've retired from my administrative position, it is easier for me to do…I'm enjoying the clinical side even more because I don't feel responsible for all the stuff that is not going right. That is the best part of it…There is nothing wrong with finding the clinical side of emergency medicine as being the side that brings you joy and pleasure.[15]

For Bruce Janiak, even those patients who are viewed by some as undesirable came to provide a sense of satisfaction. Patients who present to EDs often with noncritical, taxing problems are dubbed "frequent flyers." Janiak notes how he came to handle frequent flyers in his ED:

> We needed to have a 180-degree turnaround on the way we think about frequent flyers. The fact that they come in three times a week is not something that is a plot against us personally. There is something else going on and in some percentage of them if we take the time and don't act so angry when they come in and evaluate them in such a superficial way, if we take the time on some of them we can get another level of reward because we can help them out of whatever it is they are in, or at least be more supportive. I began to do this a couple of years ago in which I deliberately looked for the frequent flyers and signed up for them. That's not easy to do. It's not easy to force yourself to listen to this chest pain story for the 400th time that month, but not on all of them but on some of them, you begin to develop tremendous empathy for the fact that their life is shit and yours isn't. You sit down with them and start just touching them. That's all you have to do. Their attitude changes sometimes and at the end of my tenure at Toledo Hospital when I was on, frequent flyers would ask for me and I liked it. "I want that guy to take care of me, he's the only one who listens." You don't really do anything different, all you do is you don't be angry. There is a real professional reward in that and it really hit me one day when one of my frequent flyers that happened to have sickle cell and AIDS and came in always with a fever, she was sick, and died. Nobody wanted to go in the room with her and I cried when she died. Rhonda, I'll never forget Rhonda.[10]

Robert Dailey also reflects on the importance of taking care of patients,

> The last 10 years of my career were spent outside totally outside of academic emergency medicine, totally out of the politics, and was spent, if you will, in obscurity

in a couple of little community hospitals in California, and it was one of the most grat-ifying parts of my career, because I could end my career saying that I had been truly successful as a doctor, a person who goes into a hospital and takes care of people, and that is what I had originally intended before I ever went to medical school. It ended up that it was what I did only in the fading days of my career, and left me with a very deep sense of satisfaction that I know I would never had achieved had I remained in place.[11]

Dailey's last shift as an emergency physician reinforced a career of lessons about the challenges, uncertainty and surprises involved in emergency care. He recalls,

I saw a guy with intrascapular back pain that was related to exercise, only upon careful questioning, and he was a really nice guy and he wasn't that old. He had coro-nary precursors and I realized that he was there, that God had put him in the emer-gency department to get me on my last shift. Low and behold he didn't because I picked it up. Only when he wheeled his golf cart up the hill, then did he get pain and then it promptly went away. Not anterior, no neck, no shoulder pain, no nothing, but it was clearly exercise related and clearly relieved by rest. We called the cardiologist, got him admitted, and secure in the knowledge that I had picked up a case of very occult coro-nary pain. Now to end my story, I can tell you that it came to my knowledge some days later that...he had undergone coronary stress testing and subsequently coronary angiography and was found out to have perfectly normal arteries![11]

The fact that he was wrong on this case, on his last shift, does not dampen Dailey's enthusiasm. He notes, "I couldn't imagine having a more rewarding career in medicine"[11] (see insert, Figure 29).

An example from the teaching annals of Lewis Goldfrank demonstrates the intense humanism in emergency medicine. Nicole Bouchard, M.D., an emergency medicine resident, related this story to the *NYU Physician* magazine about how Dr. Goldfrank informed the residents of a patient who was coming in by ambulance to the ED:[31]

One by one, Dr. Goldfrank approached us and told us there was a VIP patient coming in, someone he would like us to personally take care of. Each of us beamed for having been chosen, not knowing in fact we all had been chosen.

The VIP patient turned out to be a septic, delirious, homeless, drug-addicted woman with HIV/AIDS who "clutched a dead baby, the placenta not yet delivered." She had been found in the tunnels under Grand Central Terminal. Goldfrank took his residents through the resuscitation of this patient. He helped them bath and comfort her. Dr. Bouchard said, "We talk about it sometimes, how it was so perfect that Dr. Goldfrank was there, and how this is what it's all about. Excellence in medi-cine and love."[31]

The joy of being an emergency physician, even the humanistic aspects would not mean much to society if emergency care was not improved by the presence of emer-gency physicians. Numerous studies of traumatic injury, head injury, myocardial infarction, and other acute diseases provide evidence that emergency care has been a factor in improved patient outcomes. When compared with the level of care found in EDs in the 1950s and 1960s, it can be argued that the expertise of emergency physi-cians has increased more than in any other field in medicine. The ability of a trained emergency physician to act decisively in a moment of crisis for the patient can deter-mine life or death, disability, or a productive life. This point is reinforced by a story from John Wiegenstein's early days in emergency practice. Wiegenstein lacked formal training in emergency medicine, but he had actively sought courses and procedural training in trauma, airway management, and acute cardiac care. He related this story:

I was in my first year at St. Lawrence and a nurse called and said, "Hurry out to the parking lot. A man is bringing in his child who looks dead." I rushed out and this child was blue–black and the father was trying to breathe for him. I looked in the baby's throat and he had epiglottitis, from an illness, blocking his throat.

And I thought, "I've never done a tracheostomy on a child before," but it was the only way. I put in a tube and he survived.[32]

Over 20 years later Wiegenstein was chief of emergency medicine at Ingham County Medical Center when a new orderly named Robert Prodinger introduced himself to Wiegenstein. Prodinger said, "Actually, I met you once before." He pulled down his shirt collar to reveal the tracheostomy scar on his neck. The young man whose life was saved by Wiegenstein later went on to medical school and now is an emergency department director in Western Michigan.[32,33]

For emergency medicine it has always been about the patients. While all of the specialties in medicine can claim to have patients as their focus, only one specialty has emerged—a paradoxic specialty of generality—to take care of anyone, with anything at anytime. The patients came first, in the 1950s and 1960s, like squatters, defining the emergency department as the place where they would receive care. They created a robust, new, unmet need and exposed a major clinical void in emergency care. It was natural that a system of emergency care developed along with a profession to provide the care. This movement improved the outcomes of the acutely ill and injured, and made significant advances in medical science. It was then perfectly American that a corresponding business enterprise developed from the new specialty. However with this progress some aspects of emergency medicine came to represent the failures, weaknesses, and absurdity of American health care. As a society, emergency medicine represents at the same time our finest suit of clothes and our dirty laundry. The professional story of emergency medicine is about a few passionate physicians who had a vision, stayed the course, and rode the wave of societal needs and demands to create a new medical specialty. Now the next generation of emergency physicians will tackle the new problems in emergency medicine, which are in many cases are just modernized versions of the old problems. The new emergency physicians are the progeny the early leaders hoped so desperately would emerge. Peter Rosen sums up the feelings of many of the founders of emergency medicine (see insert, Figure 29):

I think the thing that I am most proud of is my graduates. They've been better emergency physicians than I am, and they are good people, and they've been excellent leaders and they have made the field flourish. They are what it is all about...My life was being part of their life cycle.[3]

References

Chapter 1

1. Miller DT, Nowak M: *The fifties: the way we really were,* Garden City, NY, 1977.
2. Zinn H: *Postwar America: 1945–1971,* Indianapolis, 1973, The Bobbs-Merrill Company, Inc.
3. Leigh Brown P: Armageddon again: fear in the 50's and now, *New York Times* 2001.
4. Filreis A: *The literature and culture of the American 1950's,* 2003, University of Pennsylvania. www.writing.upenn.edu/~afilreis. Date accessed: March 2, 2004.
5. Blum JM: *Years of discord: American politics and society, 1961–1974,* New York, 1991, W. Norton and Company.
6. Domhoff GW, Ballard HB: *C.W. Wright and the power elite,* Boston, 1968, Beacon Press.
7. A hero's great discovery is put to work, *Life* 38:105, 1955.
8. Hannas RR: Interview of R. R. Hannas, M.D., by Brian Zink. Tucson, Arizona, 2003.
9. Starr P: *The social transformation of American medicine,* New York, 1982, Basic Books.
10. Stevens R: *In sickness and in wealth: American hospitals in the twentieth century,* New York, 1989, Basic Books.
11. Stevens R: *American medicine and the public interest: a history of specialization,* Berkeley, 1998, University of California Press.
12. Terkel S. *Coming of age,* New York, 1995, The New Press.
13. Ludmerer KM: *Time to heal: American medical education from the turn of the century to the era of managed care,* Oxford/New York, 1999, Oxford University Press.
14. Kendall PL, Selvin HC: Tendencies toward specialization in medical training. In Merton RK, Reader GG, Kendall PL, editors: *The student physician,* Cambridge, 1957, Harvard University Press.
15. Green JJ: Here's the new family doctor: your friendly emergency room, *The Detroit News,* 16:1972.
16. House calls, *Time,* December 30, 1957:46.
17. Wharton D: How to get a doctor in a hurry, *Reader's Digest,* 39–41, March, 1958.
18. Burden at night, *Time,* March 23, 1953.
19. Night Man. *Newsweek* 45:61, 1955.
20. Fishbein M: *Doctors at war,* New York, 1945, E.P. Dutton and Company.
21. Engleman RC, Joy RJ: *Two hundred years of military medicine,* Fort Detrick, Maryland, 1975, The Historical Unit, U.S. Army Medical Department.
22. Risse GB: *Mending bodies, saving souls: a history of hospitals,* New York, 1999, Oxford University Press.
23. Condon-Rall ME, Cowdrey AE: *The medical department: medical service in the war against Japan: United States Army in World War II—technical services,* Washington, DC, 1998, Center of Military History.
24. Whitehead IR: *Doctors in the great war,* Barnsley, S. Yorkshire: L. Cooper, 1999.
25. Gabriel RA, Metz KS: *A history of military medicine, vol II: from the Renaissance through modern times,* New York, 1992, Greenwood Press.
26. Weldon C: *Tragedy in paradise,* Bangkok, 1999, Asia Books.
27. Cooter R, Harrison M, Sturdy S: Medicine and modern warfare/and Steve Sturdy. Clio Medica (Amsterdam, The Netherlands); 55 Wellcome Institute series in the history of medicine. Amsterdam/Atlanta, 1999, Rodopi.
28. Mellor WF: *History of the second World War: casualties and medical statistics,* London, 1972, Her Majesty's Stationery Office.
29. Emergency-ward service (editorial), *N Engl J Med* 258(1):47–48, 1958.
30. Wagner D: Interview of David Wagner, M.D., by Brian Zink. Philadelphia, Pennsylvania, 2003.
31. Dowling HF: *City hospitals: the undercare of the underprivileged,* Cambridge, Massachusetts, 1982, Harvard University Press.
32. Petersen JR: Telephone interview of John R. Petersen, M.D., by Brian Zink. Ann Arbor, Michigan, 2003.
33. U.S. Department of Health, Education and Welfare. Report to the President and Congress: The Allied Health Professionals Personnel Training Act of 1966 as Amended. Bethesda, Maryland: National Institutes of Health, 1966.
34. U.S. Department of Health, Education and Welfare. Hospital Outpatient Services: Facts and Trends. Washington, DC: Public Health Service, 1964.
35. President's Commission on Heart Disease, Cancer and Stroke. A National Program to Conquer Heart Disease, Cancer, and Stroke. Washington, DC: U.S. Government Printing Office, 1964.

36. Worman LW, Cook HE, King JM: The trauma patient vs. emergency care: the role of the emergency hospital, *J Trauma* 3(4):340–348, 1963.
37. Wailoo K: *Dying in the city of the blues: sickle cell anemia and the politics of race and health—studies in social medicine,* Chapel Hill, 2001, University of North Carolina Press.
38. Wiegenstein J: Interview of John Wiegenstein, M.D., by Brian Zink. Naples, Florida, 2002.
39. Hospitals: guide issues, hospital statistics, *AHA* 1954–2004.
40. Shortliffe EC, Hamilton TS, Noroian EH: The emergency room and changing pattern of care, *N Engl J Med* 258(1):20–25, 1958.
41. American Medical Association: *Emergency department. A handbook for the medical staff,* Chicago, 1966, American Medical Association, Department of Hospitals and Medical Facilities.
42. American Hospital Association, *Emergency services: the hospital emergency department in an emergency care system,* Chicago, 1972, American Hospital Association.
43. Barry RM, Shortliffe EC, Wetstone HJ: Hospital emergency departments: two surveys—case study predicts load variation patterns, *Hospitals JAHA* 34:35, 1960.
44. McCarroll JR, Skudder PA: Hospital emergency departments: two surveys: conflicting concepts of function shown in national survey, *Hospitals JAHA* 34:33, 1960.
45. American Hospital Association: Outgrown central supply now smooth-functioning emergency room, *Hospitals JAHA* 31(6):48–52, 1957.
46. McDade J: Interview of John McDade, M.D., by Brian Zink. Rockledge, Florida, 2002.
47. Shortliffe EC: Emergency rooms…weakest link in hospital care? *Hospitals JAHA* 34:32–34, 107, 1960.
48. Stevens R, Goodman LW: The alien doctors: foreign medical graduates in American hospitals. Louis Wolf Goodman, Stephen S. Mick. New York, 1978, John Wiley & Sons, Inc., xvi, 365 ill.
49. Mamot PR: *Foreign medical graduates in America,* Springfield, Illinois, 1974, Charles C Thomas.
50. As Medicare nears—a crisis in hospital care, *U.S. News and World Report* 58:50, 1965.
51. Saunders R: The university hospital internship in 1960, *J Med Educ* 36:642, 1961.
52. Kennedy RH: Our fashionable killer: the oration on trauma, *Bull Am Coll Surg* 40:73–81, 1955.
53. Mills F: Interview of Frances Mills, wife of James Mills Jr., M.D. (deceased) by Brian Zink. Alexandria, Virginia, 2003.
54. Iserson K: Interview of Kenneth Iserson, M.D., by Brian Zink. Tucson, Arizona, 2003.
55. Leidelmeyer R: Interview of Reinald Leidelmeyer, M.D., by Brian Zink. Fairfax, Virginia, 2003.
56. Podgorny G: Interview of George Podgorny, M.D., by Brian Zink. Winston-Salem, North Carolina, 2003.
57. Birch CA: *Emergencies in medical practice,* Edinburgh/London, 1960, E. & S. Livingstone Ltd.
58. Cullen SC, Gross EG: *Manual of medical emergencies,* Chicago, 1949, The Year Book Publishers.
59. Flint T: *Emergency treatment and management,* Philadelphia, 1954, WB Saunders.
60. Kennedy RH: *Bull N Y Acad Med* 13:61, 1937.
61. Lindquist CA: Hospital facilities required for emergency care, *Bull Am Coll Surg* 38:378, 1953.
62. Howell JT, Buerki RC: The emergency unit in the modern hospital, *Hospitals JAHA* 31:37, 1957.
63. Rosen P: Interview of Peter Rosen, M.D., by Brian Zink. Jackson, Wyoming, 2002.
64. Krome R: Interview of Ronald Krome, M.D., by Brian Zink. Naples, Florida, 2002.
65. Kobler J: Why Mac isn't dead, *Saturday Evening Post* 229:28, 1956.
66. Patterson N: Emergency room, *Coronet* 36:53–56, August, 1954.
67. The crisis in American medicine, *Harper's* 221:121–168, October, 1960.

Chapter 2

1. Kennedy JF: *Speeches of John F. Kennedy,* 1961, John F. Kennedy Library. Available at: www.csumb.edu/jfklibrary. Date accessed: August 20, 2003.
2. *Chronology of Dr. Martin Luther King, Jr.* 2003. Available at: www.thekingcenter.org/mlk/chronology.html. Date accessed: April 24, 2002.
3. Blum JM: *Years of discord: American politics and society, 1961–1974,* New York, 1991, W.W. Norton and Company.
4. Ferber S: Practice limited to the emergency room, *Medical Economics* 76–85, July 15, 1963.
5. Hospital statistics, *Hospitals JAHA* 36:232, 1962.
6. *Emergency department: a handbook for the medical staff,* Chicago, 1966, American Medical Association, Department of Hospitals and Medical Facilities.
7. McDade J: Interview of John McDade, M.D., by Brian Zink. Rockledge, Florida, 2002.
8. Mills JD: *The Alexandria Plan—Emergency department: a handbook for the medical staff,* Chicago, 1966, American Medical Association, Department of Hospitals and Medical Facilities.
9. Maisel AQ: Emergency service: medicine's newest specialty, *Reader's Digest* 86(518):96–100, 1965.
10. American Medical Association: The emergency department problem—an overview, *JAMA* 198(4):146–149, 1966.
11. Green JJ: *Here's the new family doctor—your friendly emergency room,* 16:1972, The Detroit News, Sunday News Magazine.
12. Mills F: Interview of Frances Mills, wife of James Mills Jr., M.D. (deceased). Alexandria, Virginia, 2003.
13. *Contract for the Alexandria Hospital Emergency Department,* Alexandria, Virginia, 1961, Alexandria Hospital.
14. Porter R: Our enemy: the emergency room, *Medical Economics* 71–75, July 15, 1963.
15. Boom in emergency rooms, *Time* 33–34, 1963.
16. Mills JD: A method of staffing a community hospital emergency department, *Virginia Medical Monthly* 90:518–519, 1963.

17. As Medicare nears—a crisis in hospital care, *U.S. News and World Report* 50, 1965.
18. Knowles JH: The emergency ward, *Atlantic Monthly* 218:116–121, 1966.
19. Hannas RR: Interview of R. R. Hannas, M.D., by Brian Zink. Tucson, Arizona, 2003.
20. Leidelmeyer R: Interview of Reinald Leidelmeyer, M.D., by Brian Zink. Fairfax, Virginia, 2003.
21. Abbott VC: How to staff a hospital emergency department, *Bull Am Coll Surg* 47(4):137, 1962.
22. Leichtman RR, Maraveleas MF: *The Pontiac Plan—emergency department: a handbook for medical staff,* Chicago, 1966, American Medical Association.
23. Abbott VC: Emergency department staffing: five year experience with the Pontiac Plan, *Bull Am Coll Surg* 11, January/February, 1966.
24. Wagner D: Interview of David Wagner, M.D., by Brian Zink. Philadelphia, Pennsylvania, 2003.
25. Wiegenstein J: Interview of John Wiegenstein, M.D., by Brian Zink. Naples, Florida, 2002.
26. Mangold K: Interview of Karl Mangold, M.D., by Brian Zink. Oakland, California, 2002.
27. Reddy J: Meet the collegiate whiz kids. *Reader's Digest* 463:253–256, 1960.
28. Berry FB: The story of "the Berry Plan," *Bull N Y Acad Med* 52(3):278–282, 1976.
29. Haeck W: Interview of William Haeck, M.D., by Brian Zink. Boca Raton, Florida, 2003.
30. Rosen P: Interview of Peter Rosen, M.D., by Brian Zink. Jackson, Wyoming, 2003.
31. Krome R: Interview of Ronald Krome, M.D., by Brian Zink. Naples, Florida, 2002.
32. Podgorny G: Interview of George Podgorny, M.D., by Brian Zink. Winston-Salem, North Carolina, 2003.

Chapter 3

1. Kearns Goodwin D: *Lyndon Johnson and the American dream,* New York, 1991, St. Martin's Griffin.
2. Starr P: *The social transformation of American medicine,* New York, 1982, Basic Books.
3. Blum JM: *Years of discord: American politics and society, 1961–1974,* New York, 1991, W.W. Norton and Company.
4. Burner D: *Making peace with the 60s,* Princeton, New Jersey, 1996, Princeton University Press.
5. Mangold K: Interview of Karl Mangold, M.D., by Brian Zink. Oakland, California, 2002.
6. Wiegenstein J: Interview of John Wiegenstein, M.D., by Brian Zink. Naples, Florida, 2002.
7. Wagner D: Interview of David Wagner, M.D., by Brian Zink. Philadelphia, Pennsylvania, 2003.
8. American Hospital Association: *Emergency services: the hospital emergency department in an emergency care system,* Chicago, 1972, American Hospital Association.
9. Abbott VC: Emergency department staffing: five-year experience with the Pontiac Plan, *Bull Am Coll Surg* January/February, 11, 1966.
10. Leichtman RR, Maraveleas MF: *The Pontiac Plan—emergency department: a handbook for medical staff,* Chicago, 1966, American Medical Association, Department of Hospitals and Medical Facilities.
11. Green JJ: *Here's the new family doctor—your friendly emergency room,* The Detroit News, Sunday News Magazine 16, 1972.
12. Ludmerer KM: *Time to heal: American medical education from the turn of the century to the era of managed care,* Oxford/New York, 1999, Oxford University Press.
13. Krome R: Interview of Ronald Krome, M.D., by Brian Zink. Naples, Florida, 2002.
14. Rupke J: Interview of John Rupke, M.D., by Brian Zink. Lansing, Michigan, 2003.
15. President's Commission on Heart Disease, Cancer and Stroke: *A national program to conquer heart disease, cancer, and stroke,* Washington, DC, 1964, U.S. Government Printing Office.
16. McWilliams JC: The 1960s cultural revolution. Miller RM, editor. In *Greenwood Press guides to the historic events of the twentieth century,* Westport, Connecticut, 2000, Greenwood Press.
17. American Medical Association: *Emergency department: a handbook for the medical staff,* Chicago, 1966, American Medical Association, Department of Hospitals and Medical Facilities.
18. Krome R: Telephone interview with Ron Krome, M.D., by Brian Zink. Ann Arbor, Michigan, 2003.
19. Committee on Trauma and Committee on Shock, Division of Medical Sciences, National Academy of Sciences, National Research Council: *Thirty-seventh Meeting, Committee on Trauma.* Washington, DC, 1966, Academy-Research Council Building.
20. Committee on Trauma and Committee on Shock, Division of Medical Sciences, National Academy of Sciences, National Research Council: *Accidental death and disability: the neglected disease of modern society,* Washington, DC, 1966, National Academy of Sciences.
21. Eiseman B: Combat casualty management in Vietnam, *J Trauma* 7(1):53–63, 1967.
22. National Highway Traffic and Safety Administration: *Motor vehicle crash statistics: 2001.* Available at: www.nhtsa.dot.gov/people/Crash/crashstatistics. Date accessed: November 13, 2003.
23. Seely SF: *Lettter from Sam Seely,* Alan P. Thal, M.D., Editor. Washington, DC, 1966.
24. Committee on Emergency Medical Services, Division of Medical Sciences: *Roles and Resources of Federal Agencies in Support of Comprehensive Emergency Medical Services.* Washington, DC, 1972, National Academy of Sciences-National Research Council.
25. Kennedy RH: Our fashionable killer: the oration on trauma, *Bull Am Coll Surg* 40:73–81, 1955.
26. Committee on Trauma, American College of Surgeons: Standards for emergency departments in hospitals, *Bull Am Coll Surg* May–June, 112, 1963.
27. Hampton OP: The Hartford Foundation and College's program in trauma and Robert H. Kennedy, *Bull Am Coll Surg* March–April, 105–108, 1968.
28. Kennedy RH, editor: *Emergency care of the sick and injured: a manual for law-enforcement officers, fire-fighters, ambulance personnel, rescue squads and nurses,* Philadelphia, 1966, W.B. Saunders.
29. Noer RJ: Emergency care of the critically injured, *J Trauma* 3(4):331–339, 1963.

30. Noer RJ: But critical surgery belongs in the operating room—not in the emergency department, *Bull Am Coll Surg* May–June, 127, 1966.

31. Avellone JC: Emergency services for the severely injured, *J Trauma* 5(3):436–437, 1965.

32. Cassebaum WH: Does the injured patient receive optimal care? *J Trauma* 1(4):442–443, 1961.

33. Brown KL, Brown GL: An efficient emergency department with expanding facilities for disaster, *J Trauma* 1(3):217–225, 1961.

34. Curry GJ: Responsibility to the injured, *J Trauma* 1(5):549–551, 1961.

35. Stack JK: Trauma news, *J Trauma* 1(5):547–548, 1961.

36. Skudder PA, Wade PA: The organization of emergency medical facilities and services, *J Trauma* 4(3):358–372, 1964.

37. Clough WP: Problems common to emergency departments, *Bull Am Coll Surg* May–June, 125, 1966.

38. Hampton OP: Present status of ambulance services in the United States, *Bull Am Coll Surg* July–August, 177–178, 1965.

39. Kennedy RH: *The Emergency Department Situation: Agenda Item VIII.* Washington, DC: National Academy of Sciences–National Research Council, Committee on Trauma Meeting, 1966.

40. Kennedy RH: A dilemma in emergency department coverage, *J Trauma* 9(9):821–822, 1969.

41. Hampton OP: Emergency department physicians: their capabilities, contributions, education, and future status, *J Trauma* 14(10):894–901, 1974.

42. Heaton LD: Army medical services activity in Viet Nam, *Military Medicine* 131:646–647, 1966.

43. McNabney WK: Telephone interview of Kendall McNabney, M.D., by Brian Zink. Ann Arbor, Michigan, 2003.

44. Gabriel RA, Metz KS: *A History of Military Medicine, vol. II: from the Renaissance through modern times.* New York, 1992, Greenwood Press.

45. Heaton LD, Hughes CW, Rosegay H, et al: Military surgical practices of the United States Army in Viet Nam, *Curr Probl Surg* November, 1–59, 1966.

46. Winchester JH: Medical miracles in South Vietnam. *Popular Science* 191:70, July 1967.

47. Heisterkamp C: *Activities of the U.S. Army Surgical Team WRAIR—Vietnam.* Washington, DC, 1968, U.S. Army Medical Research and Development Command.

48. Otten E: Telephone interview of Mel Otten, M.D., by Brian Zink. Ann Arbor, Michigan, 2003.

49. Haeck W: Interview of William Haeck, M.D., by Brian Zink. Boca Raton, Florida, 2003.

50. A young doctor's dilemma—the draft. *Medical World News* 1968.

51. Morgan EP: *The 60s Experience—Hard Lessons about Modern America,* Philadelphia, 1991, Temple University Press.

52. Goldfrank LR: Interview of Lewis Goldfrank, M.D., by Brian Zink. Orlando, Florida, 2004.

53. Fine S: *Violence in the Model City.* Ann Arbor: University of Michigan Press, 1989.

54. Anderson GV: Interview of Gail V. Anderson, M.D., by Brian Zink. Los Angeles, California, 2002.

55. Podgorny G: Interview of George Podgorny, M.D., by Brian Zink. Winston-Salem, North Carolina, 2003.

56. Janiak B: Interview of Bruce Janiak, M.D., by Brian Zink. Maumee, Ohio, 2002.

57. Levy R: Interview of Richard Levy, M.D., by Brian Zink. Cincinnati, Ohio, 2002.

58. Levy R: E-mail from Richard Levy, M.D., to Brian Zink. Ann Arbor, Michigan, 2003.

59. Buttaravoli P: Interview of Phillip Buttaravoli, M.D., by Brian Zink. West Palm Beach, Florida, 2003.

60. Buttaravoli P: *The University Hospital Emergency Department Unwittingly Exploited: A Possible Solution,* Burlington, 1970, University of Vermont Medical School.

61. Buttaravoli P: Photographs for medical records, *N Engl J Med* 282(21):1216, 1970.

62. O'Neill WL: *Coming apart: an informal history of America in the 1960s,* New York, 1971, Times Books.

Chapter 4

1. Rupke J: Interview of John Rupke, M.D., by Brian Zink. 2003, Lansing, Michigan.

2. Rupke J: Telephone interview with John Rupke, M.D., by Brian Zink. 2003, Ann Arbor, Michigan.

3. Wiegenstein J: Interview of John Wiegenstein, M.D., by Brian Zink. 2002, Naples, Florida.

4. Committee on Injuries and Surgeons, American Academy of Orthopaedic Surgeons: *Emergency care and transportation of the sick and injured,* 1971, American Academy of Orthopaedic Surgeons.

5. American College of Emergency Physicians: *Stories from the past: emergency medicine founders speak—Rupke and Wiegenstein,* Naples, Florida, 2003, ACEP.

6. American College of Emergency Physicians: Minutes of organizational meeting, Birmingham, Michigan, 1968, ACEP.

7. Mills JD: A method of staffing a community hospital emergency department, *Virginia Medical Monthly* 90:518–519, 1963.

8. Kennedy RH: A dilemma in emergency department coverage, *J Trauma* 9(9):821–822, 1969.

9. Hannas RR: Interview of R. R. Hannas, M.D., by Brian Zink. 2003: Tucson, Arizona.

10. Thurlow RM: Better E.R. treatment for patients and doctors, *Medical Economics* 1969.

11. Haeck W: Interview of William Haeck, M.D., by Brian Zink. 2003: Boca Raton, Florida.

12. Does it take a specialist to run emergency room? *Medical World News* 1968.

13. Pulaski County Medical Society: Emergency room problems—April topic meeting. *Pulaski County Medical Society Bulletin* 1, 1966.

14. Leidelmeyer R: The emergency room: how to cope with this new challenge, *Virginia Medical Monthly* 93:504–511, 1966.

15. McDade J: Interview of John McDade, M.D., by Brian Zink. 2002: Rockledge, Florida.

16. Leidelmeyer R: The birth of emergency medicine: a retrospective, *Virginia Medical Quarterly* 124:176–177, 1997.
17. Leidelmeyer R: Interview of Reinald Leidelmeyer, M.D., by Brian Zink. 2003: Fairfax, Virginia.
18. Rupke J: *Twenty-five years on the front line*, Dallas, Texas, 1993, American College of Emergency Physicians.
19. American College of Emergency Physicians: Minutes of the first national meeting of emergency physicians, Arlington, Virginia, 1968, ACEP.
20. National Library of Medicine Web site: *Finding aid to Ward Darley, M.D.* Available at http://www.nlm.nih.gov/hmd/manuscripts/ead/darley.html 2003. Date accessed: December 27, 2003.
21. Leidelmeyer R: Letter to those who attended the national organizational meeting at Marriott Twin Bridges Motel. December 12, 1968: Fairfax, Virginia.
22. Personique Web site: Biographical description of Robert Ersek, M.D. 2003. Available at http://www.plasticsurgeryexperts.com/index.html. Date accessed: December 27, 2003.
23. Early letters and correspondence to John Wiegenstein, President, 1969–1970, Dallas, Texas, 1969, American College of Emergency Physicians Archives.
24. Collection of letters to ACEP from individuals, organizations, government and industry, 1969–1970, Dallas, Texas, American College of Emergency Physicians.
25. American College of Emergency Physicians: Minutes of the ACEP board meeting, February 7, 1969. Lansing, Michigan, 1969, ACEP.
26. Basch B: The amazing psychic doctor. Newspaper clipping, c. 1976, unknown source.
27. American College of Emergency Physicians: Minutes of ACEP board meeting, March 3, 1969, East Lansing, Michigan, 1969, Michigan State Medical Society.
28. Jenkins AL: *Time line: ACEP's 25 years, 1968–1993*, American College of Emergency Physicians, 1993.
29. American College of Emergency Physicians: Minutes of ACEP Board meeting, May 12, 1969. East Lansing, Michigan, 1969, ACEP.
30. American College of Emergency Physicians: Minutes of the ACEP Board of Directors Meeting, Hotel Sahara. Las Vegas, Nevada, 1970, ACEP.
31. American College of Emergency Physicians: ACEP winter workshop: workshop session reports, February 11–13, 1971. ACEP Winter Workshop. Sarasota, Florida, 1971, ACEP.
32. American College of Emergency Physicians: Constitution and by-laws, revised June 1969, East Lansing, Michigan, 1969, ACEP.
33. Wiegenstein J: Chairman's comments. East Lansing, Michigan, 1970, ACEP.
34. Podgorny G: Interview of George Podgorny, M.D., by Brian Zink. 2003: Winston-Salem, North Carolina.
35. American College of Emergency Physicians: Minutes of ACEP Board Meeting, February 13–14, 1970, New Orleans, 1970, ACEP.
36. Auer A: Activity report—planning trip to Hotel Sahara, Las Vegas. Lansing, Michigan, 1970, ACEP.
37. American College of Emergency Physicians: Minutes of the ACEP Publications Committee Meeting. Chicago, 1970, ACEP.
38. American College of Emergency Physicians: Minutes of Committee meetings, ACEP Winter Workshop, Sarasota, Florida, 1971, ACEP.
39. Mangold K: ACEP News: Dallas Convention Center to host first joint meeting of ACEP/EDNA, *JACEP* Sept/Oct:349, 1973.
40. Krome R: Interview of Ronald Krome, M.D., by Brian Zink. 2002, Naples, Florida.
41. American College of Emergency Physicians: Minutes of the ACEP Board of Directors Meeting, February 26, 1972. Las Vegas, Nevada, 1972, ACEP.
42. American College of Emergency Physicians: Revised constitution and by-laws. Lansing, Michigan, 1972, ACEP.
43. American College of Emergency Physicians: Minutes of the ACEP Board of Directors Meeting, November, 1972. San Francisco, 1972, ACEP.
44. Mangold K: Interview of Karl Mangold, M.D., by Brian Zink. 2002, Oakland, California.
45. Mills F: Interview of Frances Mills, wife of James Mills, Jr., M.D. (deceased). 2003, Alexandria, Virginia.

Chapter 5

1. Haeck W: Interview of William Haeck, M.D., by Brian Zink. 2003: Boca Raton, Florida.
2. Mangold K: Interview of Karl Mangold, M.D., by Brian Zink. 2002: Oakland, California.
3. Knowles JH: The emergency ward, *Atlantic Monthly* 218:116–121, 1966.
4. Dineen J: University Association for Emergency Medical Services first annual meeting—the need for training physicians in emergency medicine, *J Trauma* 2(5):378–384, 1972.
5. Goldfinger S, Federman D: Postgraduate education of community physicians. *JAMA* 206(13):2883–2884, 1968.
6. Bouzarth W: Training the "second-career" emergency physician. In Jelenko CI, Frey C, editors: *Emergency medical services: an overview,* Bowie, Maryland, 1976, Robert J. Brady Co.
7. Flessa H: Interview of Herbert Flessa, M.D., by Brian Zink. 2002: Cincinnati, Ohio.
8. University of Cincinnati, Department of Emergency Medicine: *Emergency medicine: 30th anniversary,* Cincinnati, Ohio, 2001, University of Cincinnati Medical Center, Video Services.
9. Levy R: Interview of Richard Levy, M.D., by Brian Zink. 2002: Cincinnati, Ohio.
10. Wiegenstein J: Interview of John Wiegenstein, M.D., by Brian Zink. 2002: Naples, Florida.
11. ACEP News: First resident graduates from Cincinnati program, *JACEP* Mar/Apr:44, 1972.

12. Janiak B: Interview of Bruce Janiak, M.D., by Brian Zink. 2002: Maumee, Ohio.
13. Frey C: University Association for Emergency Medical Services first annual meeting: the need for training physicians in emergency medicine, *J Trauma* 2(5):369–384, 1972.
14. Buttaravoli P: Interview of Phillip Buttaravoli, M.D., by Brian Zink. 2003: West Palm Beach, Florida.
15. Otten E: Telephone interview of Mel Otten, M.D., by Brian Zink. 2003: Ann Arbor, Michigan.
16. Iserson K: Interview of Kenneth Iserson by Brian Zink. 2003: Tucson, Arizona.
17. Levy R: E-mail from Richard Levy, M.D., to Brian Zink. Zink B, ed. 2003: Ann Arbor, Michigan.
18. Wagner D: Interview of David Wagner by Brian Zink. 2003, Philadelphia, Pennsylvania.
19. Bensen P: Telephone interview of Pamela Bensen, M.D., by Brian Zink. 2004: Ann Arbor, Michigan.
20. Bukata R: Telephone interview of Richard Bukata, M.D., by Brian Zink. 2004: Ann Arbor, Michigan.
21. Anderson GV: Interview of Gail V. Anderson, M.D., by Brian Zink. 2002: Los Angeles, California.
22. Anderson G: Where we've been, where we are, and where we're going: emergency medicine—past present and future, *Ann Emerg Med* 17:982–989, 1988.
23. Dailey R: Interview of Robert Dailey, M.D., by Brian Zink. 2002: Jackson, Wyoming.
24. Mallon W: Interview of William Mallon, M.D., by Brian Zink. 2002: Los Angeles, California.
25. Orlinsky M: Interview of Michael Orlinsky, M.D., by Brian Zink. 2002: Los Angeles, California.
26. Callaham M: Interview of Michael Callaham, M.D., by Brian Zink. 2002: Oakland, California.
27. Hannas RR: Interview of R. R. Hannas, M.D., by Brian Zink. 2003: Tucson, Arizona.
28. Scheck A: Stress and MI lead to a career in emergency medicine, *Emergency Medicine News* 25(4):28, 2003.
29. Rosen P: Interview of Peter Rosen, M.D., by Brian Zink. 2003: Jackson, Wyoming.
30. Rosen P: The evolution of education, *J Emerg Med* 12(1):73–74, 1994.
31. Fauman B: Janssen Award—American Association for Emergency Psychiatry, *Emerg Psych* 6(4): 127–130, 2000.
32. Rosen P: Interview of Peter Rosen, M.D., by Brian Zink. 2002: Jackson, Wyoming.
33. Meislin H: Interview of Harvey Meislin, M.D., by Brian Zink. 2004: Tucson, Arizona.
34. Rosen P: New procedure for care of rape victims, personnel, 1972, Chicago, 1972, University of Chicago Hospital.
35. Curing the emergency room, *Time* 98:94–95, 1971.
36. Ludmerer KM: *Time to heal: American medical education from the turn of the century to the era of managed care,* Oxford/New York, 1999, Oxford University Press.
37. Podgorny G, Munger BS: *Certification: a decade of progress,* East Lansing, Michigan, 1980, American Board of Emergency Medicine.
38. Mills JD: Improved care is common goal, *JACEP* May/June:19, 1972.
39. Podgorny G: Interview of George Podgorny, M.D., by Brian Zink. 2003: Winston-Salem, North Carolina.
40. Council on Medical Education: *Report on the Conference on Education of the Physician in Emergency Medical Care,* Chicago, 1973, American Medical Association.
41. American College of Emergency Physicians: Minutes of the ACEP Board of Directors Meeting, November, 1972. San Francisco, 1972, ACEP.
42. Tintinalli J: Interview of Judith Tintinalli, M.D., by Brian Zink. 2003: Chapel Hill, North Carolina.
43. American College of Emergency Physicians: Emergency medicine residency newsletter, *JACEP* Jan/Feb:70, 1975.
44. University Association for Emergency Medical Services: Minutes of meeting, March 6, 1970. Birmingham, Alabama, 1970.
45. Krome R: Telephone interview with Ron Krome, M.D., by Brian Zink. 2003: Ann Arbor, Michigan.
46. University Association for Emergency Medical Services: Minutes of the Executive Council meeting, UA/EMS, May 13, 1971. Ann Arbor, Michigan, 1971, UA/EMS.
47. Schropp MA: Interview of Mary Ann Schropp by Brian Zink. 2002: Lansing, Michigan.
48. University Association for Emergency Medical Services: Minutes of the UA/EMS Executive Council meeting, December 7–8, 1972. Hamilton, Ontario, Canada, 1972, UA/EMS.
49. University Association for Emergency Medical Services: Minutes of Executive Council meeting, December 11, 1973. East Lansing, Michigan, 1973, UA/EMS.
50. Hampton OP: Emergency department physicians: their capabilities, contributions, education, and future status, *J Trauma* 14(10):894–901, 1974.
51. Johnson GJ: A new flower: is it a cactus or a daisy? *JACEP* 4(Nov/Dec):517, 1975.
52. McNabney WK: Telephone interview of Kendall McNabney, M.D., by Brian Zink. 2003: Ann Arbor, Michigan.
53. American College of Emergency Physicians: Minutes of the ACEP Board of Directors meeting, November 7, 1974, Washington, DC, 1974, ACEP.
54. American College of Emergency Physicians: Minutes of the ACEP Board of Directors meeting, October 10, 1975, Las Vegas, Nevada, 1975, ACEP.
55. Society of Teachers of Emergency Medicine: Minutes of the organizational meeting, May 23, 1975. Vancouver, British Columbia, Canada, 1975, STEM.
56. University Association for Emergency Medical Services: Minutes of the UA/EMS Executive Council meeting, May 28–29, 1974. Dallas, 1974, UA/EMS.

Chapter 6

1. Podgorny G, Munger BS: Certification: a decade of progress, East Lansing, MI, 1980, American Board of Emergency Medicine.
2. Waeckerle J: Remarks upon receiving the SAEM Leadership Award. At SAEM Annual Meeting. May, 2004. Orlando, Florida.

3. Maisel AQ: Emergency service: medicine's newest specialty, Reader's Digest 518:96–100, 1965.
4. Dailey RH: The emergency physician and his residency training. In: Jelenko CI, Frey C, editors. Emergency medical services: an overview, Bowie, Maryland, 1976, Robert J. Brady Company, a Prentice-Hall Company, 143–154.
5. Dailey R: Telephone conversation with Robert Dailey, M.D., and Brian Zink. 2004: Ann Arbor, Michigan.
6. Johnson GJ: A new flower: is it a cactus or a daisy? *JACEP* 4:517, 1975.
7. Curing the emergency room. *Time* 98:94–95, 1971.
8. Where minutes count: drive for better emergency care, *U.S. News and World Report* 72:78–81, 1972.
9. Cutler A: *Four minutes to life,* New York, 1970, Cowles Book Company, Inc.
10. Feagles AM: *Emergency room,* New York, 1970, Cowles Book Company, Inc.
11. Angeli L: Emergency! Is back on T.V. 1999. Available at www.firehouse.com /news/99/1/emergency.html. Accessed August 10, 2002.
12. Stewart R: Interview of Ronald Stewart, M.D., by Brian Zink. 2004: Boularderie Island, Nova Scotia.
13. Haeck W: Interview of William Haeck, M.D., by Brian Zink. 2003: Boca Raton, Florida.
14. Walt A: Panel: Role of the specialist in the emergency room, *J Trauma* 19:481–491, 1979.
15. McDade J: Interview of John McDade, M.D., by Brian Zink. 2002: Rockledge, Florida.
16. Nixon R: Veto message—emergency medical services systems act of 1973, Document 93-31, 93rd Congress, 1st session. Washington, DC, 1973, U.S. Government Printing Office.
17. U.S. House of Representatives. Emergency Medical Services Act of 1973, H.R. 6458. Washington, DC, 1973.
18. ACEP News: Emergency Medical Services System Act of 1973, *JACEP* May/June:194–196, 1974.
19. Mangold K: Interview of Karl Mangold, M.D., by Brian Zink. 2002: Oakland, California.
20. Rupke J: *Twenty-five years on the front line,* Dallas, TX, 1993, American College of Emergency Physicians.
21. Schropp MA: Interview of Mary Ann Schropp by Brian Zink. 2002: Lansing, Michigan.
22. Dunsmore S: Telephone conversation with Susan Dunsmore and Brian Zink. American Board of Emergency Medicine 2004: Ann Arbor, Michigan.
23. Emergency Nurse Association: ENA Web site. Available at http://www.ena.org/about/history. Accessed May 30, 2004.
24. Eisenberg M: *Life in the balance: Emergency medicine and the quest to reverse sudden death,* New York, 1997, Oxford University Press.
25. Wiegenstein J: Interview of John Wiegenstein by Brian Zink. 2002: Naples, Florida.
26. Rupke J: Telephone interview with John Rupke, M.D., by Brian Zink. 2003: Ann Arbor, Michigan.
27. ACEP: *Board reaffirms ties with Profesco, JACEP* 8:93, 1979.
28. Jenkins AL: Time line: ACEP's 25 Years, 1968–1993. 1993, American College of Emergency Physicians.
29. Stevens R: *American medicine and the public interest: a history of specialization,* Berkeley, 1998, University of California Press.
30. Mulder D: Specialization in surgery—implications for trauma-related disciplines, *ACS Bull* May:15–25, 1988.
31. Little DM, Jr.: The founding of the specialty boards, *Anesthesiology* 55:317–321, 1981.
32. Wagner D: Interview of David Wagner, M.D., by Brian Zink. 2003: Philadelphia, Pennsylvania.
33. Bock B: Interview of Brooks Bock, M.D., by Brian Zink. 2004: Detroit, Michigan.
34. Burnette WE: Historical background of the AMA Commission on Emergency Medical Services. *Emergency Medicine Today* 2:7, 1975.
35. Wiegenstein J: The 25th scientific section. *JACEP* May/June:203, 1973.
36. Hannas RR: Interview of R. R. Hannas, M.D., by Brian Zink. 2003: Tucson, Arizona.
37. ACEP: *Committee on Board Establishment document—requirements and timetable*, Lansing, Michigan, 1975, ACEP.
38. Podgorny G: Interview of George Podgorny, M.D., by Brian Zink. 2003: Winston-Salem, North Carolina.
39. ACEP: *Document detailing the residency manpower requirements from emergency medicine*, Lansing, Michigan, 1976, ACEP.
40. ACEP Committee on Board Establishment, *Recommendations for eligibility requirements*, Lansing, Michigan: 1975, ACEP.
41. Rosen P: Interview of Peter Rosen, M.D., by Brian Zink. 2003: Jackson, Wyoming.
42. American Board of Emergency Medicine: *History of certification in emergency medicine: videotape,* East Lansing, Michigan, 1989, American Board of Emergency Medicine.
43. Rosen P: E-mail from Peter Rosen to Brian Zink. 2004: Ann Arbor, Michigan.
44. ACEP: Certification examination field test dates announced. *JACEP* 6:69, 1977.
45. Meislin H: Interview of Harvey Meislin, M.D., by Brian Zink. 2004: Tucson, Arizona.
46. Testimony—Liaison Committee for Specialty Boards, October 26, 1976. Chicago, 1976, American Board of Medical Specialties.
47. Testimony submitted to the Liaison Committee for Specialty Boards, February 26, 1977.Chicago, 1977, American Board of Medical Specialties.
48. Krome R: E-mail from Ronald Krome to Brian Zink on lack of AHA support, 2004: Ann Arbor, Michigan.
49. Maclean C: American Board of Pediatrics meeting—report to ABEM. Charleston, South Carolina, 1977, ACEP/ABEM.
50. Leymaster G: Letter to Ronald Krome, ACEP President, announcing favorable LCSB decision. Chicago, 1977, Liaison Committee for Specialty Boards.
51. Krome R, Wagner D, Wiegenstein J: Letter announcing LCSB approval. Lansing, Michigan, 1977, ACEP, UAEMS, ABEM.
52. Krome R: Activity Report, March 18, 1977—Appearance before the ABMS. Lansing, Michigan, 1977, ACEP.
53. Graves H: Letter to ACEP President Ron Krome. Lansing, Michigan, 1977, ACEP.

54. Krome R: Letter to Harris Graves. Lansing, Michigan, 1977, ACEP.
55. National Library of Medicine Web site: Finding aid to Ward Darley, M.D. Available at http://www.nlm.nih.gov/hmd/manuscripts/ead/darley.html 2003. Accessed December 27, 2003.
56. Anderson GV: Interview of Gail V. Anderson, Sr., M.D., by Brian Zink. 2002: Los Angeles, California.
57. ACEP: ABMS rejects ABEM application, *JACEP* 6:88–89, 1977.
58. ACEP: Certification examination field tested (in compendium), *JACEP* 6:89–90, 1977.
59. Bukata R: Telephone interview of Richard Bukata, M.D., by Brian Zink. 2004: Ann Arbor, Michigan.
60. Munger B: Interview of Benson Munger by Brian Zink. 2002: Ann Arbor, Michigan.
61. Ismach J: Emergency medicine: how far has it come, where is it going? *Medical World News* 20;19: 65–72, 1978.
62. Committee on Certification, Subcertification and Recertification of the ABMS, Report to the interim meeting, Sept. 6, 1977. Chicago, 1977, American Board of Medical Specialties.
63. Krome R: Mailgram announcing ABMS rejection of ABEM application. East Lansing, Michigan, 1977, ACEP.
64. Establishment of specialty board and certification in emergency medicine. Letter to ABMS. Philadelphia, 1977, American Board of Surgery.
65. Wagner D, Wiegenstein J: Report of the appearance before the American Board of Obstetrics and Gynecology. Lansing, Michigan, 1977, ACEP.
66. Munger BS: Presentation before the ABMS/COCERT subcommittee—letter to ACEP. Lansing, Michigan, 1977, ABEM.
67. Munger BS: Presentation before the ABMS/COSERT subcommittee. Lansing, Michigan, 1977, ABEM/ACEP.
68. Center for Health Policy Research: *Physician supply and utilization by specialty: trends and projections.* Chicago, 1988, American Medical Association.
69. Growing crisis in health care, *U.S. News and World Report* Nov. 3:70–73, 1969.
70. Ludmerer KM: *Time to heal: American medical education from the turn of the century to the era of managed care,* Oxford/New York, 1999, Oxford University Press.
71. Rosen P: The biology of emergency medicine, *JACEP* 8:279–283, 1979.
72. Marx J: Interview of John Marx, M.D., by Brian Zink. 2002: St. Louis, Missouri.
73. Organ CA: The first 50 years of the American Board of Surgery, *Bull Am Coll Surg* April:13–17, 1988.
74. Walt A: The role of the surgeon in the emergency room, *Bull Am Coll Surg* July:14–15, 1979.
75. Starr P: *The social transformation of American medicine,* New York, 1982, Basic Books, Inc.
76. Gordon C: *Dead on arrival: the politics of health care in twentieth-century America,* Princeton, New Jersey, 2003, Princeton University Press.
77. Wiegenstein J: *American Board of Emergency Medicine application: letter to sponsoring organizations,* Lansing, Michigan, 1978, ABEM.
78. Rupke J: Interview of John Rupke, M.D., by Brian Zink. 2003: Lansing, Michigan.
79. Munger B: *Sponsoring organizations governing bodies combined organizational meetings on specialty status,* Chicago, 1978, ACEP/ABEM.
80. Mangold K: Certifying board for emergency medicine—negotiating closer to a reality, *JACEP* 7, 1978.
81. Mangold K: Comments on the board recognition for emergency medicine. Lansing, Michigan, Jan. 11, 1978, ACEP.
82. Levy R: Interview of Richard Levy, M.D., by Brian Zink. 2002: Cincinnati, Ohio.
83. Janiak B: Interview of Bruce Janiak, M.D., by Brian Zink. 2002: Maumee, Ohio.
84. Bensen P: Telephone interview of Pamela Bensen, M.D., by Brian Zink. 2004: Ann Arbor, Michigan.
85. *By-laws of the American Board of Emergency Medicine.* Lansing, Michigan, 1979, ABEM.
86. Munger BS: Telephone interview of Benson Munger by Brian Zink. 2004: Ann Arbor, Michigan.
87. American Board of Emergency Medicine: *The specialty of emergency medicine: a history,* Lansing, Michigan, March 20, 1979, ABEM.
88. Podgorny G: American Board of Emergency Medicine—progress update. *JACEP* 8:88–89, 1979.
89. Rosen P: Interview of Peter Rosen, M.D., by Brian Zink. 2002: Jackson, Wyoming.
90. Wagner D: Development and direction of the American Board of Emergency Medicine, *Ann Emerg Med* 11:573–575, 1982.
91. Downing S: The validity of clinically relevant multiple-choice items, *Ann Emerg Med* 9:554–556, 1980.
92. Hannas RR: *Spreading the specialty spectrum,* Boston, 1975, Harvard Medical School Alumni Association Bulletin.

Chapter 7

1. Anwar R, et al: A comparative study of professional socialization in residency training, phase I: report on residency director interviews, 1976–1977. Philadelphia, 1978, 49–50.
2. Rosen P: Interview of Peter Rosen, M.D., by Brian Zink. 2002: Jackson, Wyoming.
3. Podgorny G: Interview of George Podgorny, M.D., by Brian Zink. 2003: Winston-Salem, North Carolina.
4. Dailey R: Emergency medicine residencies—1984: an Orwellian warning, *JACEP* 7:342–343, 1978.
5. Keith JF: Family practice: quality and credibility, *N Engl J Med* 297:1007–1008, 1977.
6. Tintinalli J: Interview of Judith Tintinalli, M.D., by Brian Zink. 2003: Chapel Hill, North Carolina.
7. Wagner D: Interview of David Wagner by Brian Zink. 2003, Philadelphia, Pennsylvania.
8. Dailey R: Interview of Robert Dailey, M.D., by Brian Zink. 2002: Jackson, Wyoming.
9. Wentz W: Telephone conversation with Waldo Wentz, Assistant Director of the National Residency Match Program. 2004: Ann Arbor, Michigan.

10. McNabney WK: RRC (nee LREC), *Ann Emerg Med* 9:595–596, 1980.
11. SAEM, Society for Academic Emergency Medicine Web site: Residency Catalog—Introduction. Available at www.saem.org. Accessed July 7, 2004.
12. Brye PE, Reding RJ: Primer on HEW's health planning policy puzzle, *JACEP* 7:213–216, 1978.
13. Health Professions Educational Assistance Act of 1976 (PL 94-484)—Fact Sheet. Washington, DC: U.S. Department of Health Education and Welfare, Public Health Service, Health Resources Administration, Bureau of Health Manpower, 1978.
14. Meislin H: Interview of Harvey Meislin, M.D., by Brian Zink. 2004: Tucson, Arizona.
15. The Robert Wood Johnson Foundation grant/proposal summary. 2002, RWJ Foundation, 1–2.
16. Levy R: *How to survive—axioms for survival, in emergency medicine,* Cincinnati, Ohio, 1977, University of Cincinnati.
17. Levy R: Interview of Richard Levy, M.D., by Brian Zink. 2002: Cincinnati, Ohio.
18. Hedges J: Interview of Jerris Hedges, M.D., by Brian Zink. 2002: St. Louis, Missouri.
19. Iserson K: Interview of Kenneth Iserson, M.D., by Brian Zink. 2003: Tucson, Arizona.
20. Davidson S: Interview of Steven Davidson, M.D., by Brian Zink. 2004: Orlando, Florida.
21. Anwar RA, et al: A comparative study of professional socialization in residency training, Phase II: Report on residency training, 1977–78, 1978.
22. McDade J: Interview of John McDade, M.D., by Brian Zink. 2002: Rockledge, Florida.
23. Krome R: Interview of Ronald Krome, M.D., by Brian Zink. 2002: Naples, Florida.
24. Bock B: Interview of Brooks Bock, M.D., by Brian Zink. 2004: Detroit, Michigan.
25. Tomlanovich M: Telephone interview of Michael Tomlanovich, M.D., by Brian Zink. 2004: Ann Arbor, Michigan.
26. Marx J: Interview of John Marx, M.D., by Brian Zink. 2002: St. Louis, Missouri.
27. Anwar RA: Trends in training: focus on emergency medicine, *Ann Emerg Med* 9:60–71, 1980.
28. Rosen P: Telephone communication with Peter Rosen, M.D., by Brian Zink. 2004: Ann Arbor, Michigan.
29. Stewart R: Interview of Ronald Stewart, M.D., by Brian Zink. 2004: Boularderie Island, Nova Scotia.
30. Nowak R: Telephone interview of Richard Nowak, M.D., by Brian Zink. 2002: Ann Arbor, Michigan.
31. Eiseman B: The emergency department physician and university teaching hospitals, *Arch Surg* 113: 678–683, 1978.
32. Meislin HW: Trouble in paradise, *Ann Emerg Med* 11:641, 1982.
33. Gann DS: Proposal to the Robert Wood Johnson Foundation for support of an educational program in emergency medical services. Baltimore: Johns Hopkins Hospital, Feb. 4, 1974.
34. Kelen G: Telephone interview of Gabor Kelen, M.D., by Brian Zink. 2002: Ann Arbor, Michigan.
35. Eisenberg M: Interview of Mickey Eisenberg, M.D., by Brian Zink. 2002: Seattle, Washington.
36. Eisenberg MS, et al: Treatment of out-of-hospital cardiac arrests with rapid defibrillation by emergency medical technicians, *N Engl J Med* 302:1379–1383, 1980.
37. Petersdorf RG: Letter from Robert Petersdorf, M.D., AAMC President, to Henry McIntosh, M.D., supporting ABEM as a primary board. McIntosh H, ed. Washington, DC, 1987, AAMC.
38. Rothstein R: 24-hour faculty coverage, *Ann Emerg Med* 14:156–157, 1985.
39. White JD, Walters B, Janiak B: ACEP and academics, *Am J Emerg Med* 3:368, 578–580, 1985.
40. Frumkin K: The future of emergency medicine residency training, *Ann Emerg Med* 14:378–379, 1985.
41. Rosen P, Markovchick V: Attending coverage, *Ann Emerg Med* 14:897–899, 1985.
42. Rosen P: Night shift and the emergency physician, *J Emerg Med* 2:29–30, 1984.
43. Binder L, et al: 24-hour coverage in academic emergency medicine: ways of dealing with the issue, *Ann Emerg Med* 19:430–434, 1990.
44. Podgorny G. Memorandum: Residency review committee for emergency medicine and its special requirements. Lansing, Michigan, 1986, American Board of Emergency Medicine, 1–4.
45. Pointer JE, Dailey RH: Standards for attending staff in an emergency medicine residency program, *J Emerg Med* 1:271–274, 1984.
46. Tomlanovich M, Wagner D: The bases of emergency medicine residency curriculum development, *Emerg Health Serv Q* 1:77–83, 1980.
47. Stewart R, Paris PM, Heller MB: Design of a resident in-field experience for an emergency medicine residency curriculum, *Ann Emerg Med* 16:175–179, 1987.
48. Carraway RP, et al: Life Saver: a complete team approach incorporated in a hospital-based program, *Am Surgeon* 50:173–182, 1984.
49. Rose WD, et al: Field experience in aeromedical transport for an emergency medicine residency, *Am J Emerg Med* 6:82–83, 1988.
50. Carter GL, et al: Safety and helicopter-based programs, *Ann Emerg Med* 15:1117–1118, 1986.
51. Rose WD, et al: Field experience in aeromedical transport for an emergency medicine residency, *Am J Emerg Med* 6:82–83, 1988.
52. Podgorny G: Length of learning, *Ann Emerg Med* 13:203–204, 1984.
53. Barsan WG, Levy R: Duration of training in emergency medicine residencies, *Ann Emerg Med* 11:639–640, 1982.
54. Goldman GE: The need for some conformity in emergency medicine, *Ann Emerg Med* 13:212, 1984.
55. Consolidated Omnibus Budget Reconciliation Act, United States Congress, 1986.
56. Krome R: The itinerant emergency physician, *Ann Emerg Med* 15:1366–1367, 1986.
57. SAEM Position Statement: Qualifications for unsupervised emergency department care. Lansing, Michigan, 2002, Society for Academic Emergency Medicine. Available at www.saem.org. Accessed July 7, 2004.
58. Eckert C: *Emergency-room care,* Boston, 1967, Little, Brown and Company.
59. Marx J: E-mail from John Marx, M.D., to Brian Zink. 2004: Ann Arbor, Michigan.
60. Kravis T, Warner CG: *Emergency medicine,* San Diego, 1983.
61. May H: *Emergency medicine,* New York, 1984, John Wiley & Sons.

62. Mills J, Ho MT, Trunkey DD: *Current emergency diagnosis and treatment*, Los Altos, California, 1983, Lange Medical Publishers.
63. Simon R, Brenner B: *Procedures and techniques in emergency medicine*, Baltimore, 1982, Williams & Wilkins.
64. Roberts J, Hedges J: *Clinical procedures in emergency medicine*, Philadelphia, 1985, WB Saunders Company.
65. Goldfrank LR: Interview of Lewis Goldfrank, M.D., by Brian Zink. 2004: Orlando, Florida.
66. Krome R: Annals of emergency medicine. *JACEP* 8:543, 1979.
67. ABEM, American Board of Emergency Medicine: History of Certification in Emergency Medicine. (Videotape.) Lansing, Michigan, 1989, American Board of Emergency Medicine.
68. Niemann J: Fellowships in emergency medicine research: an investment in our future, *Ann Emerg Med* 13:545, 1984.
69. Wagner D: Emergency medicine as an academic discipline, *JAMA* 238:147–148, 1977.
70. Niemann J: Telephone interview of James Niemann, M.D., by Brian Zink. 2004: Ann Arbor, Michigan.
71. Anwar RA, Wagner D: The research component in the development of emergency medicine as a specialty, *J Med Educ* 52:55–58, 1980.
72. Blanda M, Gerson L, Dunn K: Emergency medicine research requirements and director characteristics, *Acad Emerg Med* 6:286–291, 1999.
73. Otten E: Telephone interview of Mel Otten, M.D., by Brian Zink. 2003: Ann Arbor, Michigan.
74. Krome R: Telephone interview with Ron Krome, M.D., by Brian Zink. 2003: Ann Arbor, Michigan.
75. White BC, Hoehner PJ, Wilson RF: Mitochondrial O_2 use and ATP synthesis: kinetic effects of Ca^{++} and HPO_4^{-2} modulated by glucocorticoids, *Ann Emerg Med* 9:396, 1980.
76. Roberts J, Greenberg M, Baskin S: Endotracheal epinephrine in cardiorespiratory collapse. *JACEP* 8:515–519, 1979.
77. Greenberg M, et al: Endotracheal epinephrine in a canine anaphylactic shock model, *JACEP* 8:500–503, 1979.
78. Anwar R: The development of emergency medicine residency programs: an overview, *Emerg Health Serv Q* 1:15–20, 1980.
79. Anwar R: Residency-trained emergency physicians: where have all the flowers gone? *JACEP* 8:84–87, 1979.
80. Schropp MA: Interview of Mary Ann Schropp by Brian Zink. 2002: Lansing, Michigan.
81. Mattox KL: What's new in academic emergency medicine, *JACEP* 8:491–492, 1979.
82. Mattox KL: Observations on emergency medicine—academic style, *Ann Emerg Med* 9:642–644, 1980.
83. McCally M, DeAtley C, Piemme TE: A course in emergency care for first-year medical students, *JACEP* 7:20–23, 1978.
84. Marshall CL, et al: A multidisciplinary clerkship in emergency medicine, *J Med Educ* 54:562–566, 1979.
85. Sanders AB, et al: Survey of undergraduate emergency medical education in the United States, *Ann Emerg Med* 15:1–5, 1986.
86. Cameron C, Gilmore E, McNeil E: History of emergency medicine in New York State, *N Y J Med* July:1176–1178, 1976.
87. Goldfrank LR: Personal and literary experiences in the development of an emergency physician: Keynote address. San Francisco, 2002, American Academy of Emergency Medicine.
88. San Augustin M, Goldfrank LR: Reorganization of ambulatory health care in an urban hospital: primary care and its impact on hospitalization, *Arch Int Med* 136:1262, 1976.
89. Opdycke S: *No one was turned away: the role of public hospitals in New York City since 1900,* New York, 1999, Oxford University Press.
90. Henry M: Telephone interview of Mark Henry, M.D., by Brian Zink. 2004: Ann Arbor, Michigan.
91. New York State, Public Health Law 2805-b. 2004.
92. Asch DA, Parker RM: Sounding board: The Libby Zion case: one step forward or two steps back? *N Engl J Med* 318:771–775, 1988.
93. Robins N: *The girl who died twice: every patient's nightmare: the Libby Zion case and the hidden hazards of hospitals,* New York, 1995, Delacorte Press.
94. Bell B: Reconsideration of the New York State laws rationalizing the supervision and the working conditions of residents, *Einstein J Biol Med* 20:36–40, 2003.
95. Scotch DS: Committee letter, Goldfrank LR. New York, 1988.
96. Bellevue Hospital Center Medical Board, Resolution on emergency medicine residency. New York: Bellevue Hospital Center, 1989.
97. Ziegler E: *Emergency doctor,* New York, 1987, Ivy Books, Ballantine Publishing Group.

Chapter 8

1. Rupke J: *Twenty-five years on the front line,* Dallas, 1993, American College of Emergency Physicians.
2. AMA Center for Health Policy Research: *Physician supply and utilization by specialty: trends and projections,* Chicago, 1988, American Medical Association.
3. Cydulka R, et al: Women in academic emergency medicine, *Acad Emer Med* 7:999–1007, 2000.
4. Hoffman G, et al: Report of the task force on residency training information (2001–2002), American Board of Emergency Medicine, *Ann Emerg Med* 39:510–527, 2002.
5. Bensen P: Telephone interview of Pamela Bensen, M.D., by Brian Zink. 2004: Ann Arbor, Michigan.
6. Tintinalli J: Interview of Judith Tintinalli, M.D., by Brian Zink. 2003: Chapel Hill, North Carolina.
7. Bensen P: Follow-up telephone interview of Pamela Bensen, M.D., by Brian Zink. 2004: Ann Arbor, Michigan.
8. Newspaper clipping on Judith Tintinalli, M.D., Detroit Michigan. July 26, 1987, The Detroit News.
9. Rosen P: E-mail from Peter Rosen, M.D., to Brian Zink. 2004: Ann Arbor, Michigan.

10. Martin ML: E-mail from Marcus Martin, M.D., to Brian Zink. 2004: Ann Arbor, Michigan.
11. Rowley B, et al: Graduate medical education in the United States, *JAMA* 264:822–832, 1990.
12. Gevitz N: *The D.O.'s: osteopathic medicine in America,* Baltimore, 1982, The Johns Hopkins University Press.
13. Becher JW, Jr: Emergency medicine: the newest osteopathic specialty, *OP/The Osteopathic Physician* September:10–11, 1979.
14. American Board of Emergency Medicine: Application to change member status conjoint (modified) to primary board. Lansing, Michigan, 1987, ABEM.
15. Wagner D: Development and direction of the American Board of Emergency Medicine, *Ann Emerg Med* 11:573–575, 1982.
16. Anwar RA: Professional career characteristics of residency trained emergency physicians, *Emerg Health Serv Q* 1:21–38, 1980.
17. Rosenbach ML, Harrow B, Cromwell J: A profile of emergency physicians 1984–1985: demographic characteristics, practice patterns, and income, *Ann Emerg Med* 15:1261–1267, 1986.
18. Janiak B: Interview of Bruce Janiak, M.D., by Brian Zink. 2002: Maumee, Ohio.
19. Gallery M, et al: A study of occupational stress and depression among emergency physicians, *Ann Emerg Med* 21:58–64, 1992.
20. Meislin HW, Munger BS: Emergency medicine 2000: Residencies, resident graduates and ABEM diplomates, *Ann Emerg Med* 22:132–134, 1993.
21. Hall K, et al: Factors associated with career longevity in residency-trained emergency physicians, *Ann Emerg Med* 21:291–297, 1992.
22. ACEP: *1968–1978, ACEP's first decade of achievement,* Lansing, Michigan, 1978, ACEP.
23. Riggs L, Jr: Interview of Leonard Riggs, Jr., M.D., by Brian Zink. 2003: Dallas, Texas.
24. Wiegenstein J: Interview of John Wiegenstein, M.D., by Brian Zink. 2002: Naples, Florida.
25. Statement of activity, year ended June 30, 1981. Dallas, ACEP, 1981.
26. Schropp MA: Interview of Mary Ann Schropp by Brian Zink. 2002: Lansing, Michigan.
27. McDade J: Interview of John McDade, M.D., by Brian Zink. 2002: Rockledge, Florida.
28. Rorrie C: Interview of Colin Rorrie, Ph.D., by Brian Zink. 2003: Irving, Texas.
29. Franaszek JB: Moving to solve our manpower crisis, *Ann Emerg Med* 22:134–136, 1993.
30. Buttaravoli P: Interview of Phillip Buttaravoli, M.D., by Brian Zink. 2003: West Palm Beach, Florida.
31. Podgorny G: Interview of George Podgorny, M.D., by Brian Zink. 2003: Winston-Salem, North Carolina.
32. American College of Emergency Physicians: Revised constitution and by-laws. Lansing, Michigan: ACEP, 1972.
33. Free standing emergency care centers debated, *JACEP* 8:81–82, 1979.
34. Hellstern RA: National contract groups, *JACEP* 81:493–494, 1979.
35. Randau P: Entrepreneurial physicians seen as threat, *Ann Emerg Med* 11:336, 1982.
36. Letters E: On entrepreneurs, ethics, and leadership, *Ann Emerg Med* 11:519–521, 1982.
37. Schoenfeld E: Fast-buck medicine, *New West* 20–22, 1978.
38. Crowell RD: The organization is us, *Ann Emerg Med* 13:981, 1984.
39. McCabe JB: Turbulent times for emergency medicine: health care reform, board certification, contract management, and the growth of new organizations in emergency medicine, *Ann Emerg Med* 24:289–293, 1994.
40. Wears RL, Kamens DR, Janiak B: "Megagroups" are major problem facing emergency medicine, *Ann Emerg Med* 14:83–84, 1985.
41. Bock B: Interview of Brooks Bock, M.D., by Brian Zink. 2004: Detroit, Michigan.
42. Mueller HA, Flashner B, Rosen P: Ethics, entrepreneurs and leadership. *J Emerg Med* 1:111–118, 1983.
43. Haeck W: Interview of William Haeck, M.D., by Brian Zink. 2003: Boca Raton, Florida.
44. Web site, home page of Association of Emergency Physicians. Available at www.aep.org. Accessed Sept. 12, 2004.
45. Mangold K: Postgraduate realities: surviving in emergency medicine practice, *JACEP* 7:245–248, 1978.
46. Walt A: Panel: role of the specialist in the emergency room, *J Trauma* 19:481–491, 1979.
47. Krome R: Freestanding emergency physicians, *Ann Emerg Med* 12:188–189, 1983.
48. Gordon C: Dead on arrival: the politics of health care in twentieth-century America. Princeton, New Jersey, 2003, Princeton University Press.
49. Rupke J: Why no contracts? *JACEP* 6:510–511, 1977.
50. Mangold K: Interview of Karl Mangold, M.D., by Brian Zink. 2002: Oakland, California.
51. Callaham M: Interview of Michael Callaham, M.D., by Brian Zink. 2002: Oakland, California.
52. Williams R: Interview of Robert Williams, M.D., D.P.H., by Brian Zink. 2004: Ann Arbor, Michigan.
53. Davidson S: Interview of Steven Davidson, M.D., by Brian Zink. 2004: Orlando, Florida.
54. Page J: Emergency medicine: limited horizons? *Ann Emerg Med* 13:300–301, 1984.
55. Petersdorf RG: The place of emergency medicine in the academic community, *Ann Emerg Med* 21:193–200, 1992.
56. Advertisement. CMG adds in Annals of Emergency Medicine, *Ann Emerg Med* 17:206, 1988.
57. Keaney JK: *The rape of emergency medicine,* Mendocino, CA, 1991, Mendocino Arts & Gifts.
58. McNamara R: *Corporate practice of medicine: emergency medicine and the physician practice management industry,* Philadelphia, 1998, AAEM.
59. Larsen L, Allegra J, Franaszek JB: Equity buy-in structures of emergency medical group practice. *Am J Emerg Med* 11:28–32, 1993.
60. Meyers S: ED outsourcing: is it good for patient care? Available at http://maillists.uci.edu/mailman/public/calaaem/2004-April/000321.html2004. Accessed Sept. 21, 2004.
61. Article in *Emergency Medicine News.* 1991, p. 1, 17–18.
62. Simon R: Entrepreneurism in emergency medicine, *Ann Emerg Med* 12:722, 1983.

63. Dresnick SJ: Letter from the President. Sterling Healthcare, 2004.
64. Emedicine.com, Excerpt from American Academy of Emergency Medicine. Emedicine.com, 2004.
65. Greene J: Are docs certified? Does it make a difference? *Modern Healthcare* 32, 34–35, 1995.
66. Spectrum Emergency Care, Inc., v. St. Joseph's Health Center, et al., Civil No. 910030. Supreme Court, State of North Dakota, 1992.
67. Emergency physician staffing companies to pay $3.1 million for health care billing fraud. Washington, DC: U.S. Dept. of Justice, 1998.
68. EmCare, Inc., to pay U.S. and states $7.75 million for health care billing fraud, start integrity program. 1997. Available at www.usdoj.gov.opa/pr/1997/May97/214civ.htm. Accessed Sept. 21, 2004.
69. Norbut S: Survival skills: some PPMs have found their niche. Available at www.amednews.com. Accessed Sept. 21, 2004.
70. Munger B: Telephone conversation, Benson Munger and Brian Zink. 2004: Ann Arbor, Michigan.
71. Benson JJ: ABEM application to issue certificates of added qualifications in critical care medicine: Letter to ABMS from ABIM. Portland, OR, 1987, ABIM.
72. Meislin H: Interview of Harvey Meislin, M.D., by Brian Zink. 2004: Tucson, Arizona.
73. Benson JJ: Letter to Judith Tintinalli, ABEM President, from John Benson, ABIM President, ABEM, Editor. Portland, Oregon, 1989, ABIM.
74. Clinton JE: Mailgram from ABEM to ACEP, ACEP, Editor. East Lansing, Michigan, 1989, ABEM.
75. Associated Press: Threats force delay of test for doctors. Washington, DC, 1989, Washington Post.
76. Ludwig S, Fleisher G: *Textbook of pediatric emergency medicine*. Baltimore, Maryland, 1983, Williams & Wilkins.
77. Schafermeyer R: Letter and summary of pediatric emergency medicine development. Zink B, editor. 2002: Ann Arbor, Michigan.
78. Bukata R: Telephone interview of Richard Bukata, M.D., by Brian Zink. 2004: Ann Arbor, Michigan.
79. Petersdorf RG: An American's view of Canadian medical education, *Can Med Assoc J* 148:1550–1553, 1993.
80. Wyatt J, Weber J: A transatlantic comparison of training in emergency medicine, *J Acad Emerg Med* 15:175–180, 1998.
81. McNamara R: Impact of an emergency medicine residency program on the quality of care in an urban community hospital emergency department. *Ann Emerg Med* 21:528–533, 1992.
82. Crippen D: Emergency medicine redux: the rise and fall of a community medical specialty. *Ann Emerg Med* 13:539–542, 1984.
83. Krome R: Interview of Ronald Krome, M.D., by Brian Zink. 2002: Naples, Florida.

▌ Chapter 9

1. Leitzell J: Emergency medicine: two points of view: an uncertain future, *N Engl J Med* 304:477–480, 1981.
2. Riggs L, Jr: Emergency medicine: two points of view: a vigorous new specialty, *N Engl J Med* 304:481–483, 1981.
3. Rosen P: Interview of Peter Rosen, M.D., by Brian Zink. 2002: Jackson, Wyoming.
4. Bowles LT, Sirica C: The role of emergency medicine in the future of American medical care: a conference sponsored by the Josiah Macy, Jr., Foundation. New York, 1995, The Josiah Macy, Jr., Foundation.
5. Petersdorf RG: The place of emergency medicine in the academic community, *Ann Emerg Med* 21:193–200, 1992.
6. Goldfrank LR: Interview of Lewis Goldfrank, M.D., by Brian Zink. 2004: Orlando, Florida.
7. Rorrie C: Interview of Colin Rorrie, Ph.D., by Brian Zink. 2003: Irving, Texas.
8. ACEP: Emergency physician contractual relationships. Dallas, TX, 1999, American College of Emergency Physicians.
9. Wiegenstein J: Interview of John Wiegenstein, M.D., by Brian Zink. 2002: Naples, Florida.
10. Janiak B: Interview of Bruce Janiak, M.D., by Brian Zink. 2002: Maumee, Ohio.
11. Dailey R: Interview of Robert Dailey, M.D., by Brian Zink. 2002: Jackson, Wyoming.
12. Haeck W: Interview of William Haeck, M.D., by Brian Zink. 2003: Boca Raton, Florida.
13. Eisenberg M: Interview of Mickey Eisenberg, M.D., by Brian Zink. 2002: Seattle, Washington.
14. McDade J: Interview of John McDade, M.D., by Brian Zink. 2002: Rockledge, Florida.
15. Buttaravoli P: Interview of Phillip Buttaravoli, M.D., by Brian Zink. 2003: West Palm Beach, Florida.
16. American Hospital Association: Hospital statistics. AHA, 1974–2004.
17. Bitterman RA: Explaining the EMTALA paradox (comment), *Ann Emerg Med* 40:470–475, 2002.
18. Cunningham P, May J: Insured Americans drive surge in emergency department visits. Issue Brief No. 70. Available at http://www.hschange.org/CONTENT/613. Washington, DC, 2003, Center for Studying Health System Change.
19. Crippen D: Emergency medicine redux: the rise and fall of a community medical specialty, *Ann Emerg Med* 3:539–542, 1984.
20. Williams R: Interview of Robert Williams, M.D., D.P.H., by Brian Zink. 2004: Ann Arbor, Michigan.
21. Anderson GV: Telephone interview of Gail Anderson, Sr., M.D., by Brian Zink. 2004: Ann Arbor, Michigan.
22. Tintinalli J: Interview of Judith Tintinalli, M.D., by Brian Zink. 2003: Chapel Hill, North Carolina.
23. Stewart R: Interview of Ronald Stewart, M.D., by Brian Zink. 2004: Boularderie Island, Nova Scotia.
24. Wagner D: Interview of David Wagner, M.D., by Brian Zink. 2003: Philadelphia, Pennsylvania.
25. Anderson G, Franaszek JB, Graves HB, et al: 1920–1989. *Ann Emerg Med* 18:1007–1010, 1989.

26. Mallon W: Interview of William Mallon, M.D., by Brian Zink. 2002: Los Angeles, California.
27. Nalick J: Department of emergency medicine chair announces plan to retire, *HSC Weekly* Los Angeles, 2002:1, 4.
28. Davidson S: Interview of Steven Davidson, M.D., by Brian Zink. 2004: Orlando, Florida.
29. Anderson GV: Interview of Gail V. Anderson, Sr., M.D., by Brian Zink. 2002: Los Angeles, California.
30. Levy R: Interview of Richard Levy, M.D., by Brian Zink. 2002: Cincinnati, Ohio.
31. Dr. Lewis Goldfrank receives Distinguished Teaching Medal, *NYU Physician* 44–45, 2003.
32. The emergence of emergency medicine, *Medicine at Michigan* 2003.
33. Prodinger R: Telephone conversation with Robert Prodinger, M.D., and Brian Zink. 2004: Ann Arbor, Michigan.

Printed and bound by CPI Group (UK) Ltd, Croydon, CR0 4YY

03/10/2024

01040344-0015